OUTLINE OF *Veterinary* CLINICAL PATHOLOGY

THIRD EDITION

MAXINE M. BENJAMIN, B.S., M.S., D.V.M.

PROFESSOR OF CLINICAL PATHOLOGY
COLLEGE OF VETERINARY MEDICINE
COLORADO STATE UNIVERSITY

THE IOWA STATE UNIVERSITY PRESS *Ames*, Iowa, U.S.A.

Manufactured in the United States of America

♾ This book is printed on acid-free paper.

First edition, © 1958; second edition © 1961, carried through 11 printings

Third edition, 1978
Second printing, 1979
Third printing, 1981
Fourth printing, 1984
Fifth printing, 1986
Sixth printing, 1989

Library of Congress Cataloging in Publication Data

Benjamin, Maxine M.
Outline of veterinary clinical pathology

Includes bibliographical references and index.
1. Veterinary pathology—Handbooks, manuals, etc.
I. title.
SF769.B46 1978 636.089′3607 78-15484
ISBN 0-8138-1230-5

CONTENTS

Part One / HEMATOLOGY

1. Collection of Blood ... 5
2. Bone Marrow Examination ... 15
3. Blood Smear ... 25
4. Definitions of Hematologic Terms ... 38
5. Normal Blood Values ... 42
6. Counting of Blood Cells ... 48
7. Hemoglobin ... 60
8. Erythrocyte Sedimentation Rate ... 64
9. Packed Cell Volume (Hematocrit) ... 70
10. Interpretation of Hematologic Findings ... 76
    A. Leukocytes and Their Responses ... 76
    B. Blood Picture in Specific Conditions ... 93
11. Protein ... 108
12. Fibrinogen ... 116
13. Erythrocyte and Its Disorders ... 121
    A. Erythrocyte ... 121
    B. Recognition and Significance of Immature and Abnormal Erythrocytes ... 123
    C. Anemia ... 127
    D. Special Anemias ... 136
    E. Polycythemia ... 146
14. Leukocyte and Its Disorders ... 150
    A. Abnormal Leukocytes ... 150
    B. Leukemias, Lymphomas, and Myeloproliferative Disorders ... 151
15. Thrombocytopenia ... 158
16. Hemostatic Disorders ... 162

Part Two / CLINICAL CHEMISTRY

17. Kidney Function Tests ... 175
18. Urinalysis ... 180
19. Fluid and Electrolytes ... 213
20. Clinical Enzymology ... 229
21. Liver Function Tests ... 233
22. Pancreatic Function Tests ... 255
23. Cardiovascular Disease Tests ... 265
24. Calcium, Phosphorus, and Metabolic Bone Disorders ... 270
25. Cerebrospinal Fluid Examination ... 276
26. Serum Biochemistry Abnormalities ... 286
27. Thyroid Function ... 292

Part Three / CYTOLOGY

28. General Cytology ... 299
29. Transudates and Exudates ... 303
30. Vaginal Smears ... 308

Part Four / MYCOLOGY

31. Mycotic Skin Lesions ... 310

Glossary ... 317
References ... 319
Index ... 345

Part one
HEMATOLOGY

1 COLLECTION OF BLOOD

I. Site

A. Jugular vein—the most commonly used site in the horse, cattle, sheep, goat, and large wild mammal; used occasionally in the dog, cat, rabbit, rat, mouse, hamster, guinea pig, and bird

1. Use of the jugular vein is recommended for very small dogs or when large amounts of blood are required. With the dog in a sitting position, an assistant holds the lower jaw in one hand and turns the head upward and slightly sideways. The operator places the thumb of the left hand in the jugular furrow to occlude and anchor the jugular vein, while manipulating the syringe and needle with the right hand.(26)
   a. The dog can also be restrained in dorsal or lateral recumbency with the head extended.(35)
   b. With a puppy, it may be more convenient for the animal to be held under the assistant's right arm with the forelimbs held by the right hand.(26)
2. In the rat, guinea pig, and rabbit anesthesia and skin incision may be required.
3. Clipping the site of sampling, especially in long-haired animals, is recommended.
4. The veins are more clearly outlined when the site is rubbed with alcohol.

B. Cephalic vein—the most commonly used site for collection of small amounts of blood in the dog

1. By constricting the area on the dorsal aspect of the forelimb at the level of the elbow, the cephalic vein can be raised, beginning just above the carpal joint.

C. Ear vein—can be used in the cat, small dog, pig, rabbit, guinea pig, monkey, and chinchilla

1. A marginal ear vein on the dorsal side of the ear is usually selected.
2. Remove the hair by shaving, clipping, or application of a depilatory agent.
3. Swab the skin with alcohol or ether.
4. Place the left index finger under the ear at the point of applying a sharp razor, stylet, or syringe. This provides support and insures that a nick is made only through the skin and into the vein and not through the underlying cartilage, as notched ears and bloody fingers are to be avoided.
5. When using a syringe in a larger animal such as a rabbit, gentle aspiration is used to avoid collapse of the vein.

D. Toe or toenail—can be used in the small dog, puppy, guinea pig, and small wild mammal

1. Clipping a nail in the guinea pig will start a steady drip of blood immediately. This tapers off after 20 to 40 drops, but as many as 80 drops (4 ml) can be obtained readily. First, clip the hair away, since the presence of even a few hairs accelerates coagulation. After disinfection the capillary bed of the nail is cut into just short of the base of the nail. If bleeding stops prematurely, it may be necessary to remove the clot with gauze or clip the nail shorter.(28)
2. In the anesthetized rat or mouse, a toe may be removed with scissors or clippers and blood obtained from the site.

E. Tail—can be used in the pig, sheep, cattle, rat, mouse, hamster, and fish
   1. Venipuncture
      a. The coccygeal vein on the ventral side of the bovine tail is visible when the tail is flexed upward. The site of venipuncture is approximately 4 in. from the perineum. This site may be desirable when obtaining samples from show cattle to avoid damage to or from the horns.
      b. Rat and mouse veins can be seen with a bright light or transillumination and can be dilated for easy entry by massaging with xylene or dipping the tail in warm water.
   2. Amputation—commonest method used in the rat and mouse
      a. Amputation of a piece of the tail or a small transverse incision with a razor blade will produce drops of blood.
      b. Massaging the tail from the body to the tip can produce as much as 3 ml from a rat. Larger amounts can be obtained if the tail is warmed in water at 45° C for 1 min.
      c. If the rodent has been handled often, the above method can be used with the animal held in the hand. If it has not, place the animal in a tube of the proper size, with the tail hanging through the opening.

F. Heart—may be used in any animal, fish, reptile, or bird
   1. In all animals blood is best obtained under anesthesia, but this is not mandatory.

G. Femoral, saphenous, or tibial vessels—used in the dog, cat, primate, small mammal, and rat.(35, 50)
   1. In the cat the femoral vein is easily seen.
   2. Large quantities of blood can be obtained from the monkey at the femoral vein along the medial aspect of the leg between the knee and the abdomen.

H. Mammary vein—used for dairy cattle
   1. The vein appears at the anterior border of the mammary gland about 2 to 3 in. lateral from the linea alba and runs forward, deviating laterally and passing through a foramen in the abdominal wall posterior to the ribs.(35)
      a. Venipuncture is made in a similar manner to that of collection from the jugular; however, distention of the mammary vein is more difficult.

I. Anterior vena cava—used for the pig (25)
   1. A needle is inserted just anterior and slightly lateral to the cariniform cartilage and in a line from the cartilage to the base of the ear. The needle is directed upward, slightly backward, and medially.
      a. Large boars and brood matrons will require a 4½- to 6-in. needle, while a 17- to 20-gauge needle, 1½ to 2 in. long, will be needed for shoats.

J. Retroorbital venous plexus—used for the rat, mouse, guinea pig, and hamster (35, 42)
   1. The plexus communicates with blood vessels of the brain, and this technique is reported to be less traumatic than any other procedure.
   2. It can be repeated as often as needed and is the best method for obtaining a large quantity of blood (maximum of 0.5 to 1 ml) in the mouse.
   3. It is best performed under anesthesia but can be done without its use.
   4. The animal is held in the left hand with the thumb and index finger encircling the neck and applying slight pressure so that the veins will fill and the eyeball will protrude slightly. A blunt 20-gauge needle or a glass pipette, such as a Pasteur pipette with a fine point, is introduced at the medial or lateral canthus of the eye between the orbit and the eyeball. Drill through the conjunctiva by rotating the needle or pipette in the direction of the larynx, since the plexus is located behind the eye at a depth of 4 to 5 mm in the rat and 2 to 3 mm in the mouse. Blood will enter the needle or pipette spontaneously, and the bleeding will stop when the pressure on the neck is removed.
      a. The pipette capillary orifice for rats should be 0.6 mm in diameter with a glass wall of 0.3 mm. The wall should be thinner for use in mice.

K. Wing vein or comb—used for birds
   1. After the feathers in the axillary region are plucked, the alar vein is seen running from beneath the pectoral muscle then along the ventral surface of the humerus.

L. Vein in the web between toes or footpad—used for the mink, guinea pig, and small wild mammal

II. Containers

A. For clotted blood—size depends upon the amount of blood needed
1. Container should be chemically clean and dry.

B. For whole blood or plasma—glass vials fitted with rubber or polyethylene stoppers are recommended and are available in all sizes

C. Vacutainers (Becton-Dickinson)—vacuum tubes, used with a special holder and needle, are available in a variety of sizes from 2 to 50 ml, either plain or containing an assortment of anticoagulants
1. Technique (Fig. 1.1)

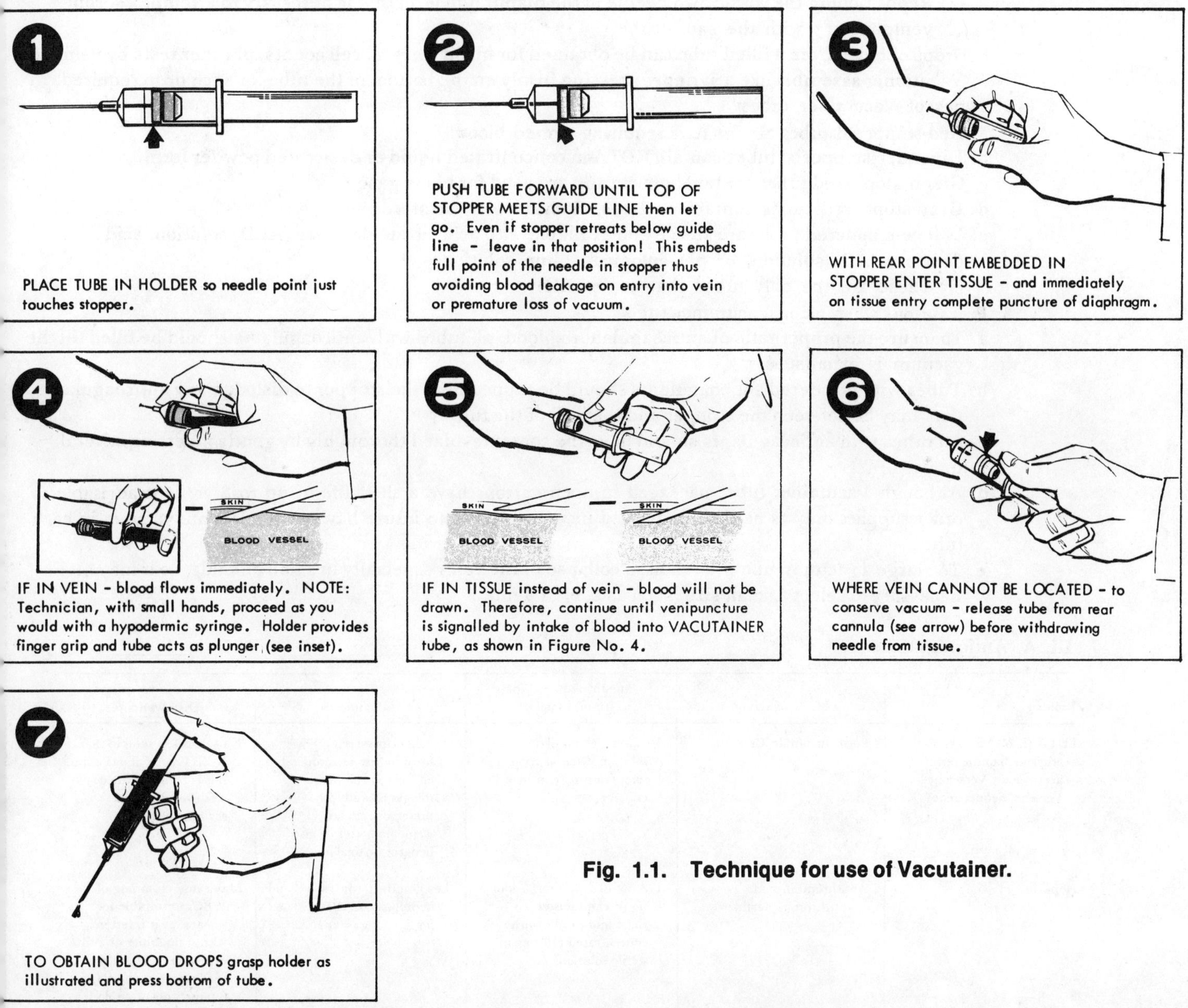

Fig. 1.1. Technique for use of Vacutainer.

a. Insert the tube in the holder onto the needle until the leading edge of the stopper meets the guideline on the holder. The stopper and tube will retract. Leave in this position, as the needle is embedded in the stopper diaphragm and a vacuum is maintained.
b. Perform venipuncture in the usual manner. With the needle under the skin, place the first two fingers behind the flange of the holder. Place the thumb of the same hand on the end of the tube. Pull with the fingers and push with the thumb until the tube is pushed onto the needle to the bottom of the holder.
c. If the needle is in the vein, blood will flow into the tube. If no blood enters the tube, probe for the vein until entry is indicated by blood flow. Relieve pressure on the vein or tourniquet while the tube is filling.
d. Multiple specimens may be obtained from one venipuncture.
   (1) For multiple filling, special needles are available that shut off blood flow while tubes are changed.
   (2) With use of regular Vacutainer needles, the blood flow can be occluded by pressing the needle bevel against the wall of the vein while tubes are changed.
e. If a vein cannot be located and it is necessary to reenter the skin, the Vacutainer tube can be released from the needle before the needle is withdrawn from the arm.
   (1) Repositioning the withdrawn needle in the diaphragm is all that is necessary to attempt a second venipuncture with the same tube.
f. Drops of blood from a filled tube can be obtained for blood smears, cell counts, or other tests by using the Vacutainer assembly like a syringe, pressing firmly on the bottom of the tube for each drop required.

2. Types of Vacutainer tubes
   a. Red-stoppered tubes are for tests requiring clotted blood.
   b. Lavender-stoppered tubes contain EDTA in concentrated liquid or desiccated powder form.
   c. Green-stoppered tubes contain heparin and are used for blood gases.
   d. Gray-stoppered tubes contain oxalates, fluorides, or citrates.
   e. Yellow-stoppered tubes are sterile and available with acid citrate dextrose (ACD) solution, acid dextrose (AD) solution, or physiological saline solution.
      (1) These are the only tubes that are sterile.
3. Precautions when using Vacutainer tubes
   a. To insure the proper ratio of anticoagulant to blood, all tubes with anticoagulants should be filled till the vacuum is exhausted.
   b. Tubes with powdered anticoagulants should be tapped near the stopper to dislodge any anticoagulant that may be between the stopper and the wall of the tube.
   c. All tubes with anticoagulants should have the contents mixed thoroughly by gently inverting several times.
   d. Although Vacutainer tubes packaged in open cartons have a shelf life of up to 3 yr, it is advisable to order supplies only as needed, or packed in vacuum cans to insure having an adequate vacuum in each tube.
   e. Too large a vacuum tube will result in collapse of the vein, especially in small animals, so it may be necessary to select a small size, such as 2, 3, or 4 ml.

III. A. Anticoagulants

Product	Mode of action	Amount required for 10 ml blood	Advantages	Disadvantages
EDTA (K or Na salts of ethylenediamine tetra-acetic acid, Versenate, Versene, Sequestrene)	Form insoluble Ca salts	10-20 mg (1 ml of 1% solution dried at room temperature or in incubator)	Excellent preserving power for 6 hours; recommended for routine hematologic procedures; preserves cellular elements better than heparin or oxalates	Na salt is less soluble than K EDTA, so dipotassium salt is recommended; excess over 2 mg/ml shrinks cells
Heparin	Antithrombin and antithromboplastin	1-2 mg (0.2 ml of 1% solution); can moisten syringe and needle with concentrated (10 mg/ml) sterile solution	Least effect on size and hemolysis of RBC; used for blood gas analysis	May cause clumping of WBC; unsuitable for smears, as it interferes with stainability of WBC; expensive; will not prevent clotting longer than 8 hours; not suitable for agglutination or prothrombin time tests

Product	Mode of action	Amount required for 10 ml blood	Advantages	Disadvantages
Sodium citrate	Combines with Ca to form an insoluble salt of calcium citrate	10-20 mg; for some coagulation studies, one part of 3.8% solution to 9 parts of blood	Can be used for blood transfusions	Interferes with many chemical tests; prevents clotting for only a few hours; shrinks cells
Potassium oxalate	Unites with Ca to form insoluble calcium oxalate	20 mg or 2 drops of 20% solution dried in incubator or oven under 55° C (overheating converts oxalates to carbonates)	Very soluble	Causes 6-8% shrinkage in cell volume, thus poor for PCV and differential; in excess interferes with precipitation of proteins; glucose levels too low; alters electrolyte distribution; poisonous
Sodium oxalate	Unites with Ca to form insoluble calcium oxalate	20 mg; for prothrombin time use 0.5 ml of 0.1 M sodium oxalate in exactly 4.5 ml blood	Used mainly for prothrombin time	Same as potassium oxalate; shrinks cells
Ammonium and potassium oxalate (Heller's and Paul's double oxalate)	Unites with Ca to form insoluble calcium oxalate	1 ml or 20 mg dried at temperature no higher than 60° C (1.2 gm ammonium oxalate, 0.8 gm potassium oxalate, 100 ml distilled water)	Can be used for most hematological procedures; produces less distortion and hemolysis of RBC than other oxalates	Potassium oxalate shrinks the RBC, while ammonium oxalate causes it to swell, offsetting the effect; cannot be used for BUN determinations
Lithium oxalate	Unites with Ca to form insoluble calcium oxalate	20 mg (1 ml of 1.5% solution evaporated just to dryness in 37° C incubator)	More soluble than sodium or potassium oxalate	Same as potassium oxalate; shrinks cells
Lithium citrate	Inactivates Ca ions	30 mg	Occasionally used for mineral constituents of whole blood	Impractical for routine use
Sodium fluoride and thymol (10:1)	Forms a weakly dissociated Ca component	100 mg sodium fluoride and 10 mg thymol	Both anticoagulant and preservative; excellent preservative for blood glucose, as it interferes with enzyme system having to do with glycolysis	Interferes with enzymatic methods for glucose and BUN (urease); thymol will cause high values in ferricyanide method
ACD solution B (acid citrate dextrose)		For transfusions use 25 ml ACD solution for 100 ml blood (dextrose 14.7 gm; trisodium citrate 13.2 gm; citric acid, anhydrous 4.4 gm; distilled water q.s. to 1000 ml; autoclave)	Recommended for blood transfusions	

B. Alterations caused by anticoagulants
1. EDTA
   a. Over 2 mg EDTA/ml of blood will cause shrinkage of the erythrocytes, resulting in low packed cell volume (PCV) and mean corpuscular volume but high mean corpuscular hemoglobin concentration.
   b. One mg EDTA/ml of blood may increase the nonprotein nitrogen value by a much as 7 mg/dl. (12)
   c. EDTA should not be used in drawing blood for alkaline phosphatase determination because it will interfere with the color development.
   d. EDTA decreases the carbon dioxide combining power of blood. (57)
   e. Heavy interference will be seen in the Jaffé reaction for creatinine when EDTA is present.
2. Heparin
   a. Heparin is a poor anticoagulant for blood cell studies, as it may cause clumping of leukocytes and will interfere with stainability of leukocytes in smears.
   b. Heparin is the best anticoagulant for blood pH studies, as ammonium oxalate, sodium citrate, or disodium EDTA will decrease blood pH significantly, while it is increased by sodium or potassium oxalate. (16)

c. The sodium or ammonium salt of heparin is effective in such a minute amount that neither have a significant effect on electrolyte or blood urea nitrogen (BUN) determinations.
d. Inorganic phosphorus will be elevated when heparin is used.
e. Since heparin preparations vary in their ammonia content, they should not be used for blood ammonia determinations. (14)
f. Some enzymes, such as cholinesterase, lactic dehydrogenase, and isocitric dehydrogenase, will have slight to marked interference when heparin is used.

3. Potassium oxalate
   a. This anticoagulant produces dilution of the plasma because of shrinkage of the erythrocytes, and as a result it is unsuitable for PCV and erythrocytic indices.
   b. Oxalate will inhibit lactic dehydrogenase (11) and alkaline and acid phosphatase. (1)
   c. Oxalate and citrate inhibit amylase activity. (30)
   d. Potassium or sodium salts of anticoagulants are not suitable for sodium, potassium, or calcium determinations.
   e. Uric acid values are lowered by potassium and sodium oxalates. (53)
4. Fluoride
   a. Fluoride is used as a preservative of glucose in plasma, although it has been shown that some hemolysis occurs from its use and that there is a concomitant decrease of 10% in glucose concentration. It is a potent enzyme inhibitor and should not be used with some enzymatic methods for glucose analysis. (30)
   b. Fluoride ions are unsuitable for BUN determinations that are dependent on urease activity.(12)
   c. Fluorides inhibit alkaline and acid phosphatase. (1)
   d. Amylase activity is activated by fluoride and chloride. (44)
   e. Fluoride cannot be used as a preservative if uricase is used for uric acid determination.

IV. Errors commonly made in the collection of blood

A. Hemolysis
1. Use of a wet syringe or failure to remove the needle before filling collection tubes hemolyzes erythrocytes.
2. Serum rather than plasma is preferred for most chemical analyses because of the possible interference by various anticoagulants. However, plasma that has been carefully separated from the cellular mass will have less hemoglobin than serum; and where anticoagulants will not interfere, plasma may be the specimen of choice. (45)
3. When the concentration of hemoglobin exceeds 0.02 g/dl, serum will appear grossly hemolyzed (9), although in icteric serum much higher levels may be undetected.
4. Chemical components of the blood are often present in varying concentrations between the plasma and erythrocytes. If the concentration of the erythrocyte is less than in the plasma, hemolysis will produce a dilutional effect. If the concentration of a substance is greater in the erythrocyte than in the plasma, hemolysis is more important. Hemolysis may interfere directly with the following tests:
   a. Serum lipase—with 0.5 g hemoglobin/dl, a 50% inhibition occurs (21)
   b. Serum bilirubin—large negative errors in the presence of hemoglobin may be due to the conversion of hemoglobin to methemoglobin by nitrous acid in the test and not in the control
   c. Icterus index—abnormally increased by hemoglobin
   d. Urea nitrogen—falsely elevated by the color in the protein-free filtrate (22)
   e. Bromsulfphalein—altered in some procedures (29, 43)
   f. Inorganic phosphate—increases rapidly in hemolyzed serum, as erythocytes contain a high concentration of organic phosphate esters that are hydrolyzed by serum phosphatases (34)
   g. Serum potassium—greatly increased in hemolyzed serum, since the ratio between erythrocytes and plasma is 23:1 in man, but potassium is low in canine erythrocytes (8)
      (1) Potassium will increase in serum in contact with the clot in the absence of visible hemolysis, by diffusing into the serum. (52) This increase is less at room temperature than at 4° C. (17)
   h. Alkaline phosphatase—increased (12)
   i. Acid phosphatase—may diffuse from the erythrocytes in unseparated serum and appears to be released into the serum during the clotting process, since it is present in the thrombocytes (59)
   j. Transaminase—hemolysis will have less influence on dog serum than on serum of human origin because of the variation in the ratio of transaminase between erythrocytes and serum

(1) SGOT—the ratio is 2:70 in the dog, but is 40:1 in man (12, 58)
(2) SGPT—the ratio is 1:38 in the dog and 6.7:1 in man (12, 58)

k. Lactic dehydrogenase (LDH)—the ratio between erythrocytes and serum may vary from 160:1 in man to 1:38 in the dog (12, 58)
l. Arginase—the ratio in the erythrocytes to that of plasma is 1000:1 (48)
m. Blood pH—decreased slightly by hemolysis (41)
n. Chloride—decreased by hemolysis (53)
o. Prothrombin—hemolysis has a negligible effect on prothrombin by the one-stage technique, but it causes interference in prothrombin consumption tests (39)

B. Lipemia may result if the patient has not been fasted an adequate time before collection of blood.

1. Colorimetric methods result in elevated optical density in the presence of lipemia when the serum is present in the final test mixture but not in the blank. Depending upon the method used, lipemia may produce falsely elevated values for:
   a. Total protein
   b. Transaminase
   c. Hemoglobin—may be elevated as much as 2 g by gross lipemia (12)
   d. Icterus index
   e. Amylase

C. When serum is desired, do not place the blood in the refrigerator immediately or before good clot formation and retraction occur, since this retards serum collection.

D. A fibrin clot occurs when blood is centrifuged too soon after the sample is taken or when the speed of the centrifuge is too fast.

E. Blood should be collected when the animal is at rest and without undue excitation to avoid alterations in the hemogram and some blood chemistry values.

F. The longer whole blood is held before examination, the greater will be the deterioration.

1. The temperature and type of anticoagulant will determine the maximum time for satisfactory storage.
2. For most tests it is best to store whole blood or serum in the refrigerator.
3. Blood smears should be made within 15 min after collecting blood, but the best smears are made immediately from fresh blood. Do not store blood smears in the refrigerator.

G. Clotting of the blood sample may result from a variety of causes.

1. Taking too much time in obtaining the blood, so that the sample has already started to clot before being mixed with the anticoagulant
2. Failure to agitate the blood sample immediately after placing it in the vial and filling the vial to the top cause clotting, as the anticoagulant is not properly mixed with the blood

H. When tubes contain concentrated anticoagulant solution, care should be taken to add an adequate amount of blood to minimize the dilution factor.

V. Amount of blood required

A. The amount of blood required will depend upon the test or tests requested and the methods used in the laboratory where the tests are being conducted.

1. For automated clinical chemistry profiles on the Technicon SMA12 it is necessary to have a minimum of 2.5 ml of serum. When it is necessary to dilute the serum or plasma, abnormally low sodium and chloride values and abnormally high creatinine results are seen.
   a. If it is not noted on the report sheet that a dilution was made, it should be suspected when a normal BUN and high serum creatinine are reported.
2. For aid in diagnosis of disease the maximum amount taken should be the smallest quantity necessary for the tests to be conducted without skimping.

B. As a general rule it is usually safe to take about 0.5 ml blood/kg body weight in all species. (6)

C. Only about one-half the circulating blood can be recovered when an animal is bled out.

D. Total blood volume

Subject	No.	Body wt. (ml/kg)	Reference	Subject	No.	Body wt. (ml/kg)	Reference
Dog				Goat			
		90	(6)			70	(6)
Beagle	14	81.9	(5)		30	70	(15)
Beagle	21	94.4	(38)	Pig			
Beagle	153	102.6	(55)			65	(6)
	30	98.7		2 wk	3	74	(19)
Greyhound	4	114	(15)	4 wk	4	67	(19)
Cat				3-4 mo	8	63	(19)
		75	(6)	2 yr	4	46	(19)
	10	66.7	(46)	3 yr	3	35	(19)
Horse				Camel, Arabian	19	83	(2)
		75	(6)	Monkey			
Thoroughbred	6	109.6	(27)	Rhesus	18	54	(18)
Thoroughbred	31	103.1	(32)	Rhesus	23	75.1	(37)
Draft	14	61.4	(32)	Rabbit			
Saddle	6	77.5	(32)			70	(6)
Burro					71	57.3	(7)
One day	2	190	(20)	Guinea pig			
1-3 mo	4	95	(20)			75	(6)
4 yr	9	66	(20)		18	72	(4)
Cattle				Rat			
		60	(6)			50	(6)
Beef					50	59.3	(51)
2-6 days	2	120	(20)	Mouse			
3 wk	1	85	(20)			80	(6)
6-8 mo	5	58	(20)		5	84.8	(54)
8-12 yr	4	57	(20)	Opossum	10	57	(2)
Dairy	20	59.2	(40)	Chicken			
Sheep						60	(6)
		60	(6)		223	90	(2)
	5	66.4	(24)	Duck, Pekin	42	102	(2)

VI. Stability—information about the stability of blood constituents and the way samples are best handled and stored before analysis is necessary to avoid considerable error in results and interpretation, as blood or serum samples frequently must be sent to a distant clinical laboratory, or a busy laboratory must program its time for analyses

A. Stability of chemistry values in canine serum refrigerated or frozen for periods up to 6 wk (31)
1. Good stability—BUN, total protein, electrophoretic determination of protein fractions, cholesterol, calcium, inorganic phosphorus, and chloride
2. Unstable—glucose deteriorated rapidly in the refrigerated state and to some extent in the frozen state

B. Stability of chemical constituents in human plasma frózen and stored up to 6 mo (49)
1. Good stability—albumin, globulin, total protein, electrophoretic determination of protein fractions, urea, uric acid, creatinine, cholesterol, bilirubin, and chloride
2. Borderline stability—glucose
3. Unstable—nonprotein nitrogen

C. Enzymes—many investigations on the stability of enzymes have been made, but the results vary widely. Many of them show great instability of enzymatic activity, whereas some other reports indicate a remarkably high stability. Differences in species, treatment of blood before analysis, analytic methods, and interpretation of statistically significant changes as opposed to the importance of significant changes in diagnostic application may account for the variations in results. Most of the work in this field has been performed on human sera. With the great differences existing in normal serum activity and isoenzyme patterns among species, it is not advisable to be confident in drawing parallels from one species to another. (47)

1. Stability of some animal serum enzymes during storage at different temperatures (47)

Enzyme	Room temperature (22° C)	Refrigerator (4° C)	Freezer (−20°C)
SGOT			
Bovine	Increases	Stable for 5 days	Stable for 38 days
Ovine	Increases	Decreases	Decreases
Porcine	Increases	Decreases	Stable
SGPT			
Bovine	Increases	Increases	Increases
Ovine	Stable	Stable	Stable
Porcine	Increases	Decreases	Decreases
LDH			
Bovine	Stable	Decreases	Stable for 6 mo
Ovine	Decreases	Decreases	Decreases
Porcine	Decreases	Decreases	Stable for 2 mo

2. Stability of enzymes in human serum at different temperatures

Enzyme	Room temperature (25° C)	Refrigerator (4° C)	Freezer (−20° C)	Reference
Acid phosphatase	4 hr	14 days	115 days	(3)
		3 days	3 days	(10)
Alkaline phosphatase	May increase 5-30% in 12 hr	Several days	20 mo	(3)
			1 mo	
	2-3 days (may increase)	2-3 days		BMC
Amylase	27 days	7 mo	2 mo	(3)
Cholinesterase	10 days	7 days	Several mo	(3)
	1 wk	1 wk	1 wk	(10)
CPK—nonactivated	2 hr	6 hr		BMC
			Unstable	(23)
CPK—activated	2 days	1 wk	1 mo	BMC
G-6-phosphate dehydrogenase		7 days		(3)
G-6-phosphatase	Unstable			(3)
Glutamic dehydrogenase	1 day	2 days	1 day	(10)
ICD	5 hr	Several days	21 days	(3)
LDH	7 days	7 days	1 mo	(3)
Lipase	7 days	21 days		(3)
OCT	24 hr	7 days	3 mo	(3)
SGOT	2 days	14 days	1 mo	(3)
SGPT	2 days	1 wk		(10)
			Unstable	(23)
Sorbitol dehydrogenase	Unstable	1 day	2 days	(10)

D. Glucose
1. When serum is allowed to stand in contact with the clot at room temperature, the serum glucose decreases about 7% in 1 hr. (12)
2. When serum is separated from the clot within 30 min after the blood is drawn, the glucose will be relatively stable for several days at refrigerator temperature or in the frozen state without the addition of a preservative, providing hemolysis does not occur. (33) Glucose does not have this stability in dog serum. (31)

E. Bilirubin
1. If bilirubin is exposed to direct sunlight, loss of 50% in 1 hr can occur. (36)
2. When it is stored overnight in the refrigerator, a slight loss of bilirubin occurs. (56)

F. Inorganic phosphorus and potassium
1. The serum should be removed rapidly from the clot, or shifts between the serum and erythrocytes will occur. (33)
2. There is a tendency for inorganic phosphorus to increase on standing, especially when the serum is hemolyzed. (34)

G. Cholesterol
1. Total cholesterol is stable for 5 days at room temperature without a preservative. (33)

H. pH
1. If blood is exposed to the air, the pH increases rapidly due to the loss of carbon dioxide. (16)
   a. The speed of this increase depends upon the volume of the sample, surface area, and amount of agitation of the sample during collection and storage.

2 BONE MARROW EXAMINATION

I. Indications for bone marrow aspiration

A. To establish or confirm the diagnosis of leukemia
B. To determine if the deficiency of one or more of the blood types in the peripheral blood is due to a deficiency of precursors in the bone marrow
C. To determine the cause, if possible, of a refractory anemia, especially if interference with erythrocyte maturation is suspected (vitamin B_{12} deficiency, folic acid deficiency, lead poisoning)
D. To demonstrate a metastatic neoplasm
E. To demonstrate certain types of infections (histoplasmosis, toxoplasmosis)
F. To investigate a deficiency in body iron stores in certain cases of suspected iron deficiency anemia

II. Types of bone marrow (36)

A. Red marrow—active in the production of erythrocytes, granulocytes, and thrombocytes
   1. Normally present in:
      a. Flat bones—ribs, pelvis, cranial bones
      b. Short bones—vertebrae
      c. Long bone ends

B. Yellow marrow—nonproductive or resting
   1. Occupies the shafts of the long bones of adult animals
   2. Consists of the following cell types:
      a. Fat cells—will compensate in its space for regression or expansion of the red marrow
      b. Endothelial cells
      c. Reticular cells

III. Aspiration sites

A. Dog, cat, young pig, and laboratory animal (40)
   1. Iliac crest—preferred for the dog since it is the most convenient and there is little variation in differential cell counts between the iliac crest, rib, and sternum (17)
   2. Proximal end of the femur through the trochanteric fossa—preferred for the cat (8)

B. Horse, cattle, sheep, and goat
   1. Rib (6, 7)
   2. Tuber coxae (2)
   3. Iliac crest—not recommended in the older horse and cattle because the red marrow may have receded from the site
   4. Sternum—difficult because of the large muscle mass and density of the bone, but preferred by a few authors for the horse, cattle, and adult swine (2, 6, 7)
   5. Vertebral spines—good site in the calf (40)

IV. Technique for bone marrow aspiration

A. Cat—using the femur (8, 37, 38)
   1. The cat is placed on its side and a small area over the greater trochanter is clipped, scrubbed, and prepared for surgery.
   2. Generally a local anesthetic, 2% xylocaine or 2% procaine, will suffice.

3. A struggling cat may require a sedative dose of Surital or Ketamine.
4. A small skin incision, 0.5 cm in length is made slightly medial to the trochanter over the trochanteric fossa.
5. An aspiration needle (¾ to 1½ in., 16- to 18-gauge) is drilled into the cortical bone of the trochanteric fossa and into the femoral canal for about ½ to 1 in., using firm pressure and a rotating motion.
   a. Needles that can be used:
      (1) Rosenthal
      (2) Vim-Silverman
      (3) Spinal tap needle
      (4) Stainless steel pin (0.2 cm in diameter) introduced with a Kirschner pin chuck and replaced with a stainless steel cannula
      (5) Salah
   b. During this procedure the stylet must be kept in place to prevent the needle from becoming plugged by skin and bone.
6. After the needle is in the femoral canal, the stylet is removed and the marrow and sinusoidal blood (½ to l ml) is aspirated into a 12- or 20-ml syringe.
   a. Aspiration will cause a twinge of pain, but this is necessary in order to obtain a good marrow specimen.

B. Dog—using the iliac crest (4, 36)
1. After outlining the iliac crest, clip the hair, apply an antiseptic, and infiltrate the area with 2% xylocaine or 2% procaine as a local anesthetic.
2. With the dog in a standing position or on its side, make a small slit in the skin, usually at the antero-dorsal angle of the iliac crest.
3. The sterile aspiration needle, with a stylet in position, is passed through the slit in the skin and the muscle over the crest of the ilium and is forced firmly into the medullary cavity by using a rotating motion and pressure.
4. Remove the stylet and establish adequate vacuum on a 20-ml syringe to withdraw marrow particles. Dilution of the marrow with blood will occur if the suction process is not stopped as soon as fluid appears in the syringe.

C. Horse
1. Rib (1, 6)
   a. The dorsal portions of the 8th to the 18th ribs are covered only with skin and fascia. Palpate until the rib is located with the smallest amount of fascial covering.
   b. Clip the area over the selected area, scrub, and apply an antiseptic solution.
   c. Introduce 5 to 10 ml of a local anesthetic into the skin, fascia, and the periosteum.
   d. A small incision is made in the skin, fascia, and periosteum.
   e. Using a rotating motion with an aspiration needle (1½ to 2½ in., 16-gauge) or a drill (about 3/32 in.), bore into the marrow cavity.
      (1) The ideal spot to drill is midway between the anterior and posterior borders to lessen the hazard of penetrating the thoracic cavity.
      (2) The needle or drill will meet less resistance when it reaches the marrow cavity.
   f. Withdraw the stylet and attach a 10-ml dry syringe firmly to the aspiration needle. Quickly apply suction to remove 1 ml or less of marrow.
      (1) When a drill is used to penetrate the bone, a cannula or trochar needle can be attached to the syringe to remove the marrow sample.
2. Tuber coxae (2)
   a. Apply a local anesthetic to the skin and periosteum.
   b. After insertion, direct the point of the aspiration needle from between the two tuberosities to the hip joint on the opposite side.
      (1) Density of the bone will vary with the age of the horse.
         (a) Up to 2 yr—1 cm before penetration into the marrow cavity
         (b) 5 yr—will require 4 cm to penetrate
         (c) 10 yr or older—2 in. or more; therefore not practical
      (2) The length and gauge of the needle will vary with the age of the animal (from 1½ to 2½ in. and 16- to 18-gauge).

D. Cattle and sheep
   1. Rib—similar to that described for the horse (7)

V. Preparation of the smear

A. Removal of excess blood—will improve the quality of the bone marrow smear. Several methods for accomplishing this include:
   1. Before it clots, eject the aspirate onto a slanted slide; smears are made from particles sticking to the slanted slide after the peripheral blood has run down. (33)
   2. Place the aspirated marrow on a watch glass or coverglass and rock carefully to move the excess blood to the periphery. The concentrated fatty particles can be picked up immediately with a pipette (leukocyte or Pasteur).
   3. After a drop of aspirate is placed on a clean slide, immediately remove excess blood by using a pipette with a fine capillary bore or with a 5- to 10-ml syringe with no larger than an 18-gauge needle attached; leave the pale gray-white marrow fragments.

B. Microscope slide or coverglass smears
   1. Smears can be made immediately from fresh marrow by the same methods used for making blood smears.
   2. An alternate method is to place marrow on a clean slide and drop a spreading slide crosswise on it. Pull the spreader slide to spread the marrow.

C. Precaution
   1. The entire procedure from aspiration to making the slide should occupy less than a minute, otherwise coagulation will occur. If a large number of smears are to be prepared, it might be necessary to place the aspirated marrow in a vial containing EDTA to prevent coagulation.

VI. Imprints

A. Select a particle of marrow and make several rows of imprints by holding the marrow vertically and touching to the slide surface with a slight smearing motion.
B. The advantage of imprints over smears is that the various cells have a better relation to each other. Primitive cells tend to be in compact clusters or masses and are more easily seen in imprints, whereas they might be overlooked in smears.

VII. Staining—similar to the methods used for staining blood smears

A. Several of the stains commonly used include:
   1. Wright's
   2. May-Grünwald-Giemsa
   3. Prussian blue reaction—for iron granules
   4. Peroxidase—to differentiate the granulocytic series from the lymphocytes

VIII. Examination of the stained slide

A. Total counts—usually not performed
   1. The marrow cells tend to clump.
   2. There is dilution with peripheral blood, and the count is variable.
      a. The first drop of marrow collected contains the greatest number of cells.

B. Degree of cellularity—assessed within broad aspects under low power
   1. Increased
   2. Normal
   3. Reduced
      a. Large cells tend to resist aspiration or are ruptured in smearing and appear in disproportionate numbers, e.g., megakaryocytes.
   4. Normal or atypical clumps of cells or parasites

C. Differential cell count—count at least 500 cells
 1. Most reliable results are obtained in the tail area of the smeared marrow fragments.
 2. Normal ranges for bone marrow cell counts are presented in table form below.

D. Myeloid:erythroid (M:E) ratio—expresses the proportion of total granulocytes to nucleated erythroid cells
 1. Divide the number of nucleated erythrocytes into the total number of cells of the granulocytic series.
 2. Normal ranges for M:E ratios according to various authors:

Species	Range (M:E ratio)	Reference
Dog	0.75-2.5	(4)
	1.0-2.0	(11)
	0.5-4.0	(29)
	0.75-2.5	(36)
	0.6-2.4	(41)
Cat	0.8-3.1	(11)
	1.6	(14)
	2.8	(24)
	3.5	(35)
	0.6-3.9	(36)
	1.45	(37)
Horse	1.1-10.2	(1)
	0.94-3.76	(6)
	0.5	(19)
Cattle	0.27-2.5	(7)
	0.7	(19)
	0.31-1.85	(36)
	0.4-1.84	(46)
Sheep	0.77-1.68	(18)
	0.5	(47)
Goat	0.62	(46)
Pig	1.77	(23)
	1.7	(31)
Man	0.56-2.67	(48)

IX. Interpretation

A. Myeloid:erythroid ratio
 1. Normal M:E ratio
  a. Normal marrow
  b. Myelosclerosis
  c. Aplastic anemia—sometimes
   (1) An aspirated marrow sample is not always reliable in indicating the degree of cellularity and may be misleading.

d. Conditions where abnormal or increased numbers of certain cell types are of diagnostic significance
  (1) Multiple myeloma (26)
  (2) Lymphosarcoma and other tumor cells (42)
e. Localized marrow lesions—assuming that the sample of marrow was not representative

2. Increased M:E ratio (48)
  a. Leukocytosis—from infection or other stimuli
  b. Leukemoid reaction
  c. Granulocytic leukemia (13, 22, 25, 27, 32)
  d. Lymphosarcoma—common in dogs, occasionally in cattle
  e. Chronic interstitial nephritis (43)
  f. Erythremic hypoplasis—decrease in nucleated erythrocytes in marrow
    (1) Must be evaluated in correlation with the total peripheral blood leukocyte count
      (a) With a normal blood leukocyte count, an M:E ratio over 2.5 would suggest depressed erythropoiesis in most animals. (36)
3. Decreased M:E ratio (48)
  a. Reduction in the number of myeloid cells
  b. Hyperplasia of the erythropoietic tissue
    (1) With a normal peripheral blood leukocyte count, an M:E ratio of less than 1 would suggest active erythrogenesis in most species. (36)
    (2) Metarubricytic (normoblastic) (48)
      (a) Blood loss—hemorrhage
      (b) Hemolysis
      (c) Iron deficiency
      (d) Lead poisoning (36)
      (e) Polycythemia vera
      (f) Cirrhosis of the liver
    (3) Rubriblastic (megaloblastic) (36)
      (a) Deficiency of vitamin B_{12} and/or folic acid
      (b) Congenital porphyria—in cattle
    (4) Erythremic myelosis (49)

B. Cells not normally found in the bone marrow or not normally present in the observed numbers
1. Lymphosarcoma (3, 12, 16, 20, 39, 42)
  a. More than 15% lymphocytes in cat's marrow is usually considered sufficient for a tentative diagnosis of lymphocytic leukemia. (16)
    (1) This number must be interpreted with reservation, however, when a relative lymphocytosis is present in the peripheral blood.
  b. Immature forms of lymphocytes (lymphoblasts) would also suggest lymphosarcoma, as would a greater number of lymphocytes in those species where the normal range exceeds 15% (cattle, horse).
  c. Adult cattle—bone marrow aspirate is not especially helpful, as extensive bone marrow infiltration is not common; when present, it is more easily diagnosed by pronounced leukemia in the peripheral blood (42)
  d. Thymic form and "calf" form—bone marrow infiltration more often than in the adult (12, 39)
  e. Dog—more often has increased M:E ratio than an increased number of atypical lymphocytes in the marrow (3)
2. Multiple myeloma—increased numbers or clusters of abnormal plasmocytes (9, 26, 34)
3. Mast cell leukemia—abnormal number of mast cells in the marrow (28)
4. Metastatic tumor cells
  a. Large cell type—carcinoma of the stomach or prostate, hypernephroma
  b. Small cell type—bronchogenic carcinoma
5. Reticulum cells—undifferentiated, phagocytic, foam cells, leukemic forms
6. Reticuloendotheliosis (15)
7. Lupus erythematosus

TERMINOLOGY OF BLOOD CELLS

Series	Recommended nomenclature (ASCP)	Synonyms
Granulocytic	Myeloblast	
	Progranulocyte	Promyelocyte
	Myelocyte	"Immature"
	Metamyelocyte	Juvenile
	Band	Stab
	Segmented	Polymorphonuclear, PMN
Lymphocytic	Lymphoblast	
	Prolymphocyte	
	Lymphocyte	
Monocytic	Monoblast	
	Promonocyte	
	Monocyte	
Erythrocytic	Rubriblast	Megaloblast, pronormoblast
	Prorubricyte	Basophilic normoblast, erythroblast
	Rubricyte	Erythroblast, polychromatophilic normoblast
	Metarubricyte	Normoblast, orthochromic normoblast
	Reticulocyte	
	Erythrocyte	Red blood cell
Plasmocytic	Plasmoblast	
	Proplasmocyte	Immunocyte, virocyte
	Plasmocyte	Plasma cell
Thrombocytic	Megakaryoblast	
	Promegakaryocyte	
	Megakaryocyte	
	Metamegakaryocyte	
	Thrombocyte	Platelet

MORPHOLOGY OF PERIPHERAL BLOOD CELLS AND BONE MARROW CELLS

Cell	Size (microns)	Nucleus				Cytoplasm		
		Shape	Staining quality	Chromatin	Nucleoli	Relative amount	Color	Granules
Granulocytes								
Myeloblast	15-20	Round or oval	Light purple	Finely reticulated	Pale blue 2-5	Small	Deep blue	. . .
Progranulocyte	14-20	Round or oval	Purple	Slightly coarse	1-3	Small	Blue	Few azurophilic
Myelocyte	10-18	Round or oval	Purple	Fairly coarse	. . .	Moderate	Bluish pink	Start differentiating
Metamyelocyte	10-18	Indented oval, resembling kidney or bean	Deep purple	Coarse	. . .	Large	Pink	Neutrophilic, eosinophilic, basophilic
Band cell	10-15	Curved with parallel sides	Purplish blue	Coarse	. . .	Large	Pink	Neutrophilic, eosinophilic, basophilic
Segmented Neutrophil	10-15	Ragged or divided into lobes	Purplish blue	Coarse	. . .	Large	Faint pink	Violet or absent in animal blood
Eosinophil	10-15	2-3 lobes	Purplish blue	Coarse	. . .	Large	Bluish pink	Bright red Horse—very large Dog—varying sizes Cat—rod-shaped
Basophil	10-15	Outline covered with granules	Pale blue	Indistinct	. . .	Moderate	Bluish pink	Bluish black Coarse in horse and cattle Moderate in dog and cat
Lymphocytes								
Lymphoblast	10-18	Round or oval	Light reddish purple	Fine	Pale blue 1-2	Small	Deep blue	. . .
Prolymphocyte	10-18	Oval or slightly indented	Deep reddish blue	Fine to slightly coarse	Occasional	Large	Dark to medium blue	Few azurophilic
Lymphocyte	6-18	Round, oval or slightly indented	Deep purplish blue	Large coarse clumps	. . .	Small to moderate	Sky blue	Few large azurophilic
Monocytes								
Monoblast	14-18	Round or oval	Deep purple	Finely reticulated	1-2	Moderate	Deep blue	. . .
Promonocyte	14-18	Irregular	Purple	Finely reticulated	0-1	Moderate	Gray-blue	Few fine lilac
Monocyte	12-18	Round, indented, band, or lobed	Pale purple	Fine strands	. . .	Large	Gray or gray-blue	Fine azurophilic
Erythrocytes								
Rubriblast	14-19	Round	Purple	Finely stippled	Usually 1-2	Small	Deep blue to gray-blue	. . .
Prorubricyte	10-15	Round	Purple	Coarse	Usually 1	Moderate	Blue	. . .
Rubricyte	8-12	Round	Deep purple	Definite clumps	. . .	Moderate	Blue to pink	. . .
Metarubricyte	7-10	Pyknotic, fragmented, or partially extruded	Dense purple	Solid	. . .	Moderate	Pink	. . .
Erythrocyte	4-8					Total	Pink	. . .
Thrombocytes	2-4					Total	Pale blue	Azurophilic

MORPHOLOGY OF OTHER BONE MARROW CELLS

Cell	Size (microns)	Nucleus			Cytoplasm			
		Shape	Staining quality	Nucleoli	Shape of cell	Relative amount	Color	Granules
Megakaryoblast	15-50	Oval or kidney-shaped, as many as 16 or more due to multiple division	Fine chromatin	Numerous	Cytoplasmic tags		Basophilic	Absent
Megakaryocyte	40-160	4 or more, irregular, multilobed, ring or doughnut	Intensely blue; chromatin is linear and coarse with distinct spaces between strands	None		Large	Light blue	Numerous, fine, azurophilic; aggregated
Osteoblast	20-50	Relatively small, round; often lies eccentrically or partially extruded	Well-defined margin and chromatin strands	1-3, distinct and blue	Irregular or blurred; cytoplasmic streamers due to trauma in aspiration	Large	Blue; chromophobic area separated from nuclear margin; wavy fibrils; bubbly due to spherical bodies	
Osteoclast	Over 100	Multiple round or oval nuclei distributed separately over entire cell	Dense chromatin	Usually one per nucleus	Irregular and elongated; indistinct borders	Large	Weakly basophilic to strongly eosinophilic with ground-glass appearance	Finely granular, azurophilic
Plasmocyte (plasma cell)	15-25	Relatively small, oval or round; eccentric	Coarse and lumpy chromatin, arranged in wheel-spoke manner		Spherical or ellipsoidal; irregular margins might be produced from trauma in aspiration	Large	Purple blue or reddish; clear zone beside the nucleus; brilliant translucency	May contain round red globules called "Russell bodies"
Reticulum cell	20-30	Large round or oval	Distinct chromatin	One or several	Indistinct outline; irregular shape with long cytoplasmic streamers		Blue	Few small blue, occasionally
Fat cells (lipocytes)	50-80	Small round or oval; eccentric	Definite and linear; globular body believed to be fatty material (sometimes present)		Round; fibril may extend out from margins	Large	Globules of fat of varying size that are chromophobic or stain a light pink or blue	

BONE MARROW CELLULAR COMPOSITION OF NORMAL ADULT ANIMALS

Cell	Dog (4) Range	Dog (4) Mean	Dog (11) Range	Cat (16) Mean	Cat (24) Mean	Cat (35) Mean	Cat (37) Mean	Horse (1, 2) Range	Horse (1, 2) Mean	Horse (6) Range	Horse (6) Mean
Granulocytic											
Myeloblast	0.00-1.6	0.58	0-1	1.1	1.3	0.82	0.34	0.0-0.66	0.237	...	...
Progranulocyte			...	2.8	7.6	...	1.11	0.14-0.99	0.502	0.0-5.0	1.83
Myelocyte											
Neutrophil	0.20-7.6	3.76	1-8	5.9	4.6	5.22	6.13	11-4-28.6	17.94	26.2-56.0	38.06
Eosinophil	0.00-0.8	0.26	0-2	0.3	...	1.10	...	0.69-2.35	1.43	0.4-3.6	2.34
Basophil											
Metamyelocyte											
Neutrophil			*	15.0	9.8	7.96	16.01	17.9-29.4	21.80	...	...
Eosinophil			0-2	0.2	...	...	...	1.05-6.95	3.46	...	...
Band											
Neutrophil	16.20-29.2	23.50	8-25*	14.7	13.4	30.59	*				
Eosinophil	0.00-0.8	0.12	0-2	0.3	...	...	...				
Segmented											
Neutrophil	12.04-29.6	18.50	15-30	14.0	5.3	22.52	32.51†	7.83-25.3	14.70	1.8-20.2	13.31
Eosinophil	0.00-3.0	1.56	0-4	1.3	1.5	1.71	2.90	0.52-5.95	2.63	0.2-1.2	0.60
Basophil	0.00-0.2	0.02	0-0.5	...	...	...	0.26	0.0-0.33	0.05	0.0-1.0	0.60
Total granulocytic cells		48.32	45-60	55.6	43.5	69.9	59.32		63.73		56.74
Erythrocytic											
Rubriblast	0.00-2.8	1.02	0-2	1.2	0.7	0.35	0.62	0.0-0.87	0.34	0.4-3.4	1.6
Prorubricyte	0.80-4.0	2.50	1-4	2.8	6.3	1.24	6.74	0.16-4.35	1.88	...	...
Rubricyte	22.80-46.6	35.18	10-25	16.1	6.3	1.24	6.74	2.21-13.0	6.34	8.0-32.0	20.94
Metarubricyte			8-25	18.2	8.3	18.52	33.34	4.20-39.20	17.60	5.0-24.2	13.71
Total erythroid cells		38.70	30-45	38.4	15.3	20.1	40.70		26.16		34.66
Lymphocyte	5.80-15.2	9.80	1-5	5.1	7.8	9.05	3.51	2.46-20.9	9.71	2.0-5.6	3.91
Immature	0.00-0.2	0.04									
Plasma cell	0.00-2.2	0.82	0-3	0.5	0.3	0.75	0.62	0.0-1.66	0.50	0.0-0.8	0.63
Monocyte	0.20-5.2	1.20	0-5	...	...	...	0.56	...	...	1.2-4.8	2.46
Immature	0.00-1.0	0.14									
Megakaryocyte											
Reticulum cell	0.00-1.6	0.84		0.3	...	0.02					
Other cells	0.00-1.2	0.44			32.5		0.48				
M:E ratio		1.25:1	1-2:1	1.6:1	2.8:1	3.5:1	1.45:1	1.1-10.2		0.9-3.76	

* Includes metamyelocytes.
† Includes bands.

BONE MARROW CELLULAR COMPOSITION OF NORMAL ADULT ANIMALS *(continued)*

Cell	Cattle (6) Range	Cattle (6) Mean	Cattle (19) Range	Cattle (44, 45) Mean	Cattle (46) Range	Cattle (46) Mean	Sheep (18) Range	Sheep (18) Mean	Sheep (47) Range	Goat (46) Mean	Pig (31) Mean
Granulocytic											
Myeloblast	...	...	1.5-4.0	2.3	...	...	0.1-1.4	0.47	0.1-1.1	...	0.6
Progranulocyte	0.0-6.8	1.51	0.5-3.0	1.5	0.2-1.4	0.79	0.0-0.6	0.24	0-1.4	0.79	2
Myelocyte											
Neutrophil	10.4-32.0	19.39	3.0-9.6	6.5*	1.0-5.0	2.90	1.5-8.1	4.60	0.5-4.9	2.69	6
Eosinophil	1.8-10.4	6.69	...	4.9*	0.1-1.4	0.73	3.3-6.2	4.85	0.2-5.7	0.85	...
Basophil											
Metamyelocyte											
Neutrophil	...	...	3.0-13.5*		1.3-7.4	4.14	2.1-6.0	4.33	1.5-9.1	8.25	11
Eosinophil	...	...	...		0.7-3.4	2.09	7.8-15.0	10.84	0.4-5.0	1.67	5
Band											
Neutrophil	...	...	7.5-18.5	9.7	5.0-12.8	8.2	10.6-22.8	16.38	2.4-18.2	8.88	17
Eosinophil	...	...		3.0					*		
Segmented									...		
Neutrophil	1.2-12.2	5.73	6.5-19.5	6.2	4.9-19.0	11.46	1.4-6.9	4.58	1-19.6	9.98	21
Eosinophil	0.0-7.6	1.92	...	0.4	2.4-10.8	5.67	0.8-5.1	2.80	2-10†	1.79	
Basophil	0.0-1.0	0.34	...	0.3	0.0-0.8	0.19	0.3-2.3	1.04	0-2	0.06	0.3
Total granulocytic cells	19.6-60.4	35.59		34.8	20-55	36.60		50.13	45-55	34.95	...
Erythrocytic											
Rubriblast				2.3			0.5-1.4	0.96	1-7.2	...	0.5
Prorubricyte	...	...	0-1.0	9.0	0.6-1.7	1.23	1.5-4.9	3.30	...	1.45	3.5
Rubricyte	11.8-42.8	30.26	30-62.5	9.0	16.3-30.8	25.73	27.2-37.3	31.86	11-37.7	30.61	24
Metarubricyte	7.2-39.2	21.69	...	40.3	10.4-35.3	23.28	4.9-15.1	9.91	13-39.9	24.27	9.1
Total erythroid cells	21.0-72.2	52.66		51.6	30-60	50.24		46.03	40-50	56.33	...
Lymphocyte	1.4-17.2	6.68	5.0-20.0	7.2	5.6-16.3	10.69	0.6-3.1	1.73	1-11	7.49	...
Immature											
Plasma cell	0.2-2.0	0.79	...	0.2	0.4-2.3	0.99	0.0-1.0	0.35	0-1	0.11-0.03	...
Monocyte	0.0-7.6	2.64	0-1.0	0.4	0.00-0.4	0.16	0.0-0.7	0.26	0-4.3	0.02	...
Immature											
Megakaryocyte			...	0.1	0.0-0.2	0.05				0	...
Reticulum cell		...	...	0.9	0.2-2.9	1.27				0.52	
Other cells				4.6			0.2-1.6	0.84		0.58	
M:E ratio	0.27-2.59	0.676	0.7	0.71	0.4-1.84	0.79		1,103:1	1.59-2.35	0.62	1.7:1

*Included in myelocytes.
†Includes bands.

3 BLOOD SMEAR

I. Importance — the examination of a well-stained blood smear by a knowledgeable observer can provide more valuable information than any other single laboratory test.

II. Preparation of the blood smear
  A. Slide method (See Fig. 3.1.)
    1. New microscope slides, preferably with beveled edges, should be used.
      a. To avoid production of artifacts in the erythrocytes, the new slide should be dipped in 95% alcohol and wiped dry with a clean cloth.
    2. Ideally, smears should be made from freshly drawn blood to which no anticoagulant has been added, as anticoagulants tend to cause distortion of the cells.
      a. If EDTA is added, slides should be prepared within 15 min after obtaining the blood sample.
        (1) The blood should be well mixed by gentle agitation or with a mechanical rotator before using a capillary tube or applicator stick to place a small drop of blood near one end of the slide, which is on a solid, flat surface.
          (a) When slides with frosted ends are used, the drop should be placed on the smooth glass near the frosted end.
    3. Place the end of a second slide (spreader slide) against the surface of the first slide, holding it at a comfortable angle of about 30°.

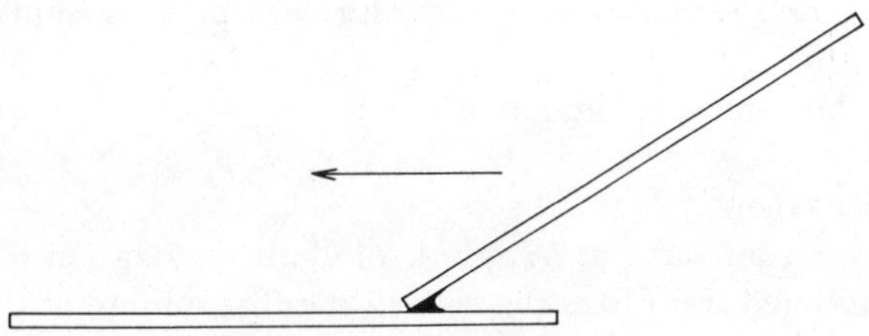

Fig. 3.1. Slide method.

    4. Draw the spreader slide gently into the drop of blood; when the blood has spread along two-thirds or more of the width by capillary action, push the spreader slide forward with a steady, even motion. The blood will follow, making a thin film.
      a. The thickness of the film should decrease from the beginning to the tail or feathered edge; that part adjacent to the tail is usually the area of ideal film thickness because the cells are not distorted in the thin area.
      b. The thickness of the smear will depend upon the size of the drop, the angle of the spreader, and the speed with which the spreader slide is pushed.
      c. If too large a drop of blood is placed on the slide, much of it can be left behind if, after the blood spreads behind the spreader slide, the slide is lifted and placed forward before spreading.
    5. Dry rapidly by waving in the air or by using a fan in humid climate.
      a. One cause of crenated erythrocytes is the slow drying of the blood film as the water moves from the erythrocyte into the plasma.
      b. Do not use heat for drying.
    6. Stain within 1 hr for best results.
      a. If the slide cannot be stained within a reasonable time, it should be preserved by fixing it in absolute methyl alcohol.

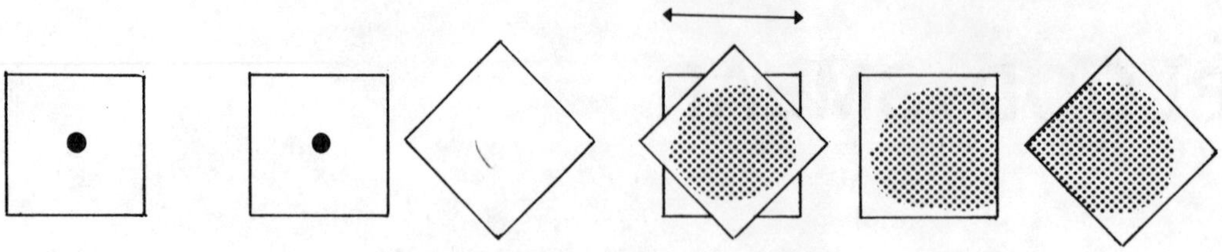

Fig. 3.2. Coverglass method.

B. Coverglass method (See Fig. 3.2.)
   1. New coverglasses (22 x 22 mm and No. 1 or No. 1.5 in thickness) can be kept in alcohol until ready to use; then dry with a clean cloth. Handle only by the edges.
   2. Place a small drop (2 to 3 mm in diameter) of blood in the center of a coverglass.
   3. Pick up a second coverglass and hold it by two adjacent corners between the thumb and index finger.
   4. Gently place the second coverglass diagonally over the first in such a manner that the two superimposed coverglasses form an octagon; the blood will spread between the two by capillary action.
   5. When the spread of blood is almost complete, grasp the protruding corners of the coverglasses and slide them apart with a steady parallel or lateral motion.
      a. There must be no upward pull or holes or an uneven distribution of cells will result.
   6. Allow the two smears to dry in the air.
   7. The coverglass with the blood may be placed in a special staining rack, in a special staining jar, or on an inverted cork fixed to the bottom of a pan by means of paraffin.
   8. Leukocytes are more evenly distributed in a good coverglass smear than in a slide smear.

III. Fixation

A. Fixatives are reagents that solidify cells and prevent them from undergoing autolytic degeneration.
B. Fixation is a preliminary step in the staining procedure except when supravital staining is carried out.
C. Types of fixatives
   1. Absolute methyl alcohol—most commonly used
   2. Ethyl alcohol
   3. Formaldehyde and its vapors
D. With a Romanowsky type stain such as Wright's, preliminary fixation of the smear is not necessary because the methanol of the undiluted stain fixes the cells in the first minute of the staining process.
E. If there is to be a long delay in staining the films, they should be immersed in methanol for up to 15 min and then allowed to air dry.

IV. Staining of blood smears

A. Romanowsky-type stains
   1. A Romanowsky-type stain is composed of polychromed methylene blue and eosin.
      a. Polychroming is the oxidation and alkalinization of methylene blue and results in the production of colored compounds known as azures.
      b. Oxidation may occur with aging or may be hastened by treatment with alkalies and by heating.
   2. Principle
      a. Acidic dyes unite with the basic parts of the cell, such as the cytoplasm.
         (1) Eosin is an acidic dye.
         (2) Cells appear red, pink, or orange in color.
         (3) The terms "eosinophilic" and "acidophilic" can be used interchangeably.
      b. Basic dyes are attracted to and combine with the acidic parts of the cell such as nucleic acids and nuclear nucleoproteins.
         (1) Methylene blue is a basic dye.
         (2) Cells appear blue, purple, or violet in color.
         (3) They are said to be "basophilic."

3. Water—good differential staining requires that the water be of the proper pH or adjusted to it
   a. Neutralization of water (5)
      (1) Water that is neutral with the use of hematoxylin as an indicator has a pH of 6.8 to 7.0.
      (2) The reaction of the water used may be tested by placing a few granules or crystals of hematoxylin in a test tube that has been previously rinsed with the water to be tested, since the tube might not be neutral. Pour about 5 ml of water into the test tube, shake, and note the color.
         (a) Neutral water—becomes pale pink within 10 sec
         (b) Acid water—becomes yellow and remains so longer than 5 min
         (c) Alkaline water—becomes reddish purple immediately, or before 1 min
      (3) If the water is acid in reaction, 1% potassium carbonate is used as a neutralizing agent, adding a drop at a time to the stock bottle; the reaction is tested until the water turns pink without a trace of yellow in 10 sec.
      (4) 1% hydrochloric or acetic acid is used as a neutralizing agent if the water is too alkaline in reaction.
      (5) Neutralize enough water for 1 day's use and store the water in a Pyrex bottle that has been used for no other purpose than to hold distilled water.
      (6) This neutral water should give satisfactory staining results with Wright's or Giemsa stain.
   b. Buffered distilled water
      (1) Prepared buffer salts may be purchased and are available over a wide pH range.
      (2) Alternately, several methods are available for preparing buffered distilled water.
         (a) pH 6.6 phosphate buffer: 5.47 g of monobasic potassium phosphate + 3.80 g of dibasic sodium phosphate q.s. with distilled water to 1000 ml in a volumetric flask.
         (b) Thoroughly mix the two salts in the proportion for the desired pH, as indicated below, in a mortar and use 1 g to 2000 ml of distilled water:

pH	$Na_2HPO_4 + 2H_2O$ (g)	KH_2PO_4 (g)
6.5	2.723	8.316
6.8	4.539	5.940
7.0	5.447	4.752
7.2	6.355	3.564

         (c) Mix stock solutions of phosphates in the proportion indicated for the desired pH:

pH	$NaH_2PO_4 \cdot H_2O$ (9.2g/L) or KH_2PO_4 (9.08 g/L in ml)	Na_2HPO_4 (anhydrous) (9.5 g/L in ml)
6.4	73.5	26.5
6.5	68.5	31.5
6.6	62.5	37.5
6.7	56.5	43.5
6.8	51.0	49.0
6.9	45.0	55.0
7.0	39.0	61.0

B. Wright's stain
   1. Forms of dye available
      a. Dry powder
         (1) Bulk
         (2) Preweighed—vials, capsules, tablets
      b. Ready-made solution—most convenient, but often has deteriorated from long storage on the distributor's shelf
   2. Preparation of stain
      a. Conventional method
         (1) Place 0.5 g of dry Wright's stain powder (certified) in a mortar.
         (2) Add 300 ml of absolute methyl alcohol (free of acetone and acetic acid) slowly to the dye in the mortar, at the same time grinding the mixture and pouring the supernate into a dry, dark bottle. Alcohol is added until all the dye is in solution and the total amount of the measured alcohol is used.
         (3) Shake the bottle each day for about 2 wk, then filter.
         (4) Aging of the stain will take 2 to 4 wk before it will be satisfactory for use.
      b. Accelerated method
         (1) Place 0.3 g of dry Wright's stain powder in a mortar and overlay with 3 ml of glycerol. Grind thoroughly.
         (2) Rinse with 100 ml of absolute methyl alcohol, added in small amounts, and place in a dark container.
         (3) Mix with magnetic stirrer about 1 wk, without heat.
         (4) Filter before use.
   3. Method of staining
      a. Cover the dried blood smear completely with Wright's stain and allow to stand for 1 to 3 min.
         (1) The undiluted alcoholic stain acts primarily as a fixative because the minimal staining properties before dilution are confined to some staining of neutral elements.
         (2) The timing will vary, depending upon the strength of each batch of stain.
         (3) The rack must be level to avoid accumulation of stain at one end of the slide.
         (4) Adjacent slides on the rack should not be touching, or the stain will flow off.
      b. Add an equal amount of buffered distilled water or ''neutral'' water (pH 6.6 to 6.8 for most animal's blood), distributing it over the entire smear and taking care that the solution does not run over the edge.
      c. Allow the mixture to stand for 3 to 5 min. A metallic scum should appear green.
         (1) Partial disassociation of the compound dye takes place upon the addition of the water, producing free acid dye (eosin) and free alkaline methylene blue and its derivatives.
         (2) The Wright's stain and the water can be evenly mixed by blowing gently on the surface.
      d. Float off the metallic scum with a stream of water form a wash bottle or from the tap. Use distilled water if the tap water is too alkaline.
         (1) Do not pour the stain off the slide before washing, as this will result in a precipitate forming on the slide.
         (2) Wash the stain off thoroughly; but avoid overwashing, as it will lighten the stain.
      e. Wipe the stain from the back of the slide or the coverglass with cleansing tissue while it is still wet. Otherwise, it will require alcohol to remove the dried stain.
      f. Stand the slide on end, wave gently in the air, or blot gently with a pad of bibulous paper to dry.
      g. Smears on stained coverglass preparations can be examined by placing a drop of oil on a slide and applying the coverglass stained side down.
         (1) If a permanent preparation is desired, the oil can be dissolved with xylene and a mounting medium applied, such as Permount or Canada balsam.
   4. Chanco modification of Wright's stain (3)
      a. Method
         (1) Use a Coplin jar containing 0.5% Wright's stain in absolute methyl alcohol for immersion of the blood films instead of flooding the slide in a horizontal position.
         (2) After immersion for 20 sec in the stain, the slides are then transferred to another Coplin jar containing ordinary tap water in which they are allowed to remain for 30 to 60 sec.
         (3) While the slides are still in the jar, flush with a strong current of tap water from the faucet to be sure all the precipitate is removed.

b. Advantages—conserves stain, methyl alcohol, and time
c. Disadvantage—more precipitate is likely to be present
d. Notes
(1) Buffered solutions or distilled water may be used if tap water does not produce proper colors.
(2) The staining solution will keep its optimum working efficiency for about 2 mo by storing it in a dark place when not in use or by keeping the top of the Coplin jar and the cover smeared with Vaseline to avoid evaporation of the alcohol.
(a) Evaporation of stain and alcohol is indicated by poor definition of the leukocyte nuclei and can be compensated for and rejuvenated by adding 5 to 10 ml of methyl alcohol to the staining solution.
(3) When the stain is used frequently, weekly filtration is desirable.

5. Wright's stain for birds (7)
a. Preparation of stain
(1) Wright's stain: 3.3 g of Wright's stain powder in 500 ml of absolute methyl alcohol
(2) Formalin solution: 0.25 ml of concentrated formalin in 500 ml of distilled water. Adjust to pH 6.8 by adding either 0.25% sodium carbonate or 0.25% hydrochloric acid as needed.
b. Method of staining:
(1) Dried smear is covered with Wright's stain and allowed to stand for 8 min.
(2) Add formalin solution slowly with a dropper, being careful not to overflow.
(3) When a metallic sheen covers the entire surface of the fluid, wash off immediately with distilled water adjusted to pH 6.8.
(4) Differentiate by dipping slides up and down 6 to 10 times in ether and absolute methyl alcohol (1:1). Blot dry.
(a) Examine under a microscope and, if too blue, differentiate further.
c. Staining characteristics

Cell	Cytoplasm	Chromatin
Erythrocytes	Yellow to pinkish	Purple
Heterophils	Yellow to brownish red rods	Light purple
Lymphocytes	Blue granules	Purplish red
Monocytes	Light blue granules	Purple
Eosinophils	Similar to heterophils	
Basophils	Dark purple granules	
Thrombocytes	Gray-blue	Purple

6. Wright's stain for cold-blooded vertebrates (7)
a. Cover with Wright's stain for 2 min.
b. Add an equal amount of citrate buffer (pH 6.7) for 3 min.
c. Wash in distilled water.

C. Giemsa stain
1. General considerations
a. Giemsa stain has various azure compounds with eosin and methylene blue, rather than empirically polychromed dyes such as provided in Wright's stain.
b. It is an excellent stain for many blood parasites and for inclusion bodies and will produce consistent results.
c. In blood smears it stains the red (azurophil) granules well, but neutrophilic granules and erythrocytes are poorly stained.
(1) For this reason, it is often incorporated in combination stains, such as Wright-Giemsa or May-Grünwald-Giemsa.
d. Commercial stock solutions of Giemsa blood stain are recommended for purchase and are stable indefinitely.

2. Method
    a. Place dried blood smear in a Coplin jar containing absolute methyl alcohol for about 3 min to fix the smear.
    b. Drain off the alcohol and allow the slide to dry.
    c. Transfer the slide to a second Coplin jar containing fresh stain and allow to stain for 15 to 60 min.
        (1) One volume of commercial stock Giemsa stain to 9 to 25 volumes of distilled water (pH6.8) can be prepared daily, depending upon the length of time desired for staining.
        (2) 12 to 18 hr may be necessary to show inclusions, while a 60-min staining period is used when blood parasites are suspected.
        (3) It is best to dilute the stain in a jar that has been used consistently for Giemsa stain, as the residual stain in the container is desirable.
            (a) Rinse the jar in hot tap water to remove the precipitate rather than using cleaning solution or detergent.
        (4) The diluted Giemsa stain must be prepared just before use; it is stable for only a few hours, after which time light stains and precipitate may result.
3. Modified Giemsa stain—for more rapid staining
    a. Fix smear in absolute methyl alcohol for 3 min.
    b. Dilute 2 ml of commercial stock Giemsa stain solution with 8 ml of distilled water or buffered water (pH 6.8) to make a more concentrated dilute stain than by the standard method.
    c. Flood the diluted stain on the smear placed on a staining rack in a manner similar to that used for the Wright's staining procedure; it is not necessary to add buffered water, as it is already incorporated in the stain.
    d. Allow to stain for 5 min, then dry and examine.

D. Leishman's stain (1)
1. Preparation
    a. Grind 0.15 g of Leishman stain powder with small amounts of absolute methyl alcohol until an even suspension is obtained. A total of 100 ml of methanol is added to produce complete solution.
    b. Pour into a dark bottle and age for a few weeks prior to use.
2. Method of staining
    a. Flood the air-dried blood film with undiluted stock Leishman's stain and leave for 1 to 2 min to fix.
    b. Dilute the stain on the smear with double the volume of buffered distilled water and stain for 5 to 15 min.
    c. Blow on the mixture or rock the slide gently to aid mixing.
    d. Wash with distilled water until the film has a pinkish tinge (0.5 to 2 min).
    e. Wipe the back of the slide to remove excess stain and allow to dry in an upright position.
3. Limitations
    a. Usually adequate for routine slides, but it will not stain the cytoplasmic granules as well as the combination stains.
    b. Leishman's stain will not differentiate the heterophils from the eosinophils of the rabbit or chicken.

E. Wright-Giemsa stain (modified Wright's stain)
1. Preparation of stain
    a. 300 mg of dry Wright's stain powder and 30 mg of Giemsa stain powder are ground in a mortar with 100 ml of absolute methyl alcohol (acetone-free).
    b. Allow to stand for 24 to 48 hr before using.
    c. Keep well stoppered to prevent evaporation of alcohol or absorption of water vapor.
    d. Commercial Wright-Giemsa solutions are available.
2. Method of staining—similar to method described for Wright's stain

F. Wright-Leishman stain (10)
1. Preparation of stain
    a. Wright's stain (solution I)
        (1) Combine 0.6 g of Wright's stain powder, 5 ml of glycerol, and 300 ml of absolute methyl alcohol in a 500-ml Pyrex Erlenmeyer flask.

(2) The mixture is heated gently to a point just below boiling, while stirring constantly.
(3) Repeat the heating process 3 or 4 times after the solution cools for a few minutes.
(4) Filter after the solution cools to room temperature. It is now ready for use.

b. Leishman's stain (solution II)
(1) Powdered Leishman's stain is substituted for Wright's stain, with the same procedure for preparation as given for solution I.

c. The staining mixture is prepared by combining 3 volumes of solution I and 1 volume of solution II; this can be stored.

2. Method of staining
a. Fix the blood smear or coverglass in absolute methyl alcohol for 5 min.
b. Transfer to the stain in a Coplin jar or flood on a horizontal slide and leave for 3 min.
c. The buffer solution (pH 6.6) should be applied for 6 min, or the smear should be placed in a Coplin jar containing 5 parts of buffer with 1 part of stain.
d. Rinse in 2 changes of distilled water.
e. Dry and examine.

G. May-Grünwald-Giemsa stain (1)
1. Method of staining
a. Fresh air-dried smears are immersed in a jar of absolute methyl alcohol for 2 to 10 min to fix.
(1) The relatively long fixation period is necessary for good staining, especially if the smears are of bone marrow.
b. Transfer to a jar containing May-Grünwald stain diluted with 1 or 2 parts of buffered distilled water (pH 6.8 to 7.2, depending upon material being stained) and leave for 3 to 15 min.
c. Without washing, transfer the slide to Giemsa stain diluted with 9 parts of buffered distilled water and leave for 7 to 30 min.
d. Differentiate in buffered distilled water for about 5 min.
e. Rinse and dry.

2. Results
a. Although more time consuming and complex than the single stains, this method will produce better stained cytoplasmic granules.

H. Staining thick blood smears for parasites
1. Giemsa stain (13)
a. In a Coplin staining jar place 1 ml of stock Giemsa solution, 2 ml of buffered distilled water (pH 7.0), and 47 ml of distilled water.
b. Immerse unfixed slides in the jar for 40 to 120 min; check at periodic intervals to determine adequacy of staining action, as the time will vary with the nature of the specimen.
(1) Trypanosomes may require as long as 2 hr for adequate staining.
c. Results
(1) The erythrocytes are hemolyzed.
(2) Blood parasites are well demonstrated in the absence of the reddish-staining hemoglobin.

2. Field's stain (7)
a. Field's stain can be obtained commercially and consists of two solutions:
(1) Solution A—methylene blue and azure A or B in phosphate buffer
(2) Solution B—eosin solution in phosphate buffer
b. Method of staining
(1) Dip slide in solution A for 1 sec.
(2) Rinse gently in distilled water for a few seconds or until stain ceases to flow from the smear.
(3) Dip slide in Solution B for 1 sec.
(a) Solution B must be used with care, as there is a tendency to decolorize the leukocytes stained with the methylene blue-azure of solution A and to hasten the dissolving of hemoglobin.
(4) Gently dip the slide 2 or 3 times in distilled water.
(5) Stand slide on end to dry. Do not blot.
c. Result
(1) The thick center of partially laked hemoglobin is not as satisfactory for examination as the surrounding area.

(2) Parasites—blue cytoplasm, purplish red or deep ruby red chromatin
(3) Thrombocytes—pale purple or lavender
(4) Leukocytes—pale blue, poorly defined cytoplasm; dark blue, well-defined nuclei; small, indistinct neutrophilic granules; bright red and well-defined eosinophilic granules; and deep blue basophilic granules with a reddish cast.

3. Modification of Field's stain for demonstration of *Babesia gibsoni* (4)
   a. Method of staining
      (1) Fix in methyl alcohol no longer than 7 min.
      (2) Place in methylene blue solution for 10 to 15 sec, stirring.
      (3) Dip the slide as follows:
         (a) 2 dips in phosphate buffer
         (b) 7 dips in eosin solution
         (c) 2 dips in phosphate buffer
         (d) 3 dips in methylene blue solution
         (e) 2 dips in water to rinse and remove precipitated stain
   b. Results
      (1) Greater contrast and variety of forms will be observed than with Giemsa stain.
      (2) Thin smears can be examined, and staining is not as time consuming as with Giemsa stain.

I. Quick stains—available from most laboratory houses
1. New methylene blue (2, 10, 11)
   a. Preparation
      (1) Dissolve 0.5 g of powdered new methylene blue in 100 ml of 0.85% sodium chloride solution.
      (2) Add 1 ml of full strength formalin (40% formaldehyde gas in solution) to each 100 ml of stain to prevent fungal growth.
      (3) Filter and store in a dark bottle.
      (4) Stain is ready for immediate use and will keep indefinitely when evaporation is prevented.
   b. New methylene blue stain in solution is also available from commercial sources.
   c. Method
      (1) Prepare the blood film on a slide or coverglass and dry.
      (2) Fixation in alcohol is not required, as this is a vital stain.
      (3) Place a drop of stain on a clean coverglass if the film is on a slide, or on a clean slide if the blood film is on a coverglass.
      (4) Place the coverglass on the slide and avoid bubble formation as the stain spreads between the glass surfaces.
      (5) The wet-mount preparation is ready for immediate examination with the low power, high dry, or oil immersion objectives.
      (6) The film is not a permanent preparation but can be preserved for several hours by ringing the edges of the coverglass with immersion oil to lessen evaporation.
   d. Advantages
      (1) Quick screening
      (2) Demonstrates structures seen only with vital or supravital stain—reticulocytes, Heinz bodies (erythrocyte refractile bodies)
      (3) Good nuclear morphology
      (4) Versatility—useful for staining urine sediment, exfoliative cytology, cerebrospinal fluid, blood parasites, smears of exudates, and all types of aspirates
   e. Disadvantages
      (1) Eosinophilic granules not well stained
      (2) *Haemobartonella* confused with reticulocytes
      (3) Not a permanent preparation
2. Camco Quik Stain (Cambridge Chemical Products Inc.)—a buffered differential Wright's stain
   a. Method
      (1) Dip the slide in stain for 5 to 10 sec.

(2) Dip the slide in distilled water for 15 to 20 sec.
(a) For darker stained leukocytes, dip the slide in distilled water for 1 min or more.
(3) Rinse by dipping in distilled water for a few seconds and dry.

3. Diff-Quik (Hartman-Leddon Co. Inc.)—claims results identical to Wright-Giemsa stain
a. Method—Diff-Quik is a dip stain, so each component should be dispensed in a Coplin jar or other dip-staining device
(1) Dip the slide in the fixative solution for 5 sec (five 1-sec dips). Allow excess fixative to drain.
(2) Dip the slide in solution I for 5 sec (five 1-sec dips). Allow excess stain to drain.
(3) Dip the stain in solution II for 5 sec (five 1-sec dips). Allow excess stain to drain.
(4) Rinse the slide with distilled or deionized water.
(5) Allow to dry; examine.
b. Notes
(1) If more intense overall stain is desired, increase the number of dips in solutions I and II.
(2) If a paler stain is desired, decrease dips in solutions I and II, but never go below 3 dips of 1 full second each.
(3) To increase eosinophilic staining, increase the number of dips in solution I.
(4) To increase basophilic staining, increase dips in solution II.
(5) Solutions should be changed every week.

4. Hemal Stain set (Hemal Stain Co.)
a. Method
(1) Fix blood film with absolute methyl alcohol and let dry.
(2) Dip slide in solution I for 6 sec.
(3) Rinse smear under tap water or in a beaker of water.
(4) Dip slide in solution II for 6 sec.
(5) Rinse smear in water.
(6) Allow to dry; examine.
b. Note
(1) Variations in time may be necessary to adjust for various species and pH of local water.
(2) Filter when the solution appears cloudy.

J. Reticulocyte stains—reticulocytes are immature nonnucleated erythrocytes still retaining basophilic material that appears as a reticulum or punctate foci with vital staining (2, 10, 11)

1. Vital stains that can be used for demonstration of reticulocytes
a. New methylene blue (basic blue 24)—0.5 g, potassium oxalate 1.6 g, and distilled water 100 ml
b. Brilliant cresyl blue—1 g in 100 ml of 0.85% sodium chloride with 0.4 g of sodium citrate added

2. Method of staining
a. Dry preparation
(1) Place equal quantities of blood and vital stain in a small test tube, in a capillary pipette, or at one end of a clean slide; mix.
(2) Allow to stand for 5 to 20 min.
(a) Cover slide with petri dish to prevent evaporation.
(3) Smear a drop of the mixture on a slide to make a thin film.
(4) Counterstain with one of the Romanowsky stains in the usual manner for staining blood smears.
b. Wet preparation
(1) Place 1 drop of blood and 2 drops of vital stain on a glass slide and mix for about 15 sec.
(2) Cover the mixture with a coverglass, apply gentle pressure on the coverglass, remove excess mixture with cleansing tissue, and seal with Vaseline or other suitable material.
(3) Allow the preparation to stand for 5 to 10 min.

3. Results—the reticulum, punctate foci, nuclei of leukocytes, and thrombocytes will stain blue

4. Counting reticulocytes
a. The proportion of erythrocytes with blue-staining threads or granules to the total erythrocyte population is determined.
(1) The percentage in 500 to 1000 erythrocytes is usually determined.

b. Laboratories performing reticulocyte counts routinely may find it helpful to use a Miller ocular micrometer in the eyepiece.
   (1) Bausch and Lomb manufactures these disks for the Kinsman Optical Co.

K. Prussian blue reaction for iron—used for demonstration of siderocytes and sideroleukocytes (1, 6, 8, 9)
1. Siderocytes—erythrocytes with iron-containing granules
   a. Prussian blue reagent is prepared just before use.

2% potassium ferrocyanide solution	25 ml
1% hydrochloric acid	75 ml

   b. Slide already stained with Wright's stain or other Romanowsky stain is immersed in Prussian blue reagent for 10 min.
      (1) Romanowsky's stain may be decolorized for several hours in methanol, but this step is not necessary before proceeding to the Prussian blue reagent.
   c. Wash under a stream of distilled water until a pink color appears.
   d. Results—the siderotic granules stain blue and vary in size from barely visible when diffuse to 2 microns in diameter when there are only a few in the cell
2. Sideroleukocytes—macrophages that have engulfed iron
   a. 9 ml of jugular blood is collected in a vial containing 1 ml of 10% sodium citrate or heparin.
   b. Allow the cells to settle for approximately 1 hr.
   c. Pipette about 5 ml of plasma into a centrifuge tube and centrifuge for 5 min at a moderate rate of speed (2000 rpm).
   d. Pour off supernatant plasma and leave just enough to suspend the concentrated leukocytes.
   e. Place a drop of the concentrated leukocytes on a slide and make an even, thick smear.
   f. Air-dry and fix with methyl alcohol for 10 min.
   g. Stain with a freshly prepared mixture of equal parts of 10 to 20% hydrochloric acid and 10% potassium ferrocyanide for 20 min.
   h. Wash with running tap water for 3 to 5 min.
   i. Counterstain with one of the following.
      (1) 0.2% pyronin for 10 min
      (2) 1% safranine for 1 min
      (3) 2% carbol fuchsin for 30 sec
   j. Under the oil immersion objective, count the number of sideroleukocytes in 100 fields, containing 300 to 400/field, to determine the number per 10,000 cells.
3. Indications
   a. Increased number of cells with ferritin granules will be seen in hemolytic anemia.
      (1) The presence of 4 circulating siderocytes per 10,000 cells is indicative of equine infectious anemia, but is not pathognomonic.
   b. Iron stain on the bone marrow is the most reliable index of an iron deficiency anemia.

L. Causes of inadequately stained blood smears
1. Anyone who has experience in staining smears will verify that the only consistent feature of staining is inconsistency in results. Analysis of the poor results will determine what modification of technique is required to correct the problem.
   a. Entire smear is too blue—granules of neutrophils overstained and larger than normal, and granules of the eosinophils deep gray
      (1) Buffered water, wash water, or stain too alkaline
      (2) Excessive thickness of the smear
      (3) Alkaline residue on the slide
      (4) Insufficient washing
      (5) Prolonged staining before diluting with buffered water
   b. Nuclei of leukocytes are pale blue, and erythrocytes and granules of eosinophils are unusually red.
      (1) Buffered water, wash water, or stain too acid
      (2) Acid residue on slide

c. Entire smear has a pale stain.
   (1) Understaining
   (2) Weak stain
   (3) Excessive washing or allowing water to stand on slide
   (4) Using warm or hot water for washing slide
d. Variation in staining on different areas of the smear
   (1) Buffered water unevenly applied and not thoroughly mixed with Wright's stain
   (2) Acid or alkaline residue on slide
   (3) Water not properly drained from slide after washing
e. Precipitated stain
   (1) Lack of thorough washing
   (2) Precipitate in Wright's stain not properly filtered
   (3) Evaporation of alcoholic stain may be due to excessive staining time, slide tilted so that stain runs to one end, or to tilting stain off slide before washing.

V. Examination of the smear (Fig. 3.3)

A. Inspect the blood smear under low power to note distribution of cells, and select a portion of the smear near the thin end where the erythrocytes do not overlap. Switch to the oil immersion objective for making the rest of the examination.

B. The erythrocytes should be inspected in regard to:
1. Size—variation (anisocytosis), normocytic, macrocytic, or microcytic
2. Shape—variation (poikilocytosis), target cells, spherocytes, acanthocytes
3. Color—normochromic, hyperchromic, hypochromic
4. Abnormal conditions—polychromasia, reticulocytes (new methylene blue stain), nucleated, Howell-Jolly bodies, basophilic stippling, parasites
5. Abnormal forms
   a. Polychromatophilia
   b. Basophilic stippling
   c. Howell-Jolly bodies
   d. Nucleated erythrocytes
   e. Reticulocytes—in brilliant cresyl blue stain or new methylene blue
   f. Parasites

C. The differential leukocyte count is done by counting and classifying at least 100 leukocytes. More should be counted when the total leukocyte count is appreciably elevated or when there is an abnormal distribution.
1. There is a tendency for the neutrophils to be more abundant along the margins of the smears made with slides, while the lymphocytes tend to be present a short distance from the margin. Monocytes and eosinophils are distributed throughout. Due to the margination of the leukocytes, the central area of the slide is usually devoid of cells except when the total count is fairly high.
   a. To give a representative sampling of all portions of the smear, examination of the feathered edge and/or the use of the Battlement method is used as follows:
      (1) Start the examination along the outer margin of the smear for about 3 fields, move inward a short distance (1 mm or 3 fields), parallel the margin for 3 fields, then move back to the edge of the smear.
      (2) Repeat the procedure for as many times as necessary to identify the required number of cells.

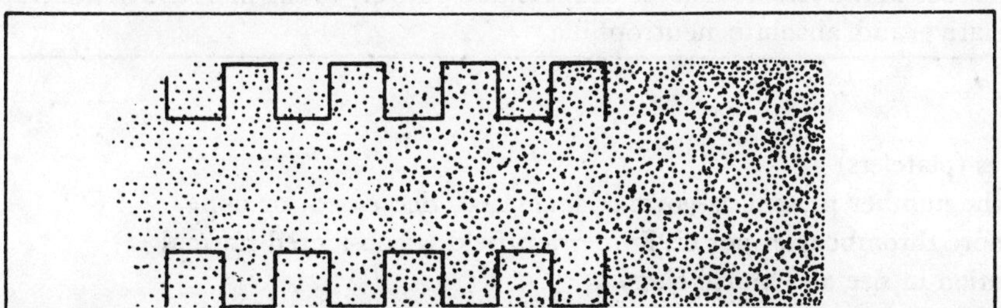

Fig. 3.3. Examination of the smear.

2. The leukocytes should be inspected in regard to:
   a. Size
   b. Cytoplasm
      (1) Color
      (2) Relative amount
      (3) Granules
   c. Nucleus
      (1) Shape
      (2) Color
      (3) Chromatin structure
      (4) Nucleoli
3. Relative and absolute values of leukocytes
   a. The leukocyte differential count expresses in percent the relative number of the different types of leukocytes present in the blood.
      (1) Relative values are often misleading; for if the percentage of one cell type is increased, it could be due to an actual increase in the number of this cell type or to a decrease in cells of another type.
   b. The absolute value for each type of leukocyte is obtained by multiplying the percent by the local leukocyte count.
      (1) If the total number of any cell per microliter is increased, it is termed an absolute increase; but if only the percentage is increased because the other types are decreased, it is a relative increase.
   c. The differential leukocyte count should be evaluated in conjunction with the total leukocyte count, so that the absolute number of each type of leukocyte can be visualized. Selected canine hemograms are presented as examples. (10, 12)

	Total WBC (thou)	Neutrophils		Lympho-cytes	Mono-cytes	Eosino-phils	Baso-phils
		Segmented	Band				
Normal (absolute)	6000-17,000	3000-11,500	0-300	1000-4800	150-1350	100-1250	
Normal (%) (relative)		60-77	0-3	12-30	3-10	2-10	
Case 1	3000	10%		69%	3%	18%	0
Absolute no.		300		2,070	90	540	0

Interpretation:

Relative and absolute neutropenia

Relative lymphocytosis and eosinophilia, but the absolute numbers of these two cell types are within normal ranges.

The relative number of monocytes is normal, but is low in respect to absolute numbers.

	Total WBC (thou)	Segmented	Band	Lympho-cytes	Mono-cytes	Eosino-phils	Baso-phils
Case 2	48,000	80%	9%	8%	1%	1%	1%
Absolute no.		38,400	4320	3840	480	480	480

Interpretation:

Although there is a relative lymphopenia, monocytopenia, and eosinopenia, the absolute numbers of these cell are within the normal limits.

The increase in the total leukocyte count is due entirely to the increase in neutrophils, with a relative and absolute neutrophilia.

D. Thrombocytes (platelets)
1. Estimate the number present as normal, increased, decreased, or none.
   a. 4 or more thrombocytes per oil immersion field is considered normal.
2. Note variation in size and morphology.
   a. Thrombocytes generally are seen in clusters consisting of a few to many, but they may occur singly or in small clumps. Always check for clumps in the feathered end.

b. giant forms are occasionally seen with a distinct cell membrane surrounding light-colored cytoplasm and deep reddish purple-staining granules.

(1) A few of these may be seen normally, especially in cattle blood; but greatly increased numbers would suggest increased activity of the bone marrow.

E. See table, Morphology of Peripheral Blood Cells and Bone Marrow Cells, at the end of Chapter 2.

4 DEFINITIONS OF HEMATOLOGIC TERMS

Acanthocyte: A spiculated or spiney erythrocyte; acanthrocyte.

Adenosine triphosphate: High-energy phosphate compound, generated by anaerobic glycolysis, which maintains the membrane of the erythrocyte.

Agranulocyte: A leukocyte without definite cytoplasmic granules.

Agranulocytosis: Nearly complete or complete absence of the granulocytes from the blood and bone marrow.

Anemia: A decrease in the hemoglobin value, the packed cell volume, or the erythrocyte count of more than two standard deviations below the mean normal.

Anisocytosis: Variation in the size of the cells, usually the erythrocytes.

Anticoagulant: A substance that prevents the coagulation of blood.

Aplastic: Cessation of blood cell formation.

Arneth's index, classification, or formula: Classification of the neutrophils according to the number of lobes their nuclei possess.

Azurophil: Applied to granules seen typically in the cytoplasm of cells of the lymphocytic and monocytic series and the progranulocytic stage of the granulocytic series. The term refers to an affinity for a particular dye and not to the color of the granules. The granules may be present or absent in any cell of the lymphocytic series and, when present, are usually coarse and in clumps. They are usually present in all cells of the monocytic series, including the monoblast. In the monocytic series they are usually fine and diffusely and uniformly scattered throughout the cytoplasm.

Band form: In the Schilling classification, a granulocyte with a nucleus that is unsegmented and ribbonlike; also called stab, nonfilamented.

Basket cell: A degenerative cell that has ruptured and in which the cell nucleus appears as a pale staining smear without prescribed form or shape.

Basophilia or **basophilic:** Terms which, when applied to a cell or cells of the erythrocytic series, indicate that the cell shows no trace of the characteristic hemoglobin color and that the cytoplasm shows a strong affinity for basophilic dyes. With the Romanowsky stains the cytoplasm of such cells stains various intensities of opaque blue.

Basophilic stippling: Erythrocyte that shows blue staining, basophilic granules scattered throughout.

Bleeding time: The time required for a small, standardized wound to stop bleeding.

Blood dyscrasia: An abnormal condition of the blood or the blood-forming organs.

Buffy coat: The layer of leukocytes, thrombocytes, and nucleated erythrocytes, if any, that collect immediately above the erythrocytes in sedimented or centrifuged whole blood.

Coagulation time: The time required for venous blood, in the absence of all tissue factors, to clot in glass tubes under controlled conditions.

Color index: The ratio between the amount of hemoglobin and the number of erythrocytes.

Crenation: Shrinkage of cells in a hypertonic solution with the formation of irregular margins and a number of prickly points. Also seen in smears caused by dirty glassware, slow drying, extreme temperatures, and poor smearing technique.

Differential count: A count of the types of leukocytes seen on a stained blood smear or bone marrow.

Disintegrated, smudge, or **basket cell:** Any cell of any series in which the cytoplasmic outline has been disrupted or the nuclear chromatin is no longer surrounded by a membrane.

Döhle bodies: Small (1 to 2 microns) round or oval, gray-blue bodies in the cytoplasm of neutrophilic leukocytes, thought to be due to incomplete utilization of RNA during maturation of the cytoplasm.

Eosinophilia: An increase in the relative or absolute number of eosinophils in the blood.

Erythrocytic hypoplasia: Hypoplasia of the erythrocytic series only; indicates a selective depression of erythrogenesis.

Erythrocytopenia: A decreased number of erythrocytes in the peripheral blood.

Erythrocytosis: The presence of an increased erythrocyte count above normal and associated with an increased total blood volume.

Erythropoiesis: The production of erythrocytes.

Erythropoietin: The hormonal or humoral substance in the plasma that regulates erythropoiesis by stimulation of the bone marrow.

Ferritin: A protein molecule that stores iron.

Fibrin: The end product of the clotting mechanism, which forms a network of fibers that enmesh the formed elements of blood.

Fragility test: A test devised to measure the resistance of the erythrocytes to break down (hemolyze) when subjected to varying concentrations of hypotonic salt solutions; osmotic fragility test.

Globin: A protein subunit of hemoglobin composed of an alpha-one and beta-one polypeptide chain.

Glucose-6-phosphate dehydrogenase (G-6-PD): An enzyme of aerobic glycolysis.

Granulocyte: A leukocyte that contains specific cytoplasmic granules (neutrophils, eosinophils, basophils) regardless of the stage of differentiation.

Granulocytosis: Presence of increased numbers of granulocytes in the blood.

Haptoglobin: A plasma beta globulin that binds the hemihemoglobin molecule.

Heinz bodies: An intraerythrocytic mass of denatured globin, irregular in shape and appearing as refractile granules when slightly out of focus. This latter property is responsible for their being called erythrocyte refractile bodies

Hemocytometer: An instrument for counting the number of cells, especially in blood.

Hemoglobinemia: A condition in which the hemoglobin is dissolved out of the erythrocytes and is in solution in the plasma.

Hemolysis: Destruction of erythrocytes by dissolution or lysis.

Hemosiderin: An insoluble form of storage iron visible microscopically.

Howell-Jolly bodies: Small, round, densely staining bodies in the erythrocytes that are considered to be nuclear remnants and are usually eccentric in location.

Hyperchromasia and **hyperchromatic:** Terms which, when applied to the microscopic appearance of a cell or cells of the erythrocytic series, indicate that the cells seem to have a more intense hemoglobin color. This is never due to an increased concentration of hemoglobin but always to an increased thickness of the observed cell.

Hyperchromic: Because a significant increase in mean corpuscular hemoglobin is not known to occur, it is recommended that this term be avoided.

Hypersegmented: A segmented neutrophil with more than the normal number of lobes in the nucleus.

Hypersplenism: The acquired hemolytic capacity of an enlarged spleen; splenic anemia.

Hypertonic: Greater than isotonic concentration.

Hypervolemia: An increased blood volume.

Hypochromasia and **hypochromatic:** Terms which, when applied to the microscopic appearance of a cell or cells of the erythrocytic series, indicate that the cells described show a significant decrease in density of the characteristic hemoglobin color for the stained or unstained cell. This may be due to either thinness of the cell, decreased concentration of hemoglobin, or both.

Hypochromic: An adjective describing a blood picture in which the erythrocytes have a mean corpuscular hemoglobin concentration or saturation index and usually a mean corpuscular hemoglobin or color index more than two standard deviations below the mean normal determined by the same method on the blood of healthy animals of the same age and sex group.

Hypoplastic anemia: Depression of all three cell types found normally in the bone marrow, namely, erythrocytes, granulocytes, and thrombocytes.

Hypotonic: Less than isotonic concentration.

Idiopathic: Of unknown cause.

Indices: Calculations of erythrocyte size, hemoglobin content, and concentration.

Iron binding capacity: Plasma transferrin binding capacity for iron.

Leptocyte: A thin erythrocyte of decreased volume in relationship to its diameter, often characterized also by abnormality of shape.

Leptocytosis: A preponderance of leptocytes. Most hypochromic microcytic anemias show the presence of leptocytes.

Leukemia: Neoplastic disease arising in hemopoietic tissue in which the type cells appear in the blood or are disseminated diffusely through the marrow.

Leukemoid: Resembling leukemia by having a marked leukocytosis or having many immature leukocytes in the peripheral blood, but not due to the same changes in the blood-forming tissues; established that the condition is not true leukemia.

Leukocytosis: An increase in the number of circulating leukocytes above the normal range.

Leukopenia: A decreased number of circulating leukocytes below the normal range.

Lupus erythematosus cell: A neutrophil that is distended by an intracytoplasmic, homogeneous, red-purple body with the lobes of its nucleus compressed at the periphery of the mass.

Lymphoma: Includes all nonleukemic malignant tumors of hemopoietic and lymphocytic tissue that are not characterized early in its course by diffuse dissemination throughout the marrow. It is recognized that transitional states may occur between many of the separate entities included in the lymphomas, that mixed types may exist, and that leukemia may develop during the course of certain lymphomas.

Macrocyte: An erythrocyte having a diameter exceeding that of the normal range.

Macrocytic: An adjective describing a blood picture in which the erythrocytes have a mean corpuscular volume or volume index exceeding by mroe than two standard deviations the mean normal determined by the same method on the blood of healthy animals of the same age and sex group when this condition is not due to reticulocytosis alone.

Mast cell: Connective tissue cell in which the basophilic granules normally stain metachromatically. The cytoplasmic granules are usually large, but may vary from large to minute rounded bodies, and tend to be uniform in size in a given cell. The granules contain heparin and histamine and seldom overlie the round, oval, or occasionally indented nucleus. The association of relatively large numbers of eosinophils with mast cells in some pathologic conditions is thought to be due to the detoxification and disposal of histamine by the eosinophils.

Megaloblast: Rubriblast, an early erythrocyte precursor.

Microcyte: An erythrocyte having a diameter below the normal range.

Microcytic: An adjective describing a blood picture in which the erythrocytes have a mean corpuscular volume or volume index more than two standard deviations below the mean normal determined by the same method on the blood of healthy animals of the same age and sex group.

Myelophthisic anemia: An anemia resulting from the displacement or crowding-out of the marrow by abnormal cells or tissue.

Neutropenia: Deficiency of neutrophilic leukocytes in the blood.

Neutrophilia: An increase in the total number of neutrophils in the blood.

Normoblast: Metarubricyte, the last stage in erythrocyte development.

Normochromasia and **normochromatic:** Terms which, when applied to the microscopic appearance of a cell or cells of the erythrocytic series, indicate that the cells described appear to have their full complement of hemoglobin and no residual basophilic material in the cytoplasm; in other words, that they show normal staining characteristics.

Normochromic: An adjective describing a blood picture in which the erythrocytes have a mean corpuscular hemoglobin or color index and a mean corpuscular hemoglobin concentration or saturation index within plus or minus two standard deviations of the mean normal determined by the same method on the blood of healthy animals of the same age and sex group.

Normocyte: An erythrocyte having a normal diameter.

Normocytic: An adjective describing a blood picture in which the erythrocytes have a mean corpuscular volume within the normal range.

Ovalocyte: An elliptical erythrocyte.

Pelger-Hüet anomaly: A rare hereditary condition associated with myeloproliferative disorder where neutrophils lack the usual nuclear segmentation.

Poikilocyte: An erythrocyte with an abnormal shape, not to be confused with distortion that results from faulty technique.

Polychromasia, polychromatic, polychromatophilia: Erythrocytes that show a faint bluish tint due to an admixture of the characteristic colors of hemoglobin and basophilic erythrocytic cytoplasm.

Polycythemia: A state of the blood characterized by an increased number of erythrocytes.

Reticulocyte: Any nonnucleated cell of the erythrocytic series containing RNA, which when supravitally stained with new methylene blue or brilliant cresyl blue will have discernible granules or a diffuse network of fibrils.

Ring sideroblast: Cell in which many iron-containing granules surround the nucleus.

Rouleaux formation: The arrangement of erythrocytes in a roll or column, with their flat surfaces facing, in which they appear as figures resembling stacks of coins.

Schilling index: A method of classifying neutrophils based on their age. The neutrophils are counted and classified as blasts, progranulocytes, myelocytes, metamyelocytes, bands, and segmented cells.

Sedimentation rate: The rate at which the erythrocytes will fall in their own plasma in a given length of time.

Shift to the left: An increase in the immature forms of the granulocytic series in the blood.

Shift to the right: An increase in the percent of older cells (hypersegmentation).

Sideroblast: Nucleated erythrocytes with iron-containing granules.

Siderocyte: An erythrocyte in which blue granules, 1 to 20 or more in number, can be demonstrated by the Prussian blue reaction. Consistently seen in equine infectious anemia.

Smudge cell: A ruptured leukocyte.

Spherocyte: A spheroid erythrocyte of decreased diameter in relationship to its volume and having the microscopic appearance of a hyperchromatic microcyte.

Splenic anemia: Anemia in which the spleen destroys normal erythrocytes.

Stab cell: Band form of granulocyte.

Stippling: Punctate, basophilic deposits within the erythrocyte seen on Romanowsky-stained blood films.

Stomatocyte: Erythrocyte with a shape deformity in which there is a linear rather than a central area of pallor.

Subacute leukemia: A leukemia in which the total leukocyte count is normal or below normal, yet the type cells of the particular variety of leukemia are present in the blood in sufficient numbers to suggest the diagnosis.

Supravital staining: Staining of cells with a stain of low toxicity that will not cause death to the living cells, so that vital and functional processes may be studied in the live cells.

Target cells: An erythrocyte with a central rounded area of pigmented material surrounded by a clear zone without pigment, with a dense ring of cytoplasm about the periphery of the erythrocyte.

Toxic neutrophil: A neutrophil characterized by toxic granules, basophilia of the cytoplasm, vacuoles, or condensation of nuclear chromatin.

5 NORMAL BLOOD VALUES

NORMAL BLOOD VALUES—EQUINE

Reference	No.	Age, breed	Erythrocytes (10^6)	Hb (g/dl)	PCV (%)	Leukocytes (10^3)	Neut., segs (%)	Neut., bands (%)	Lympho-cytes (%)	Mono-cytes (%)	Eosino-phils (%)	Baso-phils (%)
(5)		Thoroughbred										
	38	Birth-6 mo.	10.2	14.1	41.6	8.36						
			(7-13.1)	(10.5-19.2)	(31-52)	(4.5-12.95)						
	36	2 yr	9.5	14.9	40.7	9.33						
			(7.3-10.8)	(11.8-17.8)	(34.5-46)	(6.22-13.4)						
	34	Geldings	9.4	15.0	42	7.04						
			(7.5-11.4)	(11.0-17.8)	(33.5-56	(4.74-11.5)						
	24	Mares	8.0	14.5	40.3	8.45						
			(6.23-9.95)	(10.7-18.3)	(30-57)	(5.05-12.0)						
	132	Overall	9.45	14.7	41.2	8.42						
			(6.23-13.1)	(10.5-19.2)	(30-57)	(4.5-13.4)						
(8)			6.94	12.5	30-44	10-11	60-70		38	4	4	1
(9)	359	Adult	6.90	14.0	43							
		Thoroughbred	(4.50-9.63)	(9.7-18)	(30-58)							
(13)		Draft	6.5-9.4	9.0-14	30-44	5-11	56		30	8	4	0.5
							(50-65)		(20-40)	(2-12)	(1-5)	(0-1)
		Thoroughbred	8.0-13	11-17	35-58	8-15	45-60		46	6	1-5	0.5
									(35-60)	(1-8)		
(20,21,		Thoroughbred										
22,23)	70	Weanlings	11.24	11.97	36.8	13.64	45		49.7	2.72	2.3	0.1
			(9-12.81)	(10.2-13.7)	(30.2-42)	(7.62-18.57)	(20-73)		(22-79)	(.5-8)	(.5-7)	(0-1)
	36	Stallions	10.81	14.69	46.78	8.27	50.75		43.75	2	4	0.5
			(8.33-13.3)	(12-18.3)	(38-58.5)	(5.05-11.9)	(35-65)		(30-57)	(.5-7)	(.5-7)	(0-2)
	65	Mares in	10.52	14.89	45.10	10.01	49.19		43.79	2.68	3.65	0.66
		foal	(8.6-12.5)	(12.5-16.5)	(38-51)	(6.85-13.5)	(30-66)		(24-65)	(.5-6)	(.5-9)	(0-3)
	70	Barren	9.94	13.83	43.05	10.37	48.2		44.5	1.7	4.6	0.5
		mares	(8.01-11.79)	(11.9-16.0)	(35-49)	(7.10-14.1)	(25-63)		(29-71)	(.5-6)	(.5-11)	(.5-2)
(25)			7.0	10.0	28	9.0	58		29	5	7	
(38, 39)		Cold-	7.5	11.5	35	8.5	54	0.5	35	5	5	0.5
		blooded	(5.5-9.5)	(8-14)	(24-44)	(6-12)	(35-75)	(0-2)	(15-50)	(2-10)	(2-12)	(0-3)
		Hot-	9.8	13.4	42	10	49	0.5	44	2	4	0.5
		blooded	(7-13.0)	(10-18)	(32-55)	(7-14)	(30-65)	(0-2)	(25-70)	(.5-7)	(.5-11)	(0-3)
(41)	28	Thoroughbred foals	11.77	12.2	36.54	13.12	53.26		42.16	2.37	2.1	0.07
		1-26 wk	(8.52-15.21)	(9.9-16)	(23.5-49)	(4.8-21.6)	(26-82)		(15-73)	(0-13)	(0-10)	(0-1)

NORMAL BLOOD VALUES—BOVINE

Reference	No.	Age, breed	Erythrocytes (10^6)	Hb (g/dl)	PCV (%)	Leukocytes (10^3)	Neut., segs. (%)	Neut., bands (%)	Lymphocytes (%)	Monocytes (%)	Eosinophils (%)	Basophils (%)
(3)				11.5	40	5-12						
				(8.7-14.5)	(33-47)							
(7)	100	4-8 mo	8.26			9.094	26.55	0.67	61.79	7.11	3.9	0
		(Beef)	(6.3-11.55)			(4.9-19.5)	(10-52)	(0-4)	(39-77)	(1-18)	(0-14)	
(8)			6-8	12.3	30-50	7-8	20-40		64	10	5	0-1
(13)			5.4-9	8-14.5	30-40	4.5-13	30		52	9	8	0.5
							(15-55)		(40-70)	(3-15)	(1-15)	(0-1)
(16)	25	Adult	6.33			8.91	34.73		41.24	7.94	14.87	0.62
		(Holstein)										
(17)	233	Birth	7.4			8.70	45		50.8	2.8	1.1	
		1 wk	7.5				32		62.5	3.7	1.5	
		2-4 mo	8.1			9.70	37		68.6	3.4	1.9	
		4-6 mo	7.8			9.30	21.7		68.2	5.7	4.9	
		1 yr	7.5				27.7		67.0	2.2	3.0	
(25)			6.0	11.0	35	7.0	30		52	7	11	
(31)	56	Adult	6.325	12.01		8.616						
	30	Younger	6.08-13.8			8.24-13.80						
(38, 39)			7.0	11.0	35	8	28	0.5	58	58	9	0.5
			(5-10)	(8-14)	(24-48)	(4-12)	(15-45)	(0-2)	(45-75)	(2-7)	(2-20)	(0-2)
(37)	23	Adult	9.76	12	40.6	9.70	26.9		62.9	4.6	5	0.6
		(Angus)	(6.5-17.9)	(10.38-14)	(36-49)	(5.05-20.1)	(6-45)		(44-85)	(2-7)	(0-19)	(0-2)
	26	Under 1 yr		11.32	37.5	11.14	23.7		68	3.2	4.3	0.6
		(Hereford)		(9.5-13.5)	(27-50)	5.75-17.8)	(12-38)		(12-80)	(1-5)	(1-10)	(0-2)
	50	Adult		11.83	38.4	7.50	27.9		57.6	4.1	9.4	0.6
		(Hereford)		(9.63-14.25)	(31-47)	(3.20-12.0)	(8-48)		(33-87)	(2-8)	(2-30)	(0-2)
	13	Adult	8.78	10.8	38	7.84	32.5		54.3	5.7	5.2	0.6
		(Holstein)	(7.2-10.8)	(9.25-13.25)	(33-48)	(4.75-12.7)	(18-46)		(36-71)	(3-8)	(3-7)	(0-2)
	58	Adult	8.26	11.21	37.3	7.88	24.7		60	4.6	9.7	0.9
		(Jersey)	(4.63-12.5)	(7.75-14.0)	(27-50)	(3.55-17.4)	(8-51)		(33-85)	(1-15)	(0-32)	(0-2)
	23	Under 1 yr	11.2	10.9	32.5	7.76	18.3		72.2	7.6	0.9	0.3
		(Jersey)	(4.34-17.35)	(8.45-13.13)	(25-44)	(5.15-10.55)	(4-43)		(45-84)	(0-16)	(0-3)	(0-2)

NORMAL BLOOD VALUES—OVINE

Reference	No.	Age, breed	Erythrocytes (10^6)	Hb (g/dl)	PCV (%)	Leukocytes (10^3)	Neut., segs. (%)	Neut., bands (%)	Lympho-cytes (%)	Mono-cytes (%)	Eosino-phils (%)	Baso-phils (%)
(3)				12.6 (10-15.5)	32 (22-40)	4-10						
(6)	18	Mixed	11.9	12.41	37.9							
(8)			8-10	11.18	33-46	7-8	20-40		48	6	4	0-1
(10)	134	Lambs		12.2 (10-14)	29.1 (28-34)							
(13)			8.5-13.5	9-14.5	33-46	4-12	40 (20-50)		52 (40-70)	4 (1-12)	6 (0-15)	0.2 (0-2)
(18)	190	Mixed	10.97	9.94	32.8	7.62						
(24)	89		11.5 (6.2-15.5)	12.4 (8.6-15.8)	30.5 (22-39)	9.2 (1.1-17.5)	24 (11-47)		67.3 (41-83)	2.3 (0-13)	4.2 (0-15)	0.5 (0-3)
(38,39)			12 (8-16)	12 (8-16)	38 (24-50)	9 (4-12)	30 (10-50)	0.5 (0-2)	62 (40-75)	2.5 (1-6)	4.5 (1-10)	0.5 (0-3)

NORMAL BLOOD VALUES—CAPRINE

Reference	No.	Age, breed	Erythrocytes (10^6)	Hb (g/dl)	PCV (%)	Leukocytes (10^3)	Neut., segs. (%)	Neut., bands (%)	Lympho-cytes (%)	Mono-cytes (%)	Eosino-phils (%)	Baso-phils (%)
(3)				10.6	34	5-14						
(8)			13	10.90	30-40	8-9	20-40		48	5	1.5	0-1
(13)			12.5-22	9-14	28-40	5-13	36		58	2	3.5	0
(14)			13.9	10.9								
(25)			12.6	11.5	27.7	7.7	50.3		43.7	3.6	2.3	
(38,39)			15 (12-20)	11 (8-14)	35 (24-48)	12 (6-16)	36.5 (30-48)	0.5 (0-2)	55 (50-70)	2.5 (1-4)	5 (3-8)	0.5 (0-2)

NORMAL BLOOD VALUES—PORCINE

Reference	No.	Age, breed	Erythrocytes (10^6)	Hb (g/dl)	PCV (%)	Leukocytes (10^3)	Neut., segs. (%)	Neut., bands (%)	Lympho-cytes (%)	Mono-cytes (%)	Eosino-phils (%)	Baso-phils (%)
(8)			7.44	12	32-47	15	41		47	8	2.5	0-1
(12)	7	21-25 days	5.1	12.1		10.193	31.7	7.9	47.7	8	1.4	1.4
	11	32-36 days	7.0	12.7		14.273	31.5	11.5	49.6	5.7	0.8	0.8
	30	3 mo	6.6	11.1		18.265	25.2	8.9	54.8	2.7	7.3	0.5
	12	5 mo	5.1			12.871	22.2	8.3	58.7	8.9	1.7	0.6
(13)			5-9	9-16.8	32-47	8.6-20	39		52	3	4.5	1
							(30-50)		(40-60)	(1-10)	(1-10)	(0-4)
(26)	200	Birth	5.722	12.36		12.7	68.41		29.64	1.26	0.45	0.23
(30)	110	Adult				19.866	32		66.4		1.6	
(36)	215		6.7	12-13.2		8-20	39		52.1	3.3	4.5	1.2
(38,39)			6.5	13	42	16	37	1.0	53	5	3.5	0.5
			(5.8)	(10-16)	(32-50)	(11-22)	(28-47)	(0-4)	(39-52)	(2-10)	(0-11)	(0-2)
(40)	78	Birth	5.02	10.93	32.65	8.43						
(43)	300	Adult	7.93	15.0	46.3	7-20						

NORMAL BLOOD VALUES—CANINE

Reference	No.	Age, breed	Erythrocytes (10^6)	Hb (g/dl)	PCV (%)	Leukocytes (10^3)	Neut., segs. (%)	Neut., bands (%)	Lympho-cytes (%)	Mono-cytes (%)	Eosino-phils (%)	Baso-phils (%)
(2)	110	2-8 mo.	5.5	11.2		12.24	50.55	5.37	37.77	0.5	5.79	
(3)			6.3	14.8	45.5	12.00	68		21	5.2	5.1	0.7
			(4.5-8)	(11-18)	(38-53)	(8-18)	(62-80)		(10-28)	(3-9)	(2-14)	(0-2)
(4)	25	Adult	5.94	14.6	48	12.432	57.37		39.75	.05	2.12	0.12
(8)			6-8.16	13	40-58	10-12	60-70		25	8	10	0-1
(11)	34	Adult	6.45	13.56	44.28	14.18						
(13)			6.4-8	12-17.8	40-55	11.8	69		20	6	5	0.5
						(6-20)	(60-75)		(10-30)	(2-12)	(2-10)	(0-2)
(15)	158	1-3 days	3.61	10.5	39.8							
(28)	95	3-4 mo	5.00	8.92	37.82	11.89	63.61	4.37	28.13	0.7	1.81	0.03
(32)	35	2-8 mo	5.30	12.6		12.165	55.85	6.7	33.3	0.15	3.97	0
	35	Adult	6.2	15.1		11.467	65.27	6.56	21.7	0.67	5.43	0
(33)	60	Adult	6.79	14.5		13.15	73.9	4.3	17.1	1.7	3	0
			(5.22-8.46)	(11-18.8)		(5.45-28.25)	(54-91)	(.5-10)	(4.5-37)	(0-7)	(0-13)	
(34)	100	Adult	6.042			8.867	64.63		19.28	8.86	7.025	0.205
(38, 39)			6.8	14.9	45	11	70	1	20	5	4	0
			(5.5-8.5)	(12-18)	(37-55)	6-18)	(60-77)	(0-3)	(12-30)	(3-10)	(0-10)	
(43)	54	Adult	7.02	14.6	47.3							

NORMAL BLOOD VALUES—FELINE

Reference	No.	Age, breed	Erythrocytes (10^6)	Hb (g/dl)	PCV (%)	Leukocytes (10^3)	Neut., segs. (%)	Neut., bands (%)	Lymphocytes (%)	Monocytes (%)	Eosinophils (%)	Basophils (%)
(1)	20	Adult	7.24 (4.6-9.7)	11.22 (8.7-14.5)	40.15 (28.5-47)	15.0 (5.6-28.9)	59 (35-79)		32 (11-52)	0.7 (0-4)	8 (2-31)	0.01 (0-0.4)
(3)			8 (6.5-9.5)	11.2 (7-15.5)	40 (28.52)	16.0 (9-24)	59.5 (44-82)		31 (15-44)	4 (.5-7)	5.4 (2-11)	0.1 (0-0.5)
(8			7.23	10.5	30-35	12-15	60-70		20-45	0-5	6	0.2
(13)			6.2-10	8-13.8	34-46	8-35	57 (30-75)		32 (20-40)	6 (1-15)	5 (2-10)	0.1 (0-0.5)
(19)	40	Adult				17.8 (8.9-46.4)						
(27)	25	1-6 mo	6.9 (5.7-9)	10.9 (9.4-12.8)	32.6	13.0 (9.1-22)	56.7 (40-72)		32.9 (16-45)	4.5 (1-7)	5.2 (2-10)	0.68 (0-2)
(29)	52		7.24	10.5	40.2	17.2	59.3		33	0.8	6.9	0
(35)	5	8 wk	5.21 (4.3-6.2)			11.725 (8-17.5)	52.4 (40-71)		34 (23-55)	1.9 (0-5)	6.6 (0-15)	
	20	Adult	7.82 (6.17-9.8)			15.954 (10-31.2)	54.26 (26-87)		38.68 (13-70)	1.5 (0-4)	5.4 (0-15)	
(38,39)			7.5 (5.5-10)	12.0 (8-14)	37 (24-45)	17 (8-25)	59 (35-75)	0.5 (0.3)	32 (20-55)	3 (1-4)	5.5 (2-12)	0
(42)	20	Adult	7.85	12.8		9.2-24	42-84		8-45	1-3	1-18	1

6 COUNTING OF BLOOD CELLS

I. Erythrocyte count

A. Filling the pipette

1. Fresh, unclotted blood or blood with an anticoagulant may be used.
   a. The blood with an anticoagulant must be carefully mixed by inverting the vial at least 20 times. Do not shake vigorously.
   b. A tube rotator can be used to insure uniform dispersion of the blood cells, thus avoiding a common source of error.
2. After the rubber tubing is attached to a Thoma erythrocyte-diluting pipette, identified by the 101 mark above the bulb, draw the blood exactly to the 0.5 mark, using gentle suction on the mouthpiece (Fig. 6.1).

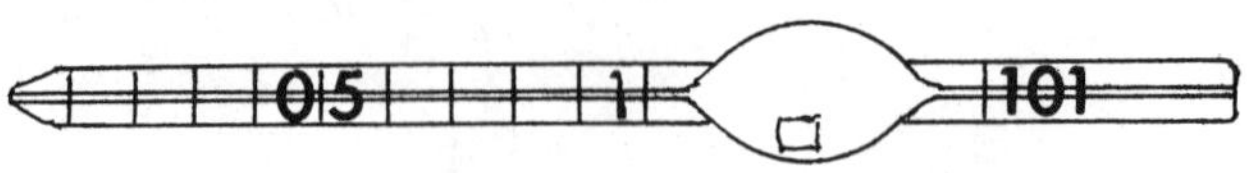

Fig. 6.1. Erythrocyte-diluting pipette.

   a. If the blood is drawn slightly past the line, it is permissible to expel the excess blood by stroking the tip of the pipette with the finger.
3. The tip of the pipette should be wiped free of blood before inserting it in one of the following erythrocyte-diluting fluids that are isotonic for erythrocytes:
   a. Isotonic salt solution—readily available; usually recommended, as it will avoid clumping associated with other diluents:

Sodium chloride	0.85 g
Distilled water	100 ml

   Should be sterile, or freshly made and filtered.

   b. Hayem's solution—(available in tablet form from Cambridge Chemical Products Co.) agglutination may result in animal blood when the fluid is more than 2 or 3 wk old or because of the effect of mercury on the plasma protein (16):

Mercuric chloride	0.5 g
Sodium chloride	1.0 g
Sodium sulfate	5.0 g
Distilled water	200 ml

   c. Gower's solution—agglutination is common and a precipitate may form on the pipette wall:

Sodium sulfate, anhydrous	12.5 g
Glacial acetic acid	33.3 ml
Distilled water	200 ml

4. The diluting fluid must be drawn into the pipette with steady suction to the 101 line above the bulb. Rotate gently while filling.
   a. The blood is diluted 1:200.
5. Bring the pipette to a horizontal position and place a finger over the tip before removing the rubber tubing.

6. The pipette must be shaken at least 2 to 3 min, preferably in a mechanical shaker.
   a. When the pipette must be shaken by hand, hold it horizontally between the thumb and middle finger, and by a simple wrist movement follow the curve of a quarter circle or a figure eight.
   b. Shaking in the direction of the longitudinal axis, either manually or with a mechanical shaker, is a serious error, as cells are forced into the stem.

B. Counting the erythrocytes (Fig. 6.2)
1. The ruled area of the hemocytometer and the special coverglass must be carefully cleaned and free from lint and grease.
2. Place the special coverglass with the longer edges parallel to and on the supporting ribs of the counting chamber while handling the coverglass only by the long edges.
3. Discard at least one-third of the contents of the pipette and wipe off the tip so that no fluid adheres. This removes the fluid in the capillary portion of the pipette that has not been mixed with blood.
4. With a forefinger over the upper end of the pipette, touch the tip to the space between the counting chamber and the coverglass. The fluid will fill the space by capillarity; when the fluid has flowed three-fourths of the way across, withdraw the pipette, as enough fluid will be left to fill the space.
   a. Any overflow will draw cells into the moat, making it necessary to clean and refill the chamber.
5. Allow about 3 min for the cells to settle; evaporation should be avoided since this will introduce a large error.
6. Under low power (x10) close to the center moat locate the central square of the 9 large squares. Observe for even distribution of cells.
7. Under high power (x45) count all the erythrocytes in 5 of the 25 small squares in the central area.
   a. Each of the 5 small squares to be counted is bordered by double or triple lines and is divided into 16 smaller squares. A total of 80 of these small squares are counted.
   b. Count the cells beginning at the left of the top row of 4 small squares, then from right to left for the next row, and so on.
   c. Avoid duplication in counting cells that touch the lines.
      (1) Triple ruling
         (a) Cells touching top and left center lines are counted.
         (b) Cells touching bottom and right center lines are not counted.
      (2) Double ruling
         (a) Cells touching top and left outer lines are counted.
         (b) Cells touching bottom and right inner lines are not counted.
   d. A variation of more than 25 cells between any of the 5 squares counted indicates an uneven distribution and would mean the count must be discarded and the hemocytometer filled with a fresh drop of fluid from the reshaken pipette.
8. Calculation
   a. Cells counted x 10 (0.1 mm depth) x 5 (1/5 of sq mm) x 200 (1:200 dilution) = erythrocytes/microliter
   b. Or, the sum of the cells in the 5 small squares x 10,000 = total erythrocytes/microliter
9. If there is a marked anemia, the blood should be drawn to the 1 mark on the pipette and then diluted to the 101 mark. The number of cells is multiplied by 5000 to obtain the number of erythrocytes per microliter.
10. Blood is drawn to the 0.3 mark rather than the 0.5 mark and the sample diluted to the 101 mark, with the resulting dilution of 1:333 used in the calculation rather than 1:2000. This is indicated under the following circumstances:
   a. When the number of erythrocytes is great and too numerous for an accurate count, as seen in some normal animals or those with polycythemia
   b. When the amount of available blood is limited

C. Unopette erythrocyte count
1. 1:200 dilution—Unopette test No. 5851
   a. 1.99 ml of 0.85% saline solution
   b. 10-microliter capillary—color code pink
2. 1:800 dilution—Unopette test No. 5801
   a. 2.397 ml of 0.85% saline solution

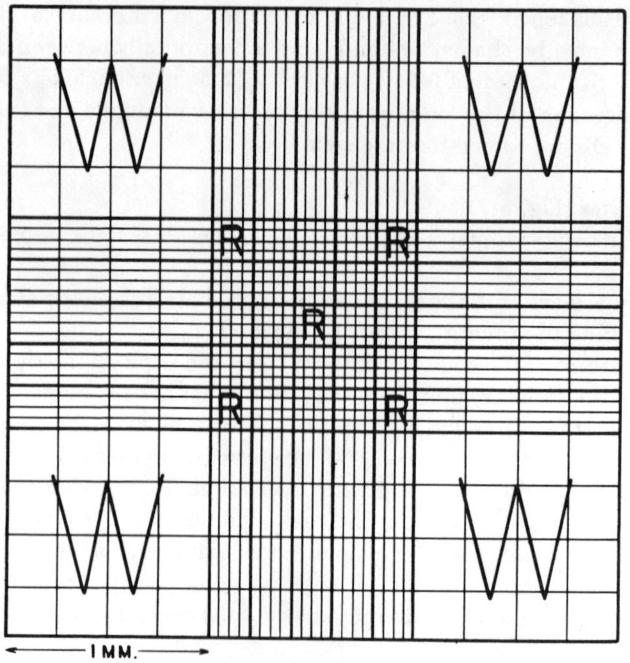

R = zones to be counted under high power for erythrocytes
W = zones to be counted under low power for leukocytes

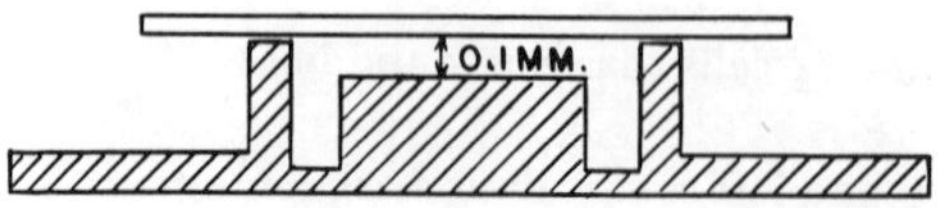

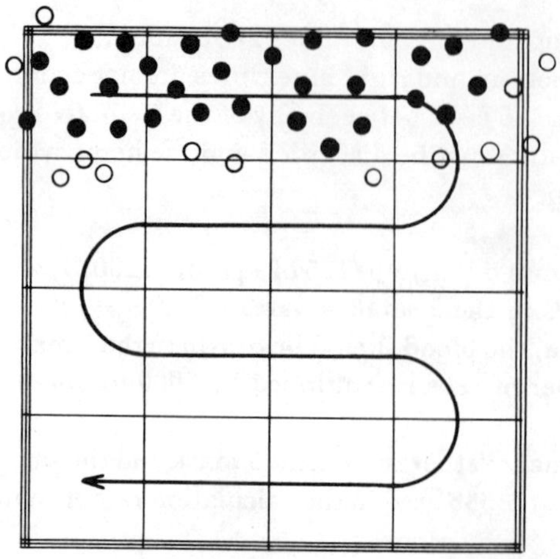

The arrow indicates the direction in which the count should be made.
Triple ruling:
Cells touching top and left center lines are counted.
Cells touching bottom and right center lines are not counted.
Double ruling:
Cells touching top and left outer lines are counted.
Cells touching bottom and right inner lines are not counted.

Fig. 6.2. Erythrocyte and leukocyte count.

b. 3-microliter capillary—color code green
3. Method
a. Add blood from the capillary to the diluent.
b. Rinse the capillary, mix by inversion, and convert to a dropper assembly.
c. Charge the hemocytometer.
d. Using the x43 objective, count cells in the 4 corner squares and the center square of the hemocytometer red cell area.
4. Calculation
a. 1:200 dilution—add 4 zeros to the total number of cells counted
b. 1:800 dilution—multiply the total number of cells counted by 4 and add 4 zeros

II. Leukocyte count

A. Filling the pipette (Fig. 6.3)
1. Follow the technique described under the erythrocyte count, except for the diluting pipette that has the mark 11 above the bulb.
a. The bore of the leukocyte pipette is larger than that of the erythrocyte pipette, making it easier to use accurately and requiring more blood.

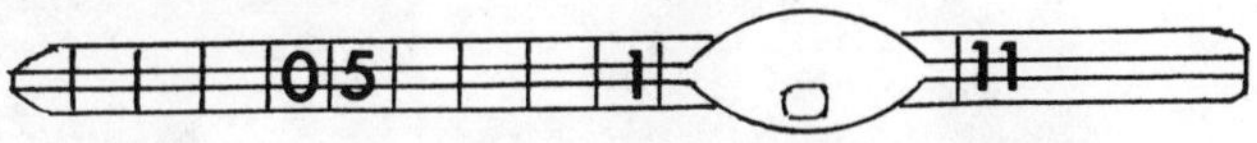

Fig. 6.3. Leukocyte-diluting pipette.

2. Draw blood exactly to the 0.5 mark and wipe blood from the outside.
3. Place the pipette in the leukocyte-diluting fluid and fill slowly to the 11 mark above the bulb. This makes a 1:20 dilution.
a. Leukocyte-diluting fluids that hemolyze erythrocytes
(1) N/10 hydrochloric acid—1 ml of concentrated hydrochloric acid in 100 ml of distilled water is approximately one-tenth normal and is sufficiently accurate
(2) Glacial acetic acid 2 ml
Gentian violet (1% aqueous) 1 ml
Distilled water 100 ml
Filter before using.
4. Shake for 3 min until well mixed.

B. Counting the leukocytes (See Fig. 6.2.)
1. Discard 2 or 3 drops from the pipette before filling the counting chamber.
2. Allow at least 1 min for erythrocytic lysis and for the leukocytes to settle.
3. Under low power (x10), count the number of cells in each of the 4 large corner squares.
a. For the leukocytes to be detectable as dark, uniform objects, it is necessary to reduce illumination as much as possible.
b. The rule for including or excluding cells touching the lines is the same as for the erythrocyte count.
c. An uneven distribution is indicated when there is a variation of more than 15 cells between any of the 4 squares counted, in which case the count must be discarded.
4. Calculation
a. $$\frac{\text{Cells counted x 20 (1:20 dilution) x 10 (0.1 mm depth)}}{\text{4 (number sq mm counted)}} = \text{leukocytes/microliter}$$
b. Or, the sum of the cells in the 4 corner squares x 50 = total leukocytes/microliter
5. If the total leukocyte count is from 50,000 to 500,000, collect the blood in an erythrocyte-diluting pipette, drawing the blood to the 1 mark. Count as an ordinary leukocyte count but multiply by 250.
6. If nucleated erythrocytes are present, the leukocyte count can be corrected according to the following formula:
$$\text{Corrected count} = \text{observed count x } \frac{100}{100 + \text{\% nucleated RBC}}$$

C. Unopette leukocyte count (See Fig. 6.4.)
  1. 1:100 dilution—Unopette test No. 5853 (5805)
    a. 1.98 ml of acetic acid
    b. 20-microliter capillary—color code yellow
  2. Method
    a. Add 20 microliters of blood to the diluent.
    b. Rinse the capillary, mix by inversion, and convert to a dropper assembly.
    c. Charge the hemocytometer.
    d. Using x100 magnification, count the cells in the nine squares of the chamber (0.9 microliter of diluted blood).
  3. Calculation
    a. Add 10% to the number of cells counted and multiply by 100.
    b. Example—if the number of cells counted in the nine 1-mm squares is 70, then the cell count is $[70 + (0.10 \times 70)] \times 100 = (70 + 7) \times 100 = 7700$ cells/microliter

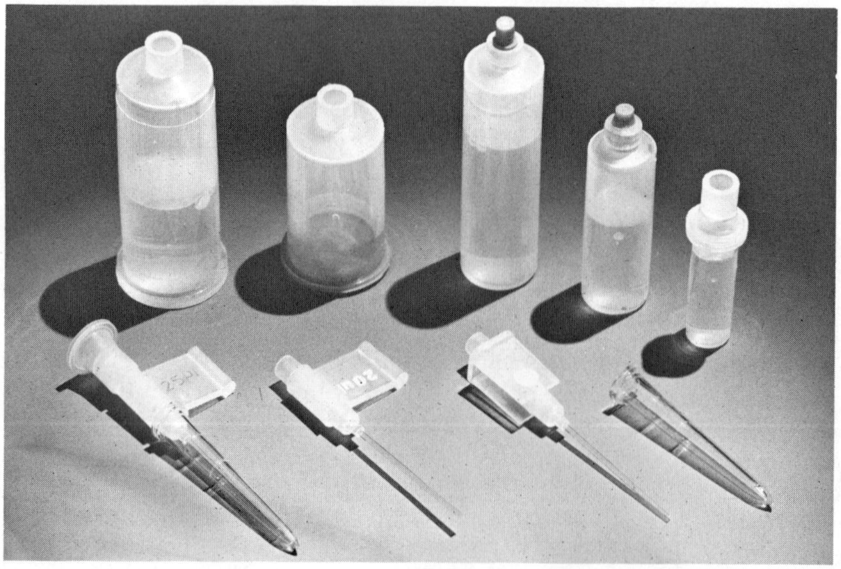

Fig. 6.4. Unopette reservoirs.

D. Unopette leukocyte and platelet count
  1. 1:100 dilution—Unopette test No. 5855
    a. 1.98 ml of 1% ammonium oxalate buffered to pH 6.5-6.8
    b. 20-microliter capillary—color code yellow
  2. Method
    a. Add 20 microliters of blood to the diluent; rinse the capillary; wait at least 10 min for hemolysis to be complete.
    b. Mix by inversion and convert to a dropper assembly.
    c. Charge the hemocytometer. If omitting the leukocyte count, cover the hemocytometer with a Petri dish to prevent dehydration, while waiting at least 10 min for the platelets to settle.
  3. Leukocyte calculation
    a. Using x100 magnification, count the cells in the 9 squares of the counting chamber (0.9 microliter of diluted blood). Add 10% to the number of cells counted and multiply by 100.
    b. Example—if 70 is the number of cells counted, then the cell count is $[70 + (0.10 \times 70)] \times 100 = (70 + 7) \times 100 = 7700$ cells/microliter
  4. Platelet calculation (Fig. 6.5)
    a. Using x430 magnification, count the platelets in the entire red cell area of the hemocytometer.
    b. Multiply the total number of platelets counted by 1000.

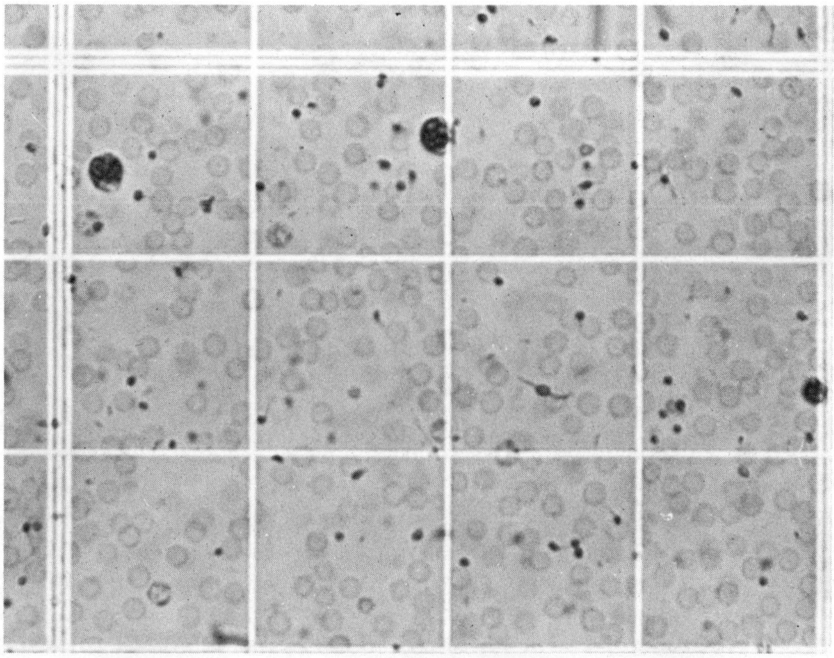

Fig. 6.5. Magnification (x430) of blood diluted 1:100 in 1% ammonium oxalate. Leukocytes, platelets, reticulocytes, and erythrocyte "ghosts" are stained with B-D platelet stain. (Before staining, the ghost cells were not visible.) Note that the filamentous appendages or tails can be seen in some of the platelets.

III. Eosinophil count

A. Indirect count

1. The number of eosinophils per microliter of blood can be estimated from the total leukocyte count multiplied by the percentage of eosinophils in the differential leukocyte count.
2. Higher numbers of eosinophils are produced by this method as compared to the direct methods; but since there is a highly significant linear relationship between the two, it is sufficiently accurate to evaluate eosinophilic responses to ACTH or disease. (4)

B. Direct count

1. Fill the leukocyte-diluting pipette to the 1 mark with blood.
2. Fill the pipette to the 11 mark with diluting fluid.

a. Pilot's solution (14):

Propylene glycol	50 ml (renders erythrocytes invisible)
Distilled water	40 ml
Phloxine (1% aqueous)	10 ml (stains eosinophils)
Sodium carbonate (10% aqueous)	1 ml (lyses all leukocytes except eosinophils)

Filter and store at room temperature. Discard after one month.

b. Hinkleman's solution (11):

Eosin yellow	0.5 g
Formalin (concentrated)	0.5 ml
Phenol (95%)	0.5 ml
Distilled water	q.s. to 100 ml

Needs no filtering and is stable for several years

c. Improved solution for dog eosinophil counts (7):

Phloxine B	0.25 g
Eosin Y	0.25 g
Water	50 ml

Mix well to dissolve, then add:

Propylene glycol	50 ml
Formalin (concentrated)	0.5 ml
Phenol (85%)	0.5 ml

No filtering is required.

3. Shake the pipette gently for 30 sec. Prolonged or harsh shaking will rupture the eosinophils.
4. It is necessary to wait 15 min for proper lysis and staining, which may take place in the chamber or the pipette.
   a. Fill both sides of two hemocytometers and place them on a damp towel and cover with Petri dish covers.
   b. Lysis may take place in the pipette rather than in the chamber if more convenient. After the 15-min wait, the pipette should be shaken again for 30 sec before discarding several drops and then filling the counting chambers. Allow several minutes for the cells to settle.
5. Under low power (x10) count the eosinophils in all 9 large squares on both sides of both counting chambers. Determine the average for the 4 counts.
6. Calculation: Ave. no. cells/9 sq mm x 11.1 = total no. eosinophils/microliter

C. Unopette eosinophil count
1. Use Unopette No. 5877 or No. 5879 (Becton-Dickinson). (9)
   a. The eosinophil Unopette comes packaged with a 25-microliter capillary pipette and a reservoir containing modified Pilot's solution (No. 5877) or bromcresol purple (No. 5879).
      (1) Modified Pilot's solution has the same ingredients as Pilot's solution except that no sodium carbonate is added and it is stable for at least 2 yr at room temperature. (5)
2. Add 25 microliters of blood to the diluent in the reservoir, using the disposable capillary pipette.
3. Rinse capillary, mix by inversion, and allow to stand 3 min.
4. Mix adequately by inversion, invert the capillary pipette, and use it as the dispenser for filling both sides of the hemacytometer.
5. Allow to stand 3 min before counting.
   a. Eosinophils appear as red granular cells or as dark purple granular cells, depending upon the Unopette selected, while the other leukocytes are unstained.
   b. Under low power (x10), count the cells in all 9 large squares on both sides of the hemocytometer, add 10%, and multiply by 16 for the total number of eosinophils per microliter.

IV. Thrombocyte (platelet) count

A. Collection of blood
1. Venous blood is preferred to capillary blood, and it should be drawn with a plastic syringe and placed in a siliconized test tube containing 2.5 to 5 mg disodium EDTA/2 ml of whole blood to eliminate clumping. (3, 18)

B. Accuracy of count
1. At best, thrombocyte counts are often unsatisfactory; the thrombocytes have their own effective characteristics that allow them to avoid being counted, or they are confused with artifacts. Their small size, irregular distribution, rapid disintegration, ready agglutination, and adhesion make accurate, reproducible counting difficult. (1)
2. The thickness of the hemocytometer does not allow the oil immersion objective to be used with the direct method, and difficulty is encountered in distinguishing thrombocytes from other particles such as dust and debris.

3. The phase microscope with appropriate equipment provides the best method but is usually not available.

C. Indirect method—the simplest and most practical for the average person
1. A stained blood smear is examined, and the number of thrombocytes is noted in several representative fields and averaged.
   a. Any of the routine blood stains, including new methylene blue, can be used.
   b. Finding 3 or less thrombocytes per oil immersion field suggests a thrombocytopenia. In some cases of thrombocytopenia it is not unusual to find only a few or no thrombocytes on the entire slide. (12)
2. The number of thrombocytes can be compared to the number of leukocytes in the smear, and this relative number may be transposed into an absolute number by the following calculation:

$$\frac{\text{No. thrombocytes}}{\text{100 leukocytes}} \times \text{total WBC count/microliter} = \text{no. thrombocytes/microliter}$$

D. Direct method
1. Blood is drawn into an erythrocyte-diluting pipette to the 0.5 mark and the diluting fluid is drawn to the 101 mark, similar to the erythrocyte count. Diluents that may be used include the following.
   a. Rees-Ecker:

Sodium citrate	3.8 g
Formaldehyde, 40%	0.2 ml
Brilliant cresyl blue	0.1 g
Distilled water	100 ml

   Keep stoppered and in refrigerator. Filter before use.
   b. 1% ammonium oxalate (3, 8):

Ammonium oxalate $1H_2O$	1.1g
Distilled water	q.s. to 100 ml

   Store in refrigerator to avoid bacterial growth.
   c. 1 or 2% disodium EDTA in 85% sodium chloride (2, 6). A crystal or two of brilliant cresyl blue can be added.
2. Mix thoroughly for 5 min, preferably in a mechanical rotator.
3. Expel and discard the first 4 drops before filling both chambers of the hemocytometer. To prevent evaporation, place the top of a Petri dish containing a wet filter paper or a wet pledget of cotton over the hemocytometer.
4. Allow 15 min for cells to settle.
5. With the illumination partially reduced, count the thrombocytes in the entire central ruled area on each side of the hemocytometer.
   a. The central ruled area is the one usually used for erythrocytes.
   b. 2 x 25 small squares or 50 groups of 16 very small squares are counted for a total of 2 sq mm.
   c. Use the fine adjustment to focus on each cell to identify the thrombocytes as lilac colored, oval, rod or comma shaped, and considerably smaller in size than the leukocytes that are also visible.
6. Calculation: No. thrombocytes x 1000 = no. thrombocytes/microliter
7. The results obtained should be checked by making a survey of the blood smear to determine if there is good correlation between the two methods.

V. Cleaning the hemocytometer and blood-diluting pipettes

A. Hemocytometer and coverglass
1. Immediately after use rinse in cold or lukewarm water and blot the etched area dry with cleansing tissue or lens paper.
2. If diluted blood has dried on the chamber, it may be washed off with soap and water, using a gentle action with the ball of the thumb.

3. Before use, the hemocytometer must be clean and free from lint, water marks, and fingerprints.
    a. After it has been cleaned, the chamber and coverglass should never be touched except at the edges.

B. Pipettes
1. An inexpensive polyethylene aspirator attached to a water faucet will provide the vacuum and suction needed for cleaning small-bore tubes efficiently.
    a. Adams Aspirator No. 1800 (Clay Adams) has a universal faucet attachment and a nonsplash screen and is easily installed and removed.
2. Attach the pipette by a rubber hose to the water-type suction pump and hold the tip of the pipette under water.
    a. To clean several pipettes at once, multiple pipette washers are available that operate from a regular tap water faucet with an Adams or other aspirator pump.
3. Blood is drawn from the pipette as water is drawn in, and water is continually aspirated until all traces of blood are removed.
4. If stains or precipitated protein remain in the bulb it will be necessary to aspirate a 50% mixture of household bleach (such as Clorox) and water and then thoroughly rinse with clean water. If this is not adequate, the pipette can be filled with bleach or cleaning solution and allowed to stand overnight.
5. Aspirate acetone into the pipette, then hold the pipette in air until dry.
6. If the pipette is properly cleaned and dried, the bead in the bulb should move freely.
7. A small stylet may be used to remove clotted blood from the bore if care is taken to prevent damage to the tip of the pipette.
8. The slightest chip that enters the bore will render the pipette unusable because of dilution inaccuracy.

VI. Special methods for blood cell counts

A. Electronic instruments for automatic counting of cells
1. Types
    a. Coulter Counter (Coulter Electronics) (Fig. 6.6) (A counter from Ab Lars Ljungberg and Co. appears to be identical to the Coulter Counter.)
    b. Celloscope (Nuclear Data Inc.)
    c. SMA4A/SMA7A and Hemalog (Technicon Instruments Corp.)
    d. Autocytometer (Fisher Scientific)
    e. Haema-Count (General Science Corp.)

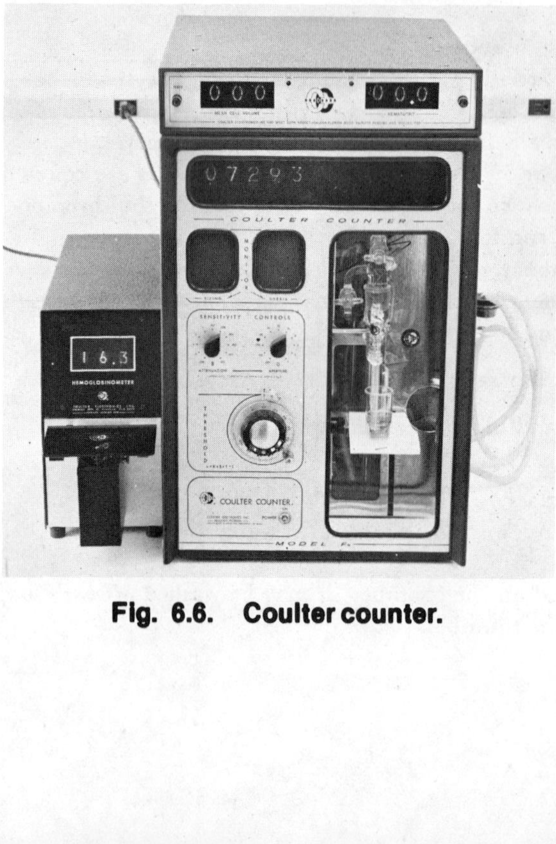

Fig. 6.6. Coulter counter.

f. Sanborn-Frommer Cell Counter (Sanborn Division, Hewlett-Packard Co.)
g. Haemoscope (Haemoscope Corp.)

2. Advantages of electronic counting
   a. Cells can be counted with greater speed than by the hemocytometer method, especially where a large volume of counts is made daily.
   b. Reproducibility is important, especially in research laboratories, and electronic counting usually results in less variation than counts performed by hand.
3. Principle and operation of the Coulter Counter, one of the most widely evaluated and accepted of the counters (Fig. 6.7)
   a. In a beaker a dilution of cells is made with a diluent.
      (1) Blood cells are insulators, while saline diluents are good conductors; the electrical conductivity differences between blood cells and the diluent is the basis of operation.
   b. The beaker is positioned on a spring platform so that the orifice tube is submerged in the sample. An electrode in the orifice tube and one in the sample beaker cause an electric current to flow through the orifice.
   c. As a cell passes through the small orifice, it raises the electrical resistance of the orifice contents.
   d. This results in a voltage pulse of short duration; this is amplified and:
      (1) Appears on the oscilloscope screen as a distinct vertical spike, with the relative size indicated by the varying height of the spike
      (2) Is fed to a threshold circuit with an adjustable threshold level, and the pulse is counted when the threshhold level is reached or exceeded
   e. The count is automatically made by actuating a vacuum control stopcock and resetting a count switch.
   f. The coincidence of two cells entering the orifice simultaneously is predictable at any given concentration and is corrected by the use of a coincidence chart.

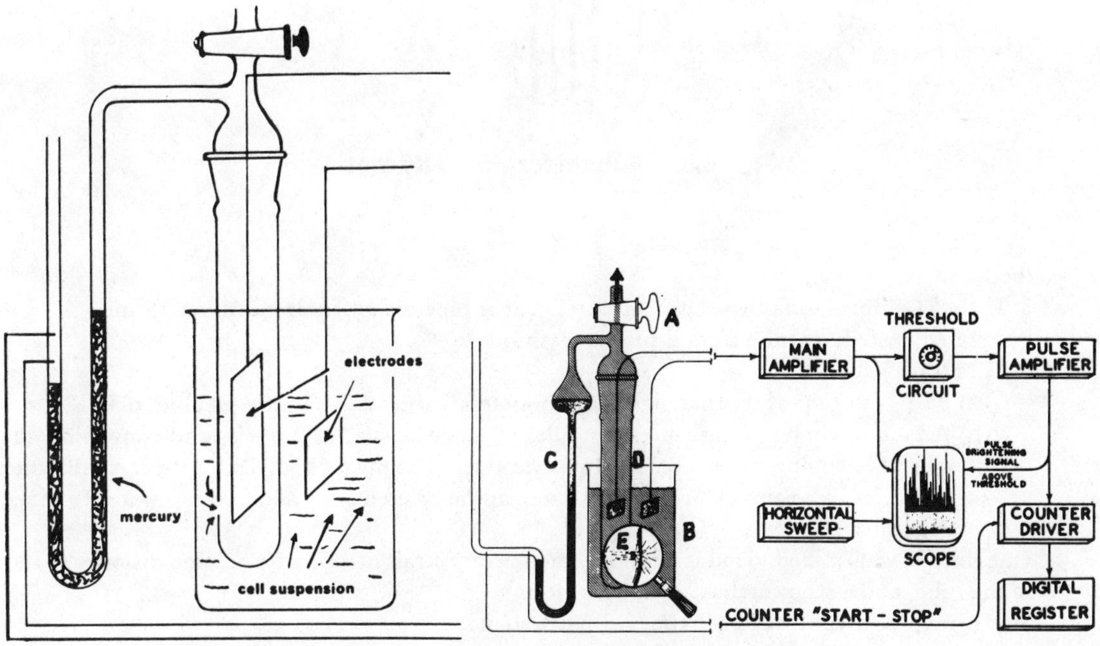

Fig. 6.7. (Left) Detail showing the principle of the Coulter counter. (Right) Electronic blood cell counter showing stopcock (A), beaker (B), mercury manometer (C), tube (D), aperture (E), and controlled external vacuum (arrow).

B. The deoxyribonucleic acid (DNA) viscosity test for indirect estimation of the leukocyte count (15, 17)

1. Principle
   a. The DNA of the leukocytic nuclei interacts with certain detergents or surface-acting reagents to produce a viscous gel.
   b. The viscosity increases in proportion to the number of cells, and the degree of viscosity is measured by the rate of flow of the mixture through the small bore of a funnel (Fig. 6.8).

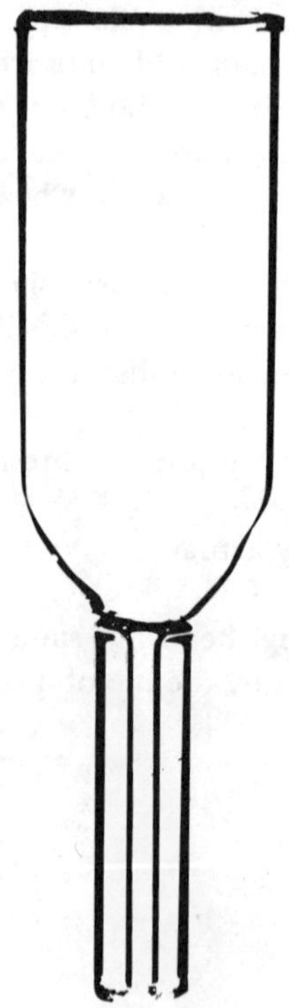

Fig. 6.8. Funnel for viscosity test.

2. Method
   a. 3.0 ml of California mastitis test (CMT) reagent is pipetted or squirted into a 15-ml graduated centrifuge tube from a plastic wash bottle.
      (1) CMT reagent
         (a) 3.0% solution of triethanolamine sulfonate at neutral to slightly alkaline pH.
         (b) A kit containing premeasured ampules of reagent, special funnels, and conversion chart is available commercially (Blood leukocyte test, Schalm method, Dairy Research Products, Inc.).
         (c) One pint of original CMT concentrate can be diluted with alkaline tap water to make 1 gal of reagent.
   b. One drop of well-mixed blood is added by means of a straight-tipped medicine dropper to the reagent in the tube, and a stopwatch is started for timing.
   c. Slowly invert the tube exactly 5 times. Do not shake.
   d. At 20 sec after the addition of the blood, pour the contents of the tube into a special funnel (4.5-ml capacity, having a calibrated stem 2.0 cm with a 1.3-mm bore) that has its stem pressed onto a large rubber stopper to close the opening.
   e. At exactly 30 sec after the addition of blood, raise the funnel, return the stopwatch to zero time, and start again.

f. Note the elapsed time in seconds when the fluid reaches the top of the funnel stem.

g. Results

(1) Leukopenia—less than 6 sec; verify by repeating with two drops of blood

(2) Normal—7 to 9 sec

(3) Beginning leukocytosis—10 sec

(4) The flow time can be converted to estimated mean leukocytes per microliter by referring to separate conversion tables for the dog, horse, cattle, and cat.

CONVERSION OF CAPILLARY FUNNEL FLOW TIMES TO ESTIMATED LEUKOCYTE NUMBERS PER MICROLITER OF BLOOD

Flow time	Mean total leukocyte number/microliter			
(sec)*	Dog (5.3)†	Cat	Horse (5.8)†	Cattle (6.4)†
6	7,500	10,000	5,500	5,500
7	12,000	14,000	8,500	8,500
8	15,000	17,000	11,000	11,000
9	17,500	20,000	13,500	13,500
10	20,000	23,000	15,000	15,000
11	21,500	26,000	16,000	16,500
12	23,500	28,000	17,000	18,000
13	25,000	30,000	18,000	18,500
14	26,000	32,000	19,000	19,500
15	27,500	35,000	20,000	20,000
16	29,000	...	21,000	21,000
17	30,000	...	22,000	21,500
18	31,500	...	23,000	22,000
19	33,000	...	24,000	23,000
20	34,000	...	25,000	23,500
21	35,500	...	26,000	24,500
22	37,000	...	27,000	25,000
23	38,000	...	28,000	26,000
24	39,000	...	29,000	26,500
25	40,500	...	30,000	27,000

Source: O. W. Schalm, Department of Clinical Pathology, University of California, Davis.

*When flow time is 5 sec or less, repeat the test with 2 drops of blood. No increase in time would be indicative of leukopenia. If an increase in flow time is obtained, one-half the estimated cell count for number of seconds recorded is used to indicate the leukocyte count.

†Reported average DNA content in micrograms x 10^{-6}/cell for the respective animal species.

7 HEMOGLOBIN

I. Functions of hemoglobin (Hb)

A. Transport of oxygen from the lungs to the tissues and of carbon dioxide in the opposite direction
   1. Within the erythrocytic membrane is a concentrated solution of hemoglobin, which is the functional unit in gas transport of oxygen and carbon dioxide.

B. Assisting in acid-base regulation by eliminating carbon dioxide in the lungs and by the buffering action of the imidazole histidine groups of hemoglobin

II. Composition of hemoglobin

A. Hemoglobin is synthesized in the immature erythrocytes in the bone marrow and consists of:
   1. Four heme molecules
      a. Heme is ferrous iron and protoporphyrin.
      b. Heme is synthesized in the mitochondria, so this must be accomplished before the nucleus is removed.
      c. The heme molecule is intimately bound to globin, as each heme group is located in a pocket or loop of one of the polypeptide chains.
      d. Heme is identical for all hemoglobin molecules, regardless of species.
   2. Globin—made up of two pairs of polypeptide chains, each with a specific amino acid sequence for each species
      a. Normal adult hemoglobin (hemoglobin A)—consists of a pair of alpha peptide chains linked with a pair of beta chains—$\alpha_2\beta_2$
         (1) Variations in hemoglobin types can result from differences in the beta polypeptide chain. With number of Hb components (separated by electrophoresis) given, these variations are:
            (a) Dog—1
            (b) Cat—2
            (c) Horse—2
            (d) Cattle—1 to 2
            (e) Sheep—1 to 4
            (f) Goat—2 to 6
            (g) Pig—1
            (h) Deer—1 to 9
      b. Fetal hemoglobin (hemoglobin F)—consists of a pair of alpha chains linked with a pair of gamma chains—$\alpha_2\gamma_2$
         (1) Disappears at or near birth
         (2) Not all species have fetal hemoglobin.
            (a) Species that have fetal hemoglobin—cattle, sheep, goat, pig, deer, man
            (b) Species that do not have fetal hemoglobin—dog, cat, horse
      c. Embryonic hemoglobin (hemoglobin E)—consists of a pair of alpha chains linked with a pair of epsilon chains—$\alpha_2\epsilon_2$
         (1) Disappears as fetal hemoglobin appears
         (2) Present in all animals

III. Methods of hemoglobin determination

A. Oxyhemoglobin
   1. Colorimeter—no longer in wide use
   2. Spencer Hb—Meter (American Optical Co.)

a. Principle:
   (1) Measures oxyhemoglobin directly by its light absorption in the green portion of the spectrum, using a suitable filter and matching the color with a colored glass standard
b. Procedure
   (1) Place a large drop of blood on the exposed chamber plateau.
      (a) Either fresh whole blood or blood with an anticoagulant may be used.
   (2) Agitate the blood gently with a hemolysis applicator containing saponin on its end until the blood loses its cloudy appearance and becomes a clear red solution.
   (3) Push the chamber into a clip, where it is held firmly against the coverglass as one unit.
   (4) Insert the complete unit into the slot in the instrument.
   (5) Press the illuminating thumb button, observe through the eyepiece, and move the lever on the side until the two fields of green match.
   (6) Hemoglobin in grams per deciliter of blood is read directly from the graduated scale.
      (a) Disregard the scales reporting results in percent, as they are confusing due to the different standards for percent.
   (7) If the hemoglobin is low, use a second chamber instead of the coverglass to provide a double depth of blood and increase the sensitivity of the reading. Divide the result by 2.
c. Comments
   (1) For use in the field, the Spencer Hb-Meter is the instrument of choice because determinations are quick, it does not require pipettes or solutions, and the accuracy achieved (± 5 to $\pm 10\%$) is within the range of clinical significance.
   (2) Methemoglobin and carboxyhemoglobin are not converted to oxyhemoglobin by the oxyhemoglobin method, but this is not a serious objection.

B. Cyanmethemoglobin
1. Principle:
   a. Ferricyanide converts hemoglobin iron from the ferrous to the ferric state to form methemoglobin in an alkaline solution. Methemoglobin then combines with potassium cyanide to produce the stable pigment cyanmethemoglobin.
2. Preparation of the calibration curve
   a. Using Ortho Acuglobin Hemoglobin Standard at room temperature, make 1:3 (25%), 1:1 (50%), 3:1 (75%), dilutions with Drabkin's reagent. Read the optical density (OD) of these along with an undiluted standard at 540 nm.
   b. The concentration of hemoglobin in the undiluted standard is equal to the assay value on the vial times the dilution.
      (1) For procedures that require 0.02 ml of whole blood and 5 ml of diluent, 1:251 is the dilution.
   c. These values should form a straight line when plotted on ordinary (straight-line) graph paper.
3. Procedure
   a. A blank of either Drabkin's solution or distilled water may be used to set 100 on the transmittance scale (T) or zero on the OD scale.
   b. Place 5 ml of Drabkin's diluent solution in a colorimeter cuvette.
      (1) Drabkin's diluent solution:

Sodium bicarbonate	1.0 g
Potassium cyanide (KCN)	50 mg
Potassium ferricyanide [$K_3Fe(CN)_6$]	200 mg
Distilled to	1000 ml

   c. Add 0.02 ml of blood with a Sahli pipette, rinsing the pipette at least three times with the diluent.
   d. Mix thoroughly and let stand at least 10 min before reading.
   e. Read the OD in the spectrophotometer at the 540 nm wavelength.
   f. Read equivalent hemoglobin from the calibration curve.
4. Comments
   a. The cyanmethemoglobin method in a correctly calibrated and maintained spectrophotometer has an error as low as 1 to 2% in automated systems and 2 to 5% in standard manual methods.

b. The U. S. National Research Council has recommended the cyanmethemoglobin method as the one of choice for calibration of instruments because solutions of standards can be prepared simply and are stable for years when maintained under proper conditions.

c. Drabkin's solution, the diluent, should be made at least once a month and kept in a brown bottle.

(1) A dry form of the reagent mixture can be purchased commercially from a number of laboratory supply houses.

(2) The concentration of cyanide in the reagent is so small that as much as four liters would be required for a lethal dose, but care should be exercised in handling.

d. The cyanmethemoglobin method measures all forms of hemoglobin likely to be in blood—oxyhemoglobin, reduced hemoglobin, and methemoglobin, but not sulfhemoglobin.

e. Besides the obvious sources of error in measurement and quality of reagents, values may be erroneously increased with:

(1) Lipemic blood

(2) Cat blood containing a large number of ER bodies—these should be removed from the diluted blood by centrifuging before the reading is made in the spectrophotometer

C. Acid hematin

1. Principle:

a. Erythrocytes are laked in dilute hydrochloric acid to form acid hematin, which is brown in color and matched with color standards.

2. Instruments based on the acid hematin principle are:

a. Sahli instruments—with a number of modifications

b. Haden-Hausser

c. Osgood-Haskins

d. Newcomer

e. Photoelectric colorimeter—using 0.1 N hydrochloric acid as a diluent

3. Comments

a. Outmoded

b. The error in the acid hematin method is up to $\pm 15\%$ due to:

(1) The rate of conversion of hemoglobin to acid hematin varying with time and temperature

(2) Interference by plasma proteins, lipids, and pigments with color matching

(3) The inactive forms, mainly carboxyhemoglobin, methemoglobin, and sulfhemoglobin, which total 2 to 12% of the total hemoglobin, are not converted to hemoglobin in an acid solution.

D. Direct matching

1. Principle:

a. Hemoglobin is determined by comparing the red color of whole fresh blood with color standards.

2. Instruments

a. Tallqvist

b. Dare

3. Comments

a. None are satisfactory.

IV. Normal ranges of hemoglobin in grams per deciliter of blood (according to Schalm) (See table.)

V. Abnormal hemoglobin pigments due to environmental agents

A. Methemoglobin

1. It does not function in oxygen or carbon dioxide transport, but is an inert true oxide of hemoglobin, containing ferric iron rather than ferrous iron.

2. The blood will be chocolate or dark brown in color, while blue to dark mucous membranes will be seen.

3. Causes

a. Oxidant drugs

b. Nitrites

NORMAL RANGES OF HEMOGLOBIN

Species	Range	Average
Dog	12-18	15
Cat	8-15	12
Horse		
Warm-blooded	11-19	14.4
Cold-blooded	8-14	11.5
Cattle	8-15	11
Sheep	9-15	11.5
Goat	8-15	10
Pig	10-16	13
Man		
Adult male	14-18	
Adult female	12-16	
Children	10-14	

c. Congenital from a variety of abnormal hemoglobins
d. Hereditary NADH-MR deficiency

4. For collection of a specimen for testing, heparin is the anticoagulant of choice.

B. Carboxyhemoglobin

1. Hemoglobin can combine with carbon monoxide in the same proportion as with oxygen, but the affinity of the hemoglobin molecule for carbon monoxide is 210 times greater.
2. Carboxyhemoglobin cannot bind oxygen and is not available as an oxygen carrier.
3. Blood has a typical cherry-red color, and discolors the mucous membranes.
4. The anticoagulant of choice for collecting a specimen for testing is sodium citrate in dry form, using a small well-stoppered tube, but heparin may also be used.
5. Simple tests may be used if spectrophotometric methods are not available.
   a. Alkali test
      (1) Two drops each of normal blood and the patient's blood are placed on a spot plate. Two drops of 25% sodium hydroxide are added to each.
      (2) Carboxyhemoglobin remains unchanged. The normal control should turn brown.
   b. Katayama's test
      (1) Place about 10 ml of water in each of two test tubes.
      (2) To one tube add 5 drops of the suspected blood and to the other add 5 drops of normal blood to serve as a control.
      (3) To each tube add 5 drops of fresh orange-colored ammonium sulfide.
      (4) Mix gently and make faintly acid with acetic acid.
      (5) The color of the blood containing carbon monoxide hemoglobin will become more or less rose-red, depending upon the concentration of the gas, while normal blood becomes dirty greenish brown.

C. Sulfhemoglobin

1. Hemoglobin reacts with hydrogen sulfide to form a greenish derivative of hemoglobin.
2. It cannot transport oxygen, but it can combine with carbon monoxide to form carboxysulfhemoglobin.
3. Sulfhemoglobin cannot be reduced back to hemoglobin but remains in the cell until it is destroyed.
4. The color of the blood is mauve-lavender.

8 ERYTHROCYTE SEDIMENTATION RATE

I. Principle

A. A tube containing blood to which an anticoagulant has been added is placed in a vertical position, and the distance that the erythrocytes fall during a given period of time is measured in millimeters.

B. Factors influencing the erythrocyte sedimentation rate (ESR)

1. Tendency of erythrocytes to form rouleaux (having the appearance of stacked coins)
   a. Varies tremendously among the different species (25, 27)
      (1) Horse—intense rouleaux formation causes the most rapid ESR
      (2) Dog and cat—moderately rapid ESR (26)
      (3) Pig—moderately rapid, but quite variable
      (4) Cattle, sheep, and goat—rouleaux absent in health
   b. Rouleaux formation can be differentiated from true agglutination.
      (1) Placing the erythrocytes in saline solution will disperse the rouleaux formation. (27)
      (2) Serum does not completely inhibit rouleaux.
   c. Factors controlling interspecies variations are still not fully known.
      (1) Differences in the plasma protein composition cannot entirely explain the variation in the tendency to form rouleaux.
         (a) Equine erythrocytes will settle rapidly in bovine or ovine plasma.
         (b) Bovine and ovine erythrocytes will settle slowly in horse plasma.
      (2) In horses, pigs, and dogs the ESR is decreased in parallel with the degree of dilution of plasma; this has been attributed to the reduction of the rouleaux-promoting factor in the plasma rather than to the decrease of specific gravity and viscosity of plasma. (27)
      (3) It appears that aggregation is affected partly by the erythrocyte and partly by plasma properties.
         (a) One theory suggests that abnormalities of plasma composition alter the electrical charges on the erythrocytes, which normally repel each other, and as a result the erythrocytes stack into rouleaux or form clumps. (18)
2. Alterations in the plasma proteins
   a. Fibrinogen—increased amounts increase the ESR (25, 27)
      (1) Corticosteroids or ACTH administered in amounts sufficient to produce a clinical remission often result in a marked reduction in both fibrinogen and the ESR. (27)
   b. Globulins—increased amounts increase the ESR
      (1) Alterations in amounts of specific globulins (beta or gamma) probably do not explain the variation of the ESR in different species. (22)
   c. Albumin—amount either has little effect or is inversely proportional to the ESR
   d. Correlations between plasma concentrations of protein-bound iodine, protein-bound carbohydrates, or sialic acid and increased ESR suggest that the asymmetric shape of these promotes the rouleaux or aggregation of the erythrocytes. (5)
3. Hypercholesterolemia increases the ESR. (19)
4. Number of erythrocytes
   a. When the number of erythocytes or the PCV is increased, the ESR is decreased.
   b. In most anemias the ESR is accelerated due to the small number of cells that can settle more easily in the large volume of fluid.
5. Size of erythocytes
   a. Macrocytosis and spherocytosis increase the rate of fall.
   b. Microcytes, leptocytes, and poikilocytes tend to retard the ESR.
6. Type and amount of anticoagulant
   a. Double oxalate, EDTA, and heparin in proper amounts will not affect the size of the erythocyte nor alter the ESR.

b. 3.8% sodium citrate in an amount of 1 volume of anticoagulant to 4 volumes of blood is the method commonly used in the Westergren method.
   (1) Increasing the amount of sodium citrate will accelerate the ESR of human and dog blood. (27)

7. Age of the blood sample
   a. After 1 hr from the time oxalated blood is drawn, the ESR will be decreased.
   b. With EDTA as an anticoagulant, the test can be delayed as long as 6 hr when the blood is stored at room temperature and 24 hr when stored at refrigerator temperature. (25)
8. Diameter and length of tube
   a. Variations in the normal values for various sedimentation rate methods are due to the differences in the height and diameter of the various tubes.
9. Position of the tube (21, 29)
   a. The tube must be kept in a vertical position, as any deviation causes an acceleration in the ESR.
   b. Modification by inclining the tube has been used to shorten the time for observation of cattle blood, as the degree of increase of the ESR is directly proportional to the inclination of the tube.
10. Temperature
   a. The ESR of blood at refrigerator temperature is decreased, but minor variations of room temperature will have little effect.

II. Methods

A. Wintrobe

1. The Wintrobe hematocrit tube is filled to the 0 mark on the left scale.
2. The tube is set in a vertical position in an appropriate rack.
   a. If the tube is at an angle of even 3%, significant acceleration (30%) of the sedimentation takes place.
3. The ESR increases with temperature and the procedure ideally should be conducted at a constant temperature, but this is usually unnecessary, as the ESR is only slightly influenced by temperatures between 22° and 27°C.
4. The upper level of sedimenting erythrocytes is read in millimeters on the left scale at the time interval best suited for the particular animal species.

Horse—10, 20, or 30 min	Pig—8 hr
Cattle—8 or 24 hr	Dog—1 hr
Sheep—24 hr	Cat—1 hr
Goat—24 hr	Man—1 hr

5. The quantity of erythrocytes in suspension influences the stability of the suspension, and it is possible to correct the ESR according to the packed cell volume (PCV) by means of a correction chart developed by Wintrobe and Landsberg. (33)
   a. When the Wintrobe chart is used, the correction is made to the following PCV (25):

      Dog—45%
      Cat—35%
      Human, male—47%
      Human, female—42%

   b. Slightly modified charts have been prepared by Schalm, with the anticipated ESR for each PCV value. (See table.) (25)

      (1) Using the chart
         (a) Observed ESR—anticipated ESR = ESR difference + or −
         (b) A horse with a PCV of 35 has an anticipated ESR of 13 to 43% (28 ± 15). If the observed ESR is 40 mm, then 40 − 28 = +12. If the observed ESR is 8 mm, then 8 − 28 = −20, which is a slow rate as compared to the anticipated ESR for that PCV.
   c. There is a difference of opinion concerning the correction for the PCV and anemia, for it has been reported that the correction is frequently misleading, is not accurate, and only lends confusion to an otherwise simple test. (19)

ANTICIPATED ESR VALUES

PCV(%)	Dog (anticipated ESR at 60 min)	Horse (anticipated ESR at 20 min)
10	79	86 ± 1
15	64	80 ± 1
20	49	70 ± 2
25	36	60 ± 3
30	26	47 ± 5
35	16	28 ± 15
40	10	11 ± 8
45	5	2.5 ± 1
50	0	0 ± 1

Cat—use table of anticipated ESR for the dog, which is significant if it varies more than ± 10%

B. Westergren
  1. The Westergren tube has a total length of 300 mm, a 2-mm diameter, a capacity of 1 ml, and graduations from 0 to 200 at 1-mm intervals.
  2. The bottom of the tube is dipped in the blood, which is drawn into the tube up to the 0 mark by aspiration, and the tube is placed in an upright position in a special rack with a soft rubber cushion at the bottom so that the tube is sealed when inserted.
  3. The fall of the erythrocytes is read in millimeters at the various time intervals best suited to the particular species.
  4. The ESR obtained by this method is not corrected for the PCV.

C. Cutler
  1. The Cutler tubes are available in 2 sizes, 1 ml and 5 ml, with markings from 0 to 50 mm. The 1-ml size is preferred because of the smaller quantity of blood required.

D. Capillary tube (3, 30)
  1. The sealed capillary tube is placed in a vertical position in a piece of clay or soap or on adhesive tape mounted on a wall surface with the sticky side out.
  2. After the appropriate time interval, the amount of erythrocyte fall must be measured and reported as normal, fast, or very fast; precise normal values have not been established for this method.
    a. A hematocrit tube reader can be used to report results in millimeters by reversing the position of the tube from that used for reading the PCV.

III. Interpretation

A. Normal ESR values (See table.)

B. General clinical applications
  1. Use in the various species
    a. It is used more extensively in human medicine than in veterinary medicine.
    b. It is more applicable to canine blood than blood of other domestic animals. (25)
    c. In the horse the ESR over a period of time shows considerable variation even in the same individual, thus making it extremely difficult to state the limits of normality. (6, 12)
    d. The ESR in cattle is so variable that a normal value cannot be given. (30)
    e. It is questionable whether the ESR of sheep could be used as a clinical diagnostic test, as the results obtained from normal sheep show marked variations not only between individual sheep but also when duplicate tests are made on the same blood. (6)
  2. The ESR is a nonspecific reaction that can be used as a diagnostic screening procedure to give informa-

NORMAL ESR VALUES

	Wintrobe (mm)						Westergren (mm)		Cutler (mm)		
Species	10 min	20 min	30 min	1 hr	8 hr	24 hr	10 min	1 hr	1 hr	7 hr	Reference
Horse	2-12	15-38									(7)
			51	59							(22)
			(24-60)	(51-63)							
							15				(12)
							(7-23)				
									18		(14)
									(0-30)		
Cattle			0	0							(7)
						2.25-4					(6)
						3					(13)
						(1-8)					
										2.4	(11)
Sheep			0	0							(7)
						3-8.25					(6)
						2-3					(15)
Goat						2-2.5					(6)
			0	0							(7)
Dog			1-6	5-25							(7)
				0-15					0-8		(16)
				18							(22)
				(7.5-26)							
				1-4							(28)
								0			(2)
								0-5			(27)
Pig			0-6	1-14							(7)
					2.25-8	5.5-11					(6)
								5-10			(27)
Human male				3.7							(33)
				(0-6.5)							
				0-9				4			(19)
								(0-15)			
Human female				9.6							(33)
				(0-15)							
				0-20				5			(19)
								(0-20)			

tion of a general character, but is not diagnostic of any one disease. It can be a measure of the presence and intensity of disease processes in the body. (33)

a. A normal ESR does not exclude the possibility of a disease process.

b. General conditions that produce an increased ESR

(1) Infections

(a) Acute generalized

(b) Acute localized infections of serosal membranes—peritonitis, pleuritis, pericarditis

(c) Chronic localized—suppurative conditions until encapsulated

(2) Skin alterations (25)

(a) Inflammation

(b) Hypothyroidism

(c) Hyperadrenocorticism

(3) Tissue injury or destruction—including surgery

(4) Malignant tumors—the ESR is not necessarily increased, even when the tumor is malignant, unless it is quite vascular, has tissue breakdown, or has a considerable reaction around it

(5) Pregnancy

3. An increased ESR directs attention to an occult disèase.

a. It may be increased when clinical and other laboratory findings are normal and should be a challenge to conduct a thorough search for the cause.

4. The ESR is a guide to prognosis, to the progress of the infection, and to the need for further treatment.
   a. In the dog, a grave prognosis is indicated when there is an increased ESR with the following. (25)
      (1) A PCV of 50% or more
      (2) Plasma protein less than 7 g/dl
5. Diphasic sedimentation rate refers to plasma with a cloudy reddish appearance that does not have a definite line of demarcation between the sedimenting erythrocytic mass and the plasma. (25)
   a. Significance
      (1) Dog—indicates the presence of immature forms of erythrocytes, including reticulocytes, or the presence of numerous erythrocytes with abnormal shapes (25)
      (2) Horse—commonly seen when the PCV is below 30% and seen less frequently when the PCV is between 30 and 38%

C. Specific conditions characterized by an increased ESR
1. Dog
   a. Distemper
      (1) There is no apparent correlation between the amount of sedimentation and the height of the fever. (4, 28)
   b. Leptospirosis (17, 20)
      (1) With *Leptospira icterohemorrhagiae* infection, the ESR increases on the 2nd day, even in subclinical cases, and the maximum ESR is reached on the 7th to 10th days.
   c. Pregnancy
      (1) A marked increase is seen as early as the 17th day in pregnancy (22) but usually is pronounced at the 6th week and returns to the normal anticipated rate by the 8th week. (1)
      (2) This increase could be related to the following.
         (a) Increased rouleaux formation caused by increased amounts of fibrinogen (25)
         (b) The anemia that develops between 7 and 9 wk after estrus (31)
         (c) A cholesterolemia that develops between the 3rd and 8th week after estrus (31)
   d. Pyometra—generally elevated
   e. Chronic interstitial nephritis
   f. Neoplasms
      (1) According to one report (8) the effectiveness of radiation of neoplasms can be evaluated by comparison of the ESR prior to and after radiation.
         (a) Little change in the ESR is noted in tumors resistant to radiation.
         (b) Radiosensitive neoplasms will have an increase in the ESR in the reading taken at 2 hr.
   g. Radiation injury (23)
   h. Filariasis (10)
   i. Acute and subacute bacterial endocarditis (9)
   j. Myocarditis and myocardial degeneration (9)
   k. Pneumonia (24)
   l. Pleuritis (24)
   m. Peritonitis (24)
   n. Infectious canine hepatitis (24)
   o. Salmon disease (28)
   p. Hypothyroidism (25)
   q. Hyperadrenocorticism (25)
   r. Bone fracture
   s. Trypanosomiasis
   t. Negative ESR—the ESR is less than the anticipated rate (25)
      (1) A significant number of cells do not become involved in the rouleaux formation
         (a) Immature erythrocytes, including reticulocytes
         (b) Leptocytes
      (2) Low plasma protein concentration
         (a) Liver disease
         (b) Poor nutrition

2. Horse
   a. Equine infectious anemia—has been attributed to changes in the PCV (12, 14)
   b. Strongyloides—usually depends upon the degree of infection
      (1) Elimination of the parasites appears to return the ESR back to normal slowly. (27)
   c. Contrary to the action in other species, hyperglobulinemia in the horse retards the ESR. (27)
3. Cattle
   a. It is necessary to have a reading over 4 mm at 7 hr (Cutler method) to indicate a disease process. (11)
   b. The ESR is normal in pregnant cows. (27)
   c. Diseases such as tuberculosis and chronic inflammation do not appear to influence the ESR of cattle as they do in man. (27)

9 PACKED CELL VOLUME (HEMATOCRIT)

I. General considerations

A. Erythrocytes, which ahve the highest specific gravity, are separated b y high-speed centrifugation from the other elements that appear from the top of the tube to the bottom in the following order:
1. Plasma—yellowish layer forced out of the layers containing cells
2. Buffy coat—white to gray layer, sometimes reddish gray
   a. Thrombocytes—uppermost cream-colored layer
   b. Leukocytes—gray layer
   c. Nucleated erythrocytes—if present, produce a reddish tinge in the buffy coat where they become trapped due to their specific gravity, which is lower than the mature erythrocytes
3. Erythrocytes—dark red layer separated from the buffy coat by a dark line produced by the reduction of hemoglobin from contact with the leukocytes

B. Whole blood is collected using an anticoagulant that does not affect the distribution of fluid between the erythrocytes and plasma.
1. This anticoagulant can be EDTA, heparin, or a mixture of ammonium and potassium oxalate.
2. The EDTA should be used in proper amounts, as an excess will cause shrinkage of the erythrocytes and a PCV that is lower than it should be.

II. Methods

A. Wintrobe method
1. The Wintrobe hematocrit is a tube of uniform bore (3 mm) and flat bottom, calibrated longitudinally into 10 cm or 100 mm (Fig. 9.1).
   a. The numbers on the right read up from 0 to 10 cm and are used for the PCV determinations.
   b. The numbers on the left of the scale read down from 0 to 10 cm and are used for the erythrocyte sedimentation rate.
   c. Since no absolute volumetric measurement is required, the volume contained within the tube is of no consequence.
2. Withdraw 1 ml of venous blood in a dry syringe and place it in a vial containing the exact amount of proper anticoagulant for the amount of blood, or fill a Vacutainer tube. Shake the tube immediately to prevent clotting.
   a. Only partially filling the Vacutainer tube produces a common source of error, as the excess EDTA shrinks the erythrocytes.
3. When the hematocrit tube is ready to be filled, the blood should be well shaken to insure a uniform suspension of cells.
4. Place the blood in a Wintrobe hematocrit tube by means of a special Wintrobe pipette or a disposable transfer pipette that is long enough to reach the bottom of the tube.
   a. First, insert the tip to the bottom of the tube, and then slowly withdraw at a rate that will avoid the formation of bubbles, by keeping the tip below the level of blood.
   b. Fill to the 10 mark on the right side; avoid filling beyond even though the marks continue above 10.
5. It is not necessary to stopper the tube if it has been filled exactly to the 10 mark since evaporation will affect only the plasma, the upper level of which has already been determined.
6. **Use a suitable centrifuge at an rpm that will provide a relative centrifugal force (RCF) of 2260 x gravity (G), which is generally adequate to provide maximum packing. (2)**
   a. The rpm necessary for a centrifuge to achieve the desired RCF will vary with the length of the radius measured from the center of the centrifuge shaft to the bottom of the hematocrit tube in the cup.

(1) Usually 3000 to 4000 rpm will suffice, but this will vary with the radius of the head that is being used.

7. The time required for maximum packing and minimum trapping of plasma between the cells will vary with the species.
   a. 30 min—dog and horse
   b. 60 min—cattle, pig, sheep, and goat
      (1) Sheep and the pig require more than 2260 RCF, since their smaller erythrocytes permit more trapping of plasma. (9)
8. Prolonging the time of centrifugation will not compensate for inadequate RCF or speed.
9. Read the scale at the top of the packed erythrocytes immediately adjacent to the buffy coat.
10. Multiply the large numbers by 10 for volume per deciliter of blood, as the PCV is reported as percent.

11. The hematocrit tube is most easily cleaned by inserting a U-shaped Wintrobe pipette cleaner into the bottom of the tube, applying suction, and simultaneously holding the tube under water. The hematocrit is then removed from the water, and the water within the tube is withdrawn by suction. If the tube is allowed to stand in an inverted position, drying will be completed; or acetone may be used to hasten the process.
    a. Disposable Wintrobe tubes are available if it is more practical to dispense with cleaning the tubes.

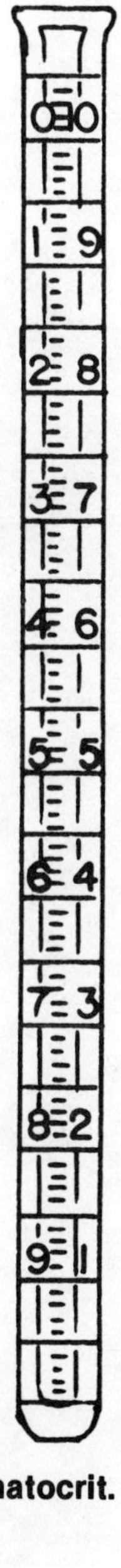

Fig. 9.1. Wintrobe hematocrit.

B. Microhematocrit method
   1. When the blood already contains an anticoagulant, use plain capillary tubes (75 mm x 1.0 mm) and fill to approximately 1 cm from the end. When the blood sample is taken directly from the ear, lip, toenail, or finger, use the heparinized tubes. Hold the tube near a horizontal plane to facilitate filling.
   2. Wipe the blood from the outside of the tube while it is still wet.
   3. Seal the vacant end of the tube with special clay or plastic, with plastic caps, or by holding it in the flame of a propane torch (using care not to heat the blood).
      a. Capillary tubes that have a fire-polished end are desirable and are usually coded by a color on that end. Sealing this end will avoid most of the leakage that occurs with an end that is not smooth.
   4. Unscrew the center knurled bolt on the head of the high-speed centrifuge and remove the cover plate.
      a. Most brands of microhematocrit centrifuges will have a cover plate, but an occasional one does not.
   5. Place the tubes on the head in the slots with open ends toward the hub and sealed ends as close as possible to the rim of the head to prevent the tubes from breaking while centrifuging.
      a. Since the tubes are too small to be marked, it is essential to keep track of their identification by noting the number of the slot for respective tubes.
   6. Replace the cover securely, and centrifuge for 5 min at 10,000 to 13,000 rpm or for 2 min at 16,000 rpm and above.
   7. Remove tubes and read percent of PCV by using any one of a variety of hematocrit tube readers.
      a. The simplest of the readers has a linear scale to compensate for the variable amount of blood in all tubes except those calibrated for use with the Clay-Adams Readacrit centrifuge.
         (1) Using the linear chart or Graphic Reader requires that the hematocrit tube be placed on the scale with the meniscus of plasma on the top line.
         (2) Slide the tube until the bottom of the erythrocyte layer corresponds with the zero line.
         (3) The line that intercepts the top of the erythrocyte layer is followed along to the point where it can be read on the scale at the end of the line.

III. Uses (Fig. 9.2)

A. Information derived from the examination of the hematocrit, together with the microscopic examination of the new methylene blue stained blood smear, provides a rapid, extremely useful hemogram of the patient. Not only is the PCV obtained but also a rough estimate of the total leukocyte count, as well as clues derived from the characteristics of the plasma.

B. Because of the better accuracy of the PCV as an indicator of the patient's erythrocytic status, the total erythrocyte count can be confined to conditions where computation of erythrocytic indices are needed. The PCV has the best sensitivity and reproducibility of the various techniques:

1. PCV error—1 to 2%
2. Erythrocyte count error—up to 40%
   a. To reduce the error in a manual count, thousands of cells would have to be counted.
   b. Even electronic counts are commonly in error.
3. Hemoglobin error—2 to 50%

C. Approximate leukocyte counts can be made from the buffy coat at the top of the packed erythrocyte layer in the Wintrobe tube.
   1. The first millimeter equals 10,000, and each 0.1 mm thereafter equals 2000 leukocytes/microliter. (13)
   2. This approximation should never be used as a substitute for a total leukocyte count, since it is possible to be misled by a marked thrombocytosis or the variability in cell size.

D. A rough approximation of the total erythrocyte count of canine blood can be obtained by dividing the PCV by 6, and the estimation of hemoglobin can be obtained by dividing the PCV reading by 3. (8)

E. The color of the plasma layer should be routinely noted; it is important to be familiar with the normal color for each of the species, as changes often give an indication of the cause of the clinical problem.
   1. Deep yellow or icteric—measured as icterus index units
      a. Ration—color of plasma is not as significant in herbivorous animals as in small animals and man, as the plant pigments that are consumed will influence the color.

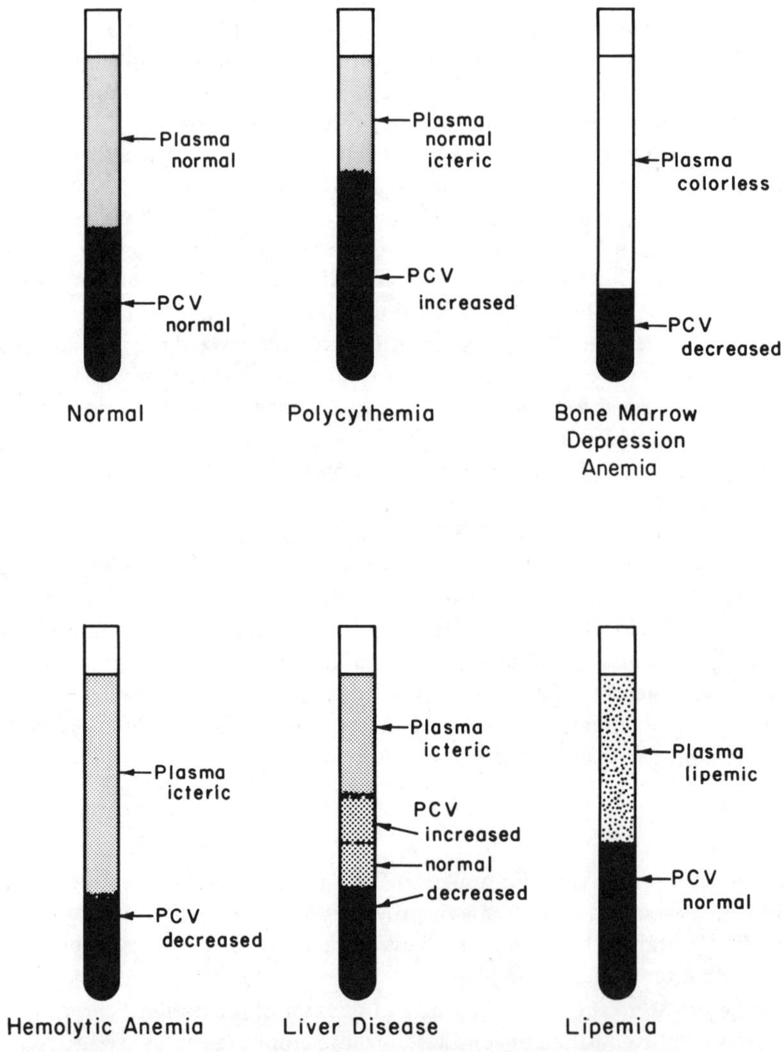

Fig. 9.2. Hematocrit readings for various conditions.

(1) Horse—normally has a higher icterus index than other species, but on a ration of alfalfa hay or pasture the index will be even higher

(2) Cattle—plasma is fairly pale on dry feed, but green feed will result in a much increased yellow color

b. Hemoconcentration—seen with an increased PCV

(1) When the hemoconcentration is from fasting, reduced fluid intake, or increased fluid loss, the color will be increased.

(a) Even a short period of water or food deprivation in the horse will have a marked effect upon the icterus index, which therefore is not a reliable indicator of the clinical problem.

(2) In the horse, a PCV increase of 50% over resting levels occurs within 10 min after racing. A transitory but pronounced hyperbilirubinemia occurs 16 to 24 hr after racing, with an increase in cell fragility during the recovery phase from splenic contraction and disintegration rather than relocation in the spleen. (11)

c. Hemolysis—increased amount of bilirubin is associated with a low PCV

d. Hepatocellular damage—increase in the bilirubin may be seen with a variety of PCV levels

(1) Normal PCV

(2) High PCV—due to hemoconcentration

(3) Low PCV—anemia may accompany this type of liver disease

e. Biliary obstruction—the markedly increased bilirubin is usually seen with a high to normal PCV and clay-colored fecal material

2. Colorless to pale plasma

a. Bone marrow depression—PCV is low and the condition is slow in developing

b. Acute hemorrhage—lighter plasma than normal may be associated with acute hemorrhage but will depend upon the extent of blood loss and fluid shifts

3. Lipemic plasma—Chylomicra in the plasma may be evident as creamlike throughout the plasma, hazy plasma, or as a creamline at the top of the plasma (especially when the microhematocrit is used)

a. Dietary

(1) Small animals that have not been fasted and have recently ingested some form of fatty food or drink will have lipemic plasma and a serum cholesterol that is usually normal to only slightly elevated.

b. Abnormal lipemia—usually associated with increased serum cholesterol levels

(1) Diabetes mellitus—consistently produces lipemic plasma

(2) Acute pancreatitis—when the islet cells are involved as well as the acinar tissue

(3) Hypothyroidism—sluggish biliary flow reduces the removal of cholesterol

(4) Hyperadrenocorticism—occasionally

(5) Liver disease

IV. Normal values

A. Adults

Species	PCV(%) (9)	PCV(%) (2)	PCV(%) (13)
Dog	45 (37 to 55)	45 (38 to 53)	
Cat	37 (24 to 45)	40 (30 to 50)	
Horse			
Hot-blooded	42 (32 to 55)	45 (36 to 52)	
Cold-blooded	35 (24 to 44)	35 (28 to 42)	
Cattle	35 (24 to 48)	37 (33 to 48)	
Sheep	38 (24 to 50)	34 (29 to 38)	
Goat	35 (24 to 48)	34 (29 to 38)	
Pig	42 (32 to 50)	40 (35 to 40)	
Rabbit		40 (30 to 50)	
Guinea pig		40 (35 to 45)	
Rat		40 (35 to 45)	
Mouse		40 (35 to 45)	
Chicken		35 (25 to 45)	
Human, male			47
Human. female			42

B. Young animals—age will influence the normal PCV range, and in many instances it is inadvisable to interpret the PCV of young animals by using the adult normal range

1. Dog—the PCV can be at the normal adult value at birth, but immediately undergoes a marked change. At 3 wk the PCV has fallen to about 32% and begins to increase when the pup starts to ingest solid food (3)—2 to 4 mo, 32 to 45%; 4 to 6 mo, 35 to 52%; 6 to 8 mo, 41 to 55%
2. Cat—8 to 30 wk, 33% (21 to 50) (6)
3. Horse
   a. The erythrocytes show a change that is most marked at from 1 to 9 mo of age. (1)
      (1) At this time the PCV, hemoglobin, mean corpuscular volume (MCV), and mean corpuscular hemoglobin (MCH) are at their lowest, the erythrocyte count is high, and the MCHC is constant.
         (a) Presumably postnatal hematopoiesis is relatively ineffective under about 2 mo of age, and these findings reflect the first influx of cells attributable to postnatal medullary hematopoiesis. In an animal over 2 mo of age, hepatic and splenic hematopoiesis is not active.
   b. There is a smooth progression of PCV, hemoglobin, MCV, and MCH from 1 to 9 mo up to 4 yr of age.
      (1) 2-year-old Thoroughbreds have lower PCV than 3-year-olds, but there is no significant difference between 3-year-olds and older except when these older horses are out of training. (4, 10)

Age	PCV(%)
Under 1 mo	37.8 ± 5.00
1 to 9 mo	35.3 ± 4.40
Yearling	37.5 ± 3.89
2-year-old	39.9 ± 3.99
3-year-old	41.4 ± 4.18
4-year-old	40.8 ± 4.65
Over 4 yr	39.8 ± 4.70

4. Cattle—the PCV and hemoglobin are high at birth but are reduced as soon as the calf begins to nurse. With the calf increasing in size and the input of iron low, the PCV and hemoglobin may continue to decline for several weeks. (5)

Age	PCV(%)	Hemoglobin
Birth	42	13.0
1 wk	35	11.0
2 mo	32	10.5
4 mo	35	11.0
24 mo	35	11.0

5. Sheep—PCV declines from 41.9% at birth to a low of 27.2% at 2 wk. These values increase to 31.5% at 1 mo and reach a maximum of 34.2% at 3 mo of age. (12)

Age	PCV(%)
Birth	41.9 ± 0.6
48 hr	33.4 ± 0.8
2 wk	27.2 ± 0.5
1 mo	31.5 ± 0.3
2 mo	34.0 ± 0.2
3 mo	34.2 ± 0.4
5 mo	31.4 ± 0.7
8 mo	31.8 ± 0.5
12 mo	33.8 ± 0.5

6. Pig—during the first 10 days, there is a marked fall in the PCV, hemoglobin, and total erythrocyte count, as the doubling of the pig's weight with its expanding blood volume exceeds the supply of iron in the sow's milk that is required for hemoglobin formation

Age	PCV(%) (9)	PCV(%) (7)
On concrete		
Birth		40
1 day	35	38
2 days		33
3 days	33	31
6 days	26.7	
7 days		34
10 days	24	38
On soil		
3 wk	37	36
5 wk	39.7	33
9 wk		35
3 mo		38
6 mo		39
9 mo		40
1 yr		39

10 INTERPRETATION OF HEMATOLOGIC FINDINGS

A LEUKOCYTES AND THEIR RESPONSES

I. General considerations

A. If the hemogram is to be used effectively as a diagnostic aid, it is important to be familiar with:
   1. Production, distribution, and fate of each type of leukocyte
   2. The functions and characteristics of each independent type of leukocyte
      a. It should be kept in mind that the mobilization and transport of leukocytes in the blood is for the purpose of carrying them to tissues where their functional capacity is utilized and is transitory, so that sequential counts may be enlightening.
   3. The normal ranges of total leukocyte counts and differential counts for each species, including not only percent distribution but also ranges for absolute numbers of each cell type
      a. Repeated clinical use will familiarize an individual with a feeling for normal values, as this is preferable to memorizing a table.
   4. The indications for requesting or conducting various blood examinations
      a. Although the hemogram should be considered part of the minimum data base, a laboratory examination should never be used as a substitute for a complete physical examination.
         (1) From the physical examination several diagnostic possibilities may come to mind, and some possible conditions may be eliminated or a suspicion may be confirmed by a particular leukocytic response.
   5. The interpretation of results, while taking into account the basic physiopathologic factors that influence alterations in:
      a. Total number of leukocytes
      b. Proportion of different types of leukocytes
      c. Morphology—especially if abnormal

B. Only after a complete history and a thorough physical examination can the blood picture be used effectively:
   1. In confirming or eliminating a tentative diagnosis
   2. As a guide to therapy
   3. As an index to prognosis

C. The leukocytic response and field of diagnosis can be divided into several general categories based upon the total leukocyte count and the differential cell pattern.
   1. Increase (leukocytosis) or decrease (leukopenia) of total leukocyte count, as well as the alteration of a particular cell type, can be significant.
      a. To achieve the maximum information, the total leukocyte count should be correlated with the distribution of cell types.
   2. Alterations may be in the form of cells not normally present in the circulating blood, such as immature or abnormal cells.
   3. Some disease conditions produce no alteration in the total or differential leukocyte counts, and in these a normal picture would be significant.

D. Alterations in the leukocyte count due to young age

1. Dog
   a. The newborn puppy has a relatively high leukocyte count (16,500/microliter), decreasing rapidly during the first few days of life, but then rising during the first week after birth. After this temporary increase, the total number reaches a low at about 2 wk of age, following which there is a gradual increase. The leukocyte count then decreases with age from a mean of 13,000/microliter at 60 days to a mean of 10,000/microliter at 4½ yr of age.
2. Cat
   a. Even though the total leukocyte count is not appreciably influenced by age, young kittens (12 wk and under) have somewhat higher mean leukocyte counts than older kittens. There are more high leukocyte counts (over 25,000/microliter) in younger kittens than in kittens 18 to 26 wk of age.
   b. Lymphocytes may dominate the differential leukocyte count up to the age of puberty.
3. Cattle
   a. Some investigators indicate higher leukocyte counts for calves than for adults, while others claim the opposite. Even when present, the differences do not vary markedly. It has also been stated that the mean average leukocyte count in calves is similar to adults, but with a higher proportion of calves producing a physiological leukocytosis; counts under 6000/microliter occur in only a few.
   b. Neutrophils are higher than lymphocytes on the day of birth due to stress, but within one day the neutrophils start to decrease, while the lymphocytes increase and continue to do so during the first year of life. During the first week of life the lymphocytes exceed the neutrophils and remain dominant throughout life.
4. Horse
   a. The total leukocyte count is at its lowest in the first month, with a range of 5000 to 11,000 and a mean of 8000/microliter. In weanlings, the total leukocyte count begins to decline slightly.
5. Sheep
   a. Total leukocyte counts rise from 3000/microliter at birth to a peak of 9500 at 3 mo.
6. Pig
   a. The total number of leukocytes decreases after birth, then an increase takes place at about 2 wk of age. From 7000/microliter at birth, the count gradually increases to 19,000 to 20,000/microliter at 5 wk. From 6 to 12 wk, the count ranges from 10,000 to 40,000/microliter, with a mean of 21,000. A leukocyte count lower than 10,000/microliter in pigs 6 wk of age or older would indicate a leukopenia.
   b. Neutrophils make up 70% of the leukocytes at birth, but within a week they decrease to the adult level.

II. Alterations in the total leukocyte count

A. Leukopenia—decrease in the total number of circulating leukocytes

1. Infection
   a. Viral—viruses must multiply in body cells with rapid RNA and DNA synthesis rates and the blast cells of the bone marrow are actively dividing cells, so virus replication in these young cells may be harmful or lethal. Destruction of the myeloid cells is usually at the blast or stem cell stage, but all stages of lymphocytes may be affected, as they are cells capable of division. After viral infection occurs, the decrease in production and cell destruction will result in a leukopenia in 3 to 8 days, depending upon the life span of the particular cell line. Not all viral infections produce a leukopenia, but the following are characterized by a leukopenia at some time in their course:
      (1) Feline panleukopenia—absolute lymphopenia is followed by an absolute neutropenia, producing a severe leukopenia
      (2) Canine distemper—in the viral stage, the total leukocyte count is generally between 6000 and 10,000, but it can be much lower
      (3) Infectious canine hepatitis—moderate to severe leukopenia due to neutropenia and lymphopenia, a relative monocytosis, and many immunocytes during the recovery phase

(4) Lymphosarcoma in cats (C-type virus)—sometimes a leukopenia, especially when the sarcomatous masses are forming
(5) Feline infectious peritonitis—sometimes a leukopenia, but quite variable
(6) Picornavirus—respiratory disease in cats with an initial leukopenia and a return to normal or high normal range
(7) Hog cholera
(8) Swine influenza
(9) Bluetongue
(10) Malignant catarrhal fever
(11) Bovine virus diarrhea
(12) Psittacosis-granuloma infection of cattle
(13) Rinderpest
(14) Viral arteritis—in horses

b. Bacterial
(1) Early stages of an infectious disease or of a localized severe infection where there is depletion of the peripheral blood of its leukocytes with concentration in the area of the infection, resulting in a leukopenia until the bone marrow catches up with the production
(a) The initial stage of a localized acute bacterial infection in cattle will produce a leukopenia due to migration from the peripheral blood with exudation in the injured tissue area, coupled with lysis of lymphocytes in the circulation (25 to 50%):
[1] 6 to 24 hr—leukopenia (2000 ±)
[2] 24 + hr—leukopenia with a shift to the left
[3] 3 to 4 days—normal leukocyte range or leukocytosis with neutrophilia
(2) Overwhelming bacterial infection—in terminal stages

c. Rickettsial
(1) Ehrlichiosis—in dogs and horses

d. Protozoan
(1) Toxoplasmosis
(2) East Coast fever

2. Sequestration of neutrophils in the capillaries of the lung, liver, and spleen
a. Shock
(1) Endotoxic
(2) Septic
(3) Anaphylactic
b. Retention in normal reservoirs—the leukocytes in the peripheral blood represent cells in temporary residence and make up a small fraction of the total population. Leukocytes move constantly from venous sinusoids, spleen, marrow, and other organs to lymphatic circulation and the bloodstream, so that census taking of this nomadic population may vary considerably.

3. Bone marrow abnormalities
a. Diminished production, normal life span
(1) Bone marrow hypoplasia
(a) Metabolic disorders
[1] Chronic nephritis
[2] Secondary nutritional hyperparathyroidism
(b) Ionizing radiation
(c) Chemical agents
(2) Bone marrow dysplasia
(a) Subleukemic or aleukemic leukemia
(b) Bone marrow displacement (myelophthisic)
[1] Myeloproliferative disorders
[2] Myelofibrosis
b. Normal production, defective maturation—vitamin B^{12} and folic acid deficiency, mild chronic leukopenia
(1) Old or debilitated animals
(2) Experimental animals on purified diets or long-term antibiotics

4. Chemical agents
   a. Mode of action:
      (1) Directly cytotoxic—usually develop slowly and are chronic in nature
      (2) Hypersensitivity—not common; acute leukopenias
         (a) The drug, usually with a benzene ring or other ring structure acts as a hapten that combines with a protein constituent of the leukocytes to form an antigen to which the patient develops antibodies. The antibody is toxic to the leukocytes and causes either lysis or agglutination.
   b. Some of the drugs listed consistently produce a leukopenia, while others cause a leukopenia only in isolated instances.
      (1) Antibiotics—chloramphenicol, streptomycin, penicillin
      (2) Antifungal—griseofulvin
      (3) Analgesics—aspirin, phenacetin, phenylbutazone, antipyrine
      (4) Antihistamines—pyribenzamine
      (5) Anticonvulsants—Primidone, Dilantin
      (6) Antithyroid drugs—thiouracil, propylthiouracil
      (7) Hemopoietic depressants—Cytoxan, 6-mercaptopurine
      (8) Arsenicals—arsphenamine, Mapharsen
      (9) Miscellaneous—DDT, barbiturates, pyrimethamine, chlorpromazine
   c. Metallic poisons
      (1) Lead
      (2) Thallium
      (3) Mercury
      (4) Arsenic

B. Leukocytosis—an increase above the accepted normal range of total leukocytes per microliter
1. As a rule, only one type of cell is responsible for the elevation, but there may be a simultaneous increase in several cell types.
   a. Absolute increases in the neutrophil count are so much more frequent than are increases in the other leukocytic types that the general term, leukocytosis, implies neutrophilia unless a qualifying term is used, such as eosinophilic leukocytosis.
2. The degree of leukocytosis depends upon several factors:
   a. Cause
   b. Severity of the infection
   c. Resistance of the animal
   d. Localization of the inflammatory response
      (1) Greater neutrophilic leukocytosis is produced by a localized disease process such as pyometra, rather than by a generalized one.
   e. Modification by therapy
   f. Species variation in response to stress—the neutrophil:lymphocyte ratio (N:L) parallels the amount of total leukocytic response

	N:L		Leukocytosis*		
Species	Ratio	Leukopenia*	Moderate	Marked	Extreme
Dog	3.5	6	18-30	30-50	50-100
Cat	1.8	8	20-30	30-50	50-75
Horse	1.1	7	15-25	25-30	35+
Cattle	0.5	4	12-20	15-25	25+

*Total leukocyte count in thousands per microliter. (Table according to Schalm.)

3. Physiologic leukocytosis
   a. Physiologic leukocytosis refers to a total leukocyte count above the normal, without the association of any known disease process. It is usually associated with conditions that result in a release of epinephrine, with the immediate mobilization of neutrophils that have marginated in small blood

vessels and are flushed into the larger vessels with the increased blood flow. As a rule, all cell types participate in the increase, but there is a tendency toward a neutrophilia without a shift to the left. Absolute numbers of lymphocytes and eosinophils remain normal except in the cat, where a mild lymphocytosis may occur.

(1) Strenuous exercise
   (a) While strenuous muscular activity increases the neutrophils, prolonged muscular activity leads to an increased number of lymphocytes. The lymphocytic increase with the greater physiologic leukocytosis is probably due to the increased lymph flow dumping more cells into the circulation.
   (b) At one time the increase was thought to be entirely the result of splenic contraction, but it has since been demonstrated in splenectomized animals.

(2) Convulsive seizures
   (a) The same effect is seen in convulsive seizures as with strenuous exercise.

(3) Excitement, fear, apprehension, or pain
   (a) This is particularly evident in the cat and horse, less so in the dog, and negligible in cattle and sheep.
   (b) A mild leukocytosis may be due to a redistribution, mainly a flushing effect. A more pronounced leukocytosis may find lymphocytes increased to a greater extent.

(4) Digestion
   (a) In the dog an increase in leukocytes begins an hour or so after eating, usually reaching a maximum in about 3 or 4 hr, and then declining.
   (b) In the pig, leukocytosis occurs within 3 to 5 hr after feeding. The count may increase more than 5000/microliter in a period of 1¾ hr.
   (c) Horses have a weak digestion leukocytosis.
   (d) Digestion leukocytosis appears to be absent in the herbivore, probably because digestion is slower and goes on constantly.

(5) Pregnancy
   (a) During pregnancy in the dog, the total leukocyte count can increase from 12,000 to 19,000/microliter.
   (b) In cats, leukocyte counts remain constant during pregnancy.
   (c) Pregnant cows have a slight increase in the total leukocyte count up to and including the third month, after which it slowly falls. The increase is usually less than 1000/microliter and would not be apparent in clinical interpretation. A second leukocytosis is noted during the 2 wk immediately prior to parturition.
   (d) During gestation in sheep, total leukocyte counts tend to rise, reaching their highest values at parturition.

4. Pathological leukocytosis
   a. Infection—localized or generalized
   b. Intoxications
      (1) Metabolic—uremia, acidosis, eclampsia
      (2) Chemical
      (3) Insect venom
      (4) Foreign protein reaction
   c. Tissue necrosis from any cause—infarction, burns, gangrene, neoplasms
   d. Acute hemorrhage
   e. Acute hemolysis
   f. Neoplasia (including leukemia)
   g. Adrenal corticosteroids—either from parenteral administration or excessive secretion
      (1) Within a few hours the characteristic hematologic response includes:
         (a) Leukocytosis, eosinopenia, and lymphopenia—in all species
         (b) Monocytosis—in dogs, cats, and cattle, but not in horses
         (c) Basopenia—seen in dogs, cattle, and horses

III. Qualitative changes in the maturation of granulocytes

A. An increase in the peripheral blood of immature cells of the granulocytic series is termed "shift to the left," and is based upon Schilling's maturation sequence, which is pictured with the more mature forms to the right and the immature forms progressing to the left (Fig. 10.1).

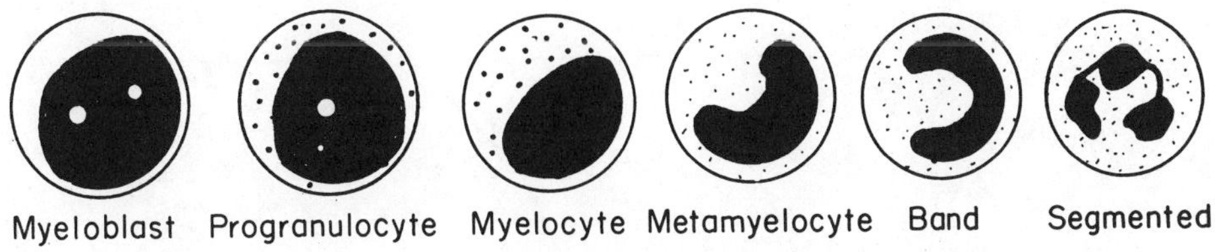

Fig. 10.1. Schilling's maturation sequence.

1. An elevated total leukocyte count with a slight to moderate increase in immature forms is considered a "regenerative shift to the left."
   a. Slight shift to the left—limited to bands
      (1) Mild stress or infection
   b. Moderate shift to the left—includes both band and metamyelocyte stages
      (1) Moderately severe to severe infection or severe stress
   c. Marked shift to the left—myelocytes and progranulocytes would be present in the peripheral blood
   d. Species differences in extreme leukocytosis:
      (1) Dog—responds well, and shift to the left includes bands or metamyelocytes (juveniles)
      (2) Cat—shift to the left is seldom more immature than the early band
2. A low, normal, or slightly elevated total leukocyte count with an increase in immature cells of the granulocytic series in the peripheral blood is called a "degenerative shift to the left."
   a. The bone marrow is unable to maintain an adequate reaction by increasing the number of mature cells.
   b. Toxic neutrophils are common.
   c. It often indicates a septicemia or bacterial sepsis.
   d. In the initial stages of the inflammatory process in cattle, marked leukopenia with an increase in immature granulocytes is common, but it is not considered degenerative for this species nor does it denote an unfavorable prognosis, as these findings would suggest in dogs, cats, and horses.
3. A "shift to the right" is an increase in the percent of the older cells (hypersegmentation) with 5 or more lobes due to aging.
   a. Some of the conditions associated with hypersegmentation:
      (1) Blood left in anticoagulant too long can produce this as an artifact.
      (2) Effect of corticosteroid released in stress, which partially prevents the diapedesis of neutrophils, with prolonged aging in the circulation
      (3) Vitamin B^{12} and/or folic acid deficiency—rare in animals
4. A normal or elevated total leukocyte count with immature granulocytes exceeding the mature forms denotes an unfavorable prognosis.

IV. Responses of individual leukocytic types

A. Neutrophil
   1. Kinetics (Figs. 10.2, 10.3.)
      a. Proliferating pool—comprises cells of the bone marrow capable of division and includes myeloblasts, progranulocytes, and myelocytes
         (1) Number of divisions:
            (a) Myeloblast—1

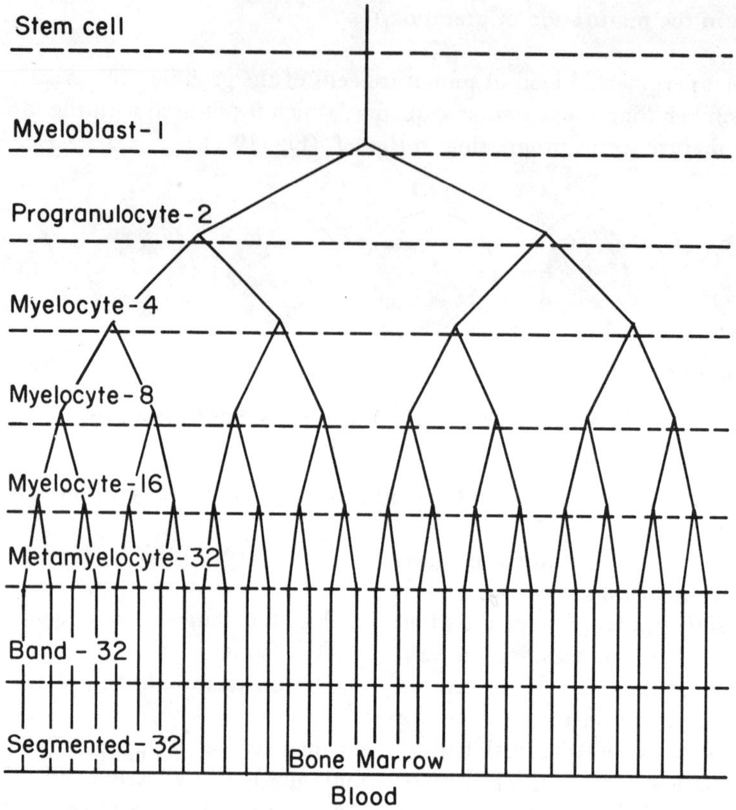

Fig. 10.2. Kinetics of the neutrophil.

(b) Progranulocyte—2

(c) Myelocyte—at least 4 times and can be more when neutrophilic production is required, as each division doubles the cell production

[1] Hyperplasia of granulocytes can occur in 72 to 96 hr.

[2] Myelocyte division has a greater effect than increased stem cell production.

b. Maturation pool—neutrophils of the bone marrow that do not divide and include metamyelocytes, bands, and segmented granulocytes

(1) Constitutes the reserve of neutrophils in the body, when in the bone marrow

(a) In man, represents 25 to 30 cells for each neutrophil in the circulating blood

(b) Cells are released from the bone marrow to the blood according to the stage of maturation, normally only mature cells, but the pool responds to disease by releasing less mature cells.

c. Marginal neutrophilic pool (MNP)—neutrophils in the small blood vessels that marginate along the walls and move at a slower rate than the other blood cells

(1) Healthy dog and man—1 neutrophil for each 1 in the circulating pool

(2) Healthy cat—2 to 3 neutrophils for each neutrophil in the circulating blood

d. Circulating neutrophilic pool (CNP)—cells in the larger blood vessels moving in the main or axial stream of blood

(1) 6 to 7 hours is the half-life of neutrophils in the blood, with replacement of the entire population occurring approximately 2½ times daily.

e. Tissues

(1) After circulating for 6 to 7 hours (dog and cat), the neutrophils migrate through the capillary wall into the surrounding tissues where they are needed.

(2) Movement of neutrophils into the tissues is not orderly in respect to the stage of maturation of the cell, and these cells do not return to the blood.

(3) Following injury, a flow of cells into exudates is evident within 2 hr.

(4) Once the neutrophils have left the blood, their fate is migration from tissues into body secretions (gut, pulmonary secretions, urine, saliva), where they may perform a protective function or die.

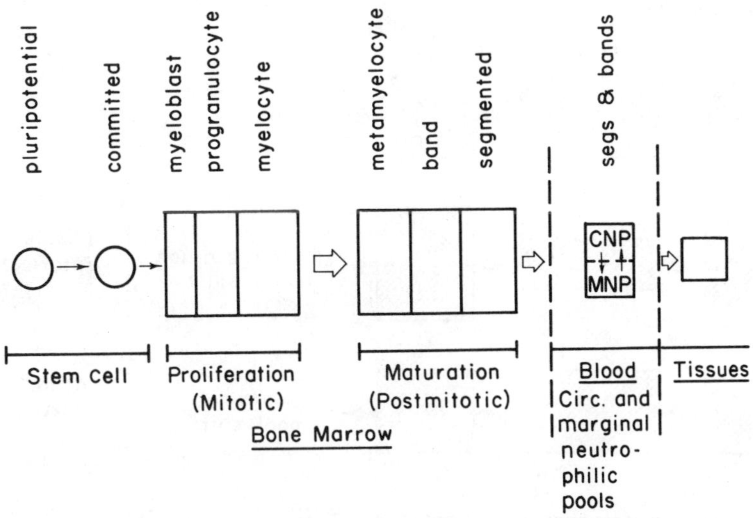

Fig. 10.3. Division and movement of neutrophils.

2. Function of neutrophils in acute inflammation and phagocytosis
   a. Margination and pavementing of neutrophils in the vessels is the initial step, and the immediate cause is poorly understood.
   b. Emigration through endothelial open cell junctions is seen, as neutrophils are motile with amoeboid movements.
   c. Chemotaxis and aggregation of neutrophils occur at the site of injury.
      (1) A substance provided by bacterial and tissue breakdown provides chemotactic stimuli and attracts neutrophils so that they will accumulate at the site of injury or infection. The complement may also attract neutrophils in certain cases.
   d. Phagocytosis
      (1) Phagocytosis and digestion of foreign material (bacteria and other particulate matter) is accomplished by neutrophils as their main function, and hence they are sometimes called microphages.
      (2) The cytoplasmic granules (lysosomes) contain digestive enzymes that unite with and kill bacteria by enzymatic hydrolysis. These enzymes are alkaline phosphatase (in some animals), acid phosphatase, RNAase, DNAase, lipase, esterase, and antibacterial protein.
      (3) The neutrophil flows around the bacterium and eventually engulfs it, incorporating it within a phagocytic vacuole. The phagocytic vacuole then fuses with lysosomes, producing a phagolysosome. The lysosomal enzymes with powerful proteolytic action are released into the vacuole, where the direct contact with the bacterium digests it.
      (4) Any stage younger than the metamyelocyte is not capable of phagocytosis.
   e. The reaction in the initial stage of an acute inflammation is alkaline, and as the reaction in the inflammatory focus becomes more acid, the neutrophils are injured and cannot survive, resulting in a suppurative reaction, and they are later replaced by macrophages.
      (1) Neutrophils are short-lived, about 4 days in the tissues, after which they will be replaced by mononuclear cells, mostly monocytes, that can withstand the falling pH.
3. Neutrophilia (See Figs. 10.4, 10.5, 10.6.)
   a. Noninflammatory neutrophilia with systemic stress associated with endogenous release of corticosteroids
      (1) Corticosteroids—produce up to a fourfold increase in mature neutrophils in the peripheral blood of dogs, cattle, and horses as:
         (a) Marginated neutrophils are mobilized to increase the circulating pool.
         (b) Neutrophils are retained in the blood as diapedesis is reduced, thus prolonging the half-life of the neutrophil.
         (c) The rate of release of neutrophils from the bone marrow may be increased. If the effect is prolonged, it may eventually result in band forms being released.

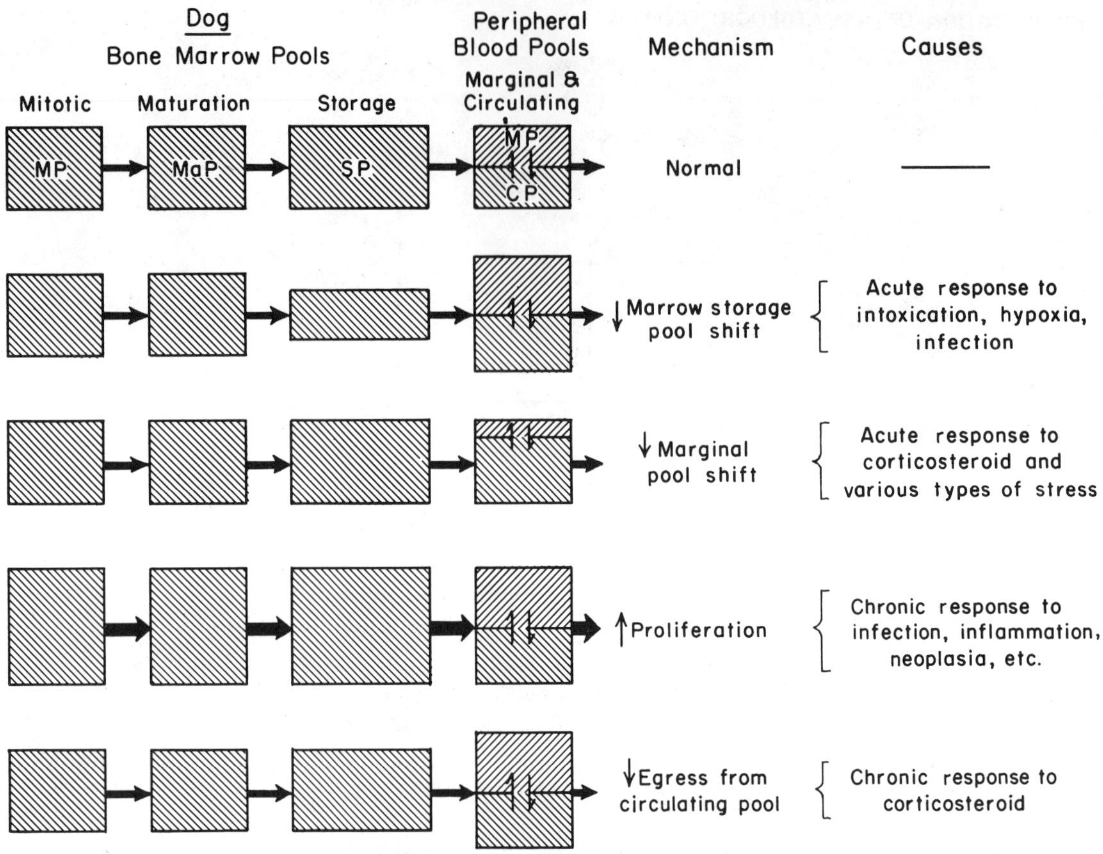

Fig. 10.4. Bone marrow pools—dog.

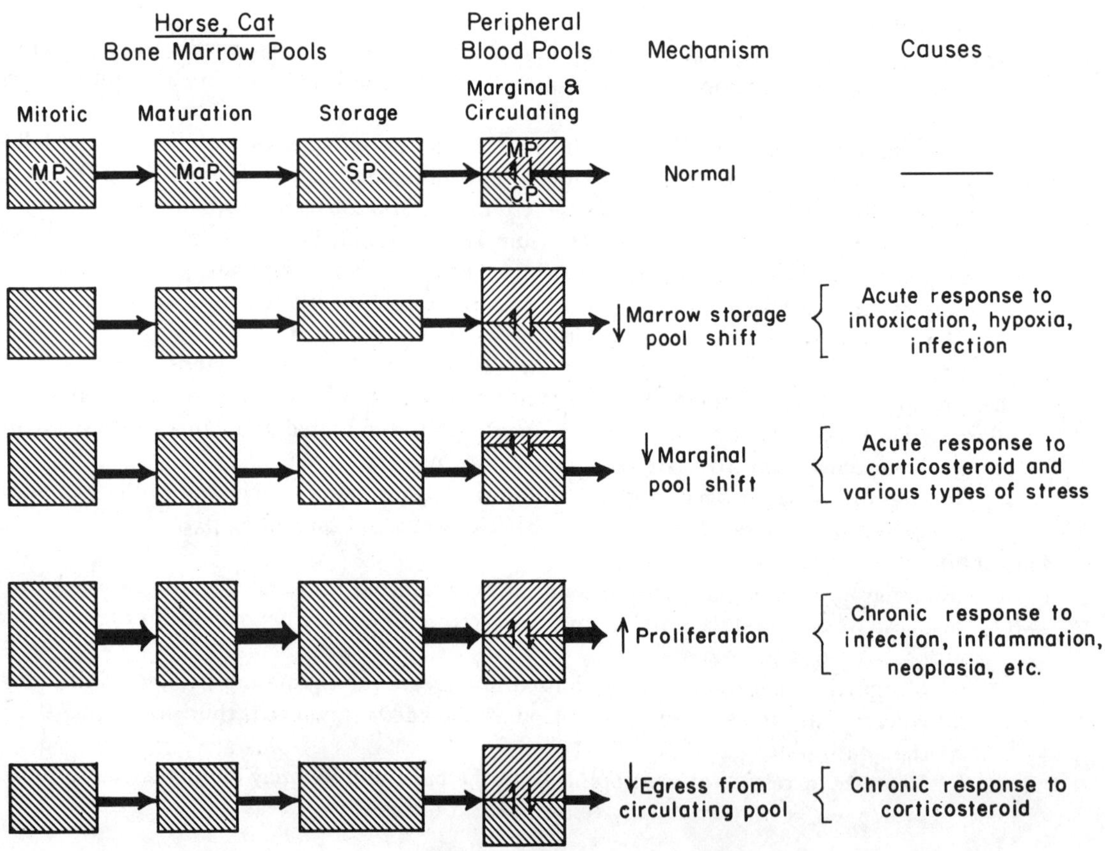

Fig. 10.5. Bone marrow pools—horse, cat.

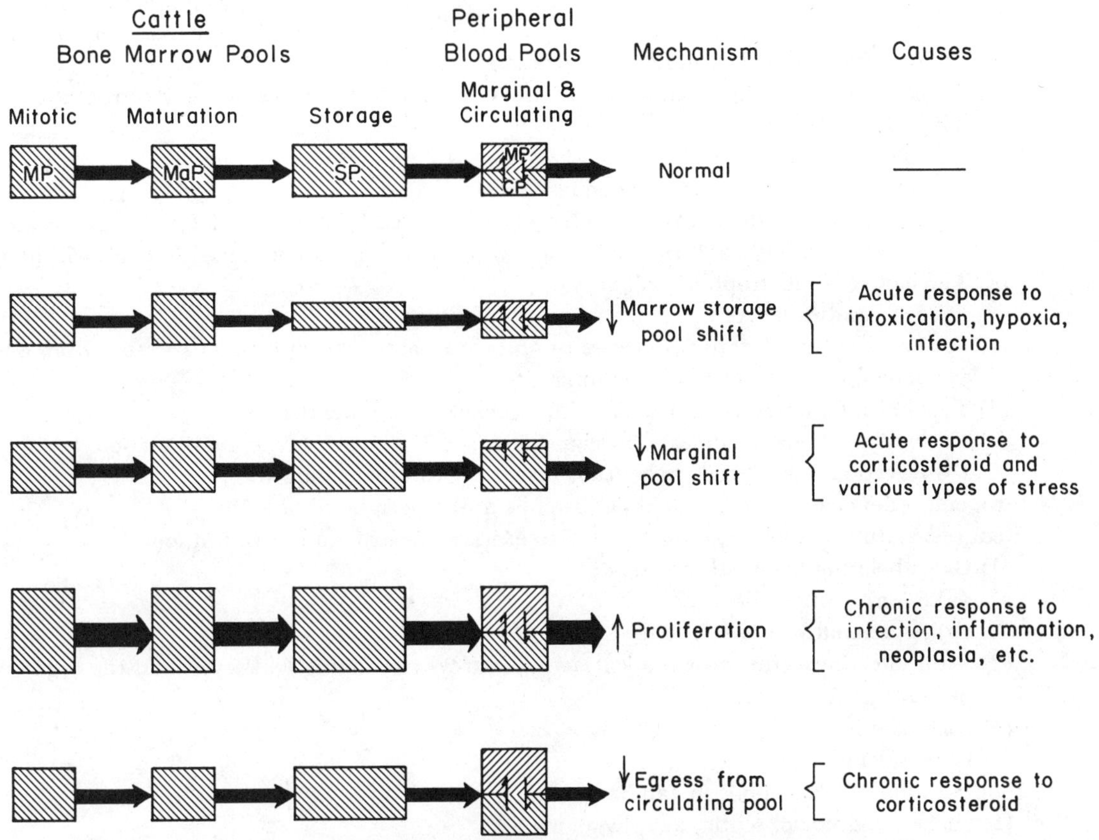

Fig. 10.6. Bone marrow pools—cattle.

(2) The mobilization of neutrophils by corticosteroids is not useful in fighting bacterial infections, due to the following effects of corticosteroids on the neutrophils with depression of:
 (a) Phagocytosis
 (b) Digestion
 (c) Ameboid activity
 (d) Diapedesis
 (e) Glycolysis

(3) Conditions associated with noninflammatory disorders
 (a) Intoxication
 (b) Trauma
 (c) Neoplasia
 (d) Surgical procedures
 (e) Anesthetics
 (f) Metabolic and endocrine disorders—sometimes
 (g) Hyperadrenocorticism
 (h) Stress—usually the cause or contributing cause if the total leukocyte count does not exceed 30,000 (in dogs and cats), with few bands and an absolute lymphopenia and eosinopenia

b. Inflammatory neutrophilia
 (1) There is a demand by the tissue for neutrophils in inflammatory disease, whether it is generalized or localized in character.
  (a) The number of neutrophils in the circulating blood will reflect the balance between demand, movement, and bone marrow release.
 (2) In acute inflammatory diseases, the total leukocyte count will increase, with a left shift, as the rate of movement of neutrophils into the blood is greater than their movement into the tissues.
  (a) In the early stages the increase in the circulating pool will be at the expense of the maturation pool.

(b) As the inflammatory state becomes established, there will be an increase in bone marrow proliferation with a subsequent increase in the maturation pool.

(3) The magnitude of the inflammation may be estimated by the degree of neutrophilia and type of left shift produced:

(a) Regenerative left shift—implies adequate release and mobilization

(b) Degenerative left shift—inadequate release

(c) Chronic suppurative diseases will be characterized by a marked left shift (bands and metamyelocytes), and the bone marrow proliferating and maturation pools will be contracted.

(4) The degree of neutrophilia will vary.

(a) Species differences

(b) Localized suppurative processes produce a greater neutrophilic leukocytosis than does a generalized infection or inflammation.

(5) Types of inflammatory disorders—either localized or generalized

(a) Noninfectious—neoplasia, foreign body, sterile abscess, tissue manipulation

(b) Infectious—bacterial, rickettsial, mycotic, protozoan, parasitic

4. Neutropenia—deficiency of functional neutrophils in the peripheral blood

a. Reduced mature granulocyte survival due to excessive destruction or utilization

(1) Overwhelming bacterial infection

(a) Severe septicemia

(b) Associated with a left shift

(2) Viral infections—the virus replicates and destroys circulating leukocytes and the organs that produce them

(3) Rickettsia

(4) Hypersplenism

b. Sequestration of neutrophils in capillary beds

(1) Shock—endotoxic, septic, anaphylactic

(2) Initial stage of an acute bacterial infection—especially in cattle

c. Reduction of granulopoiesis in the bone marrow

(1) Drug-induced

(a) Cytolytic

(b) Metabolic interference

(c) Idiosyncratic

(2) Chronic infection

(3) Malignancies causing replacement of marrow

d. Impairment of the ability of mature neutrophils to leave the bone marrow in the presence of adequate marrow reserve (myelokathaexis)

(1) Deficiencies of vitamin B^{12} and folic acid

e. Congenital defect

(1) Cyclic neutropenia in grey Collies—cyclic maturation arrest

(a) Intervals of 8 to 12 days between neutropenic stages

(b) Lethal syndrome that affects both sexes

B. Eosinophil

1. Kinetics

a. Eosinophils originate in the bone marrow and follow a maturation pattern, similar in production time (3 to 6 days), life span, and circulation to the neutrophil. Under normal conditions, eosinophils do not return to the circulation after reaching the tissues.

(1) There are 300 to 400 eosinophils in the bone marrow for every one in the circulating blood, with 75% mature, thus forming a reservoir.

(2) Eosinophils are attracted into tissues where there has been a high histamine release.

2. Functions

a. Deactivation of histamine

(1) The major source of histamine is from the disruption of tissue mast cells and basophils in the blood, with degranulation releasing their histamine-rich granules into the tissues.

(a) Injury

(b) Antigen-antibody reaction—a factor released by lymphocytes, lymphokine, is chemotactic for eosinophils following antigen-antibody complexes as well as the histaminic chemotactic effect of histamine

(2) Eosinophils neutralize histamine, serotonin, and bradykinin, resulting in an antiinflammatory effect.

(3) Glucocorticoids have a neutralizing effect on histamine, which explains the eosinopenia seen with stress and glucocorticoid or ACTH administration.

(4) Much peroxidase is present in specific eosinophilic granules and appears to exert some antiinflammatory effect at sites where antigen antibodies interact, even when histamine is not involved.

b. Fibrin degradation

(1) While developing in the bone marrow, eosinophils synthesize profibrinolysin, a fibrinolytic system, which assists in the degradation of excessive fibrin deposits produced by exudation of plasma proteins in hypersensitivity reactions.

c. Phagocytosis and detoxification

(1) Foreign substances and decomposing body protein in the body may be detoxified by eosinophils and then phagocytized.

(a) Eosinophilic granules are lysosomes that contain digestive enzymes, mainly alkaline and acid phosphatases. The granules function in phagocytosis by membrane fusion with phagosomes, similar to neutrophilic lysosomes.

(2) An eosinophilia developing in the presence of stress, as indicated by a neutrophilia and lymphopenia, is an unfavorable sign, since it denotes advancing body protein decomposition.

3. Eosinophilia— >750/microliter in dogs and cats

a. Common in diseases of tissues containing a large number of mast cells:

(1) Skin—allergies

(2) Lung—eosinophilic pneumonia

(3) Gastrointestinal tract—eosinophilic gastroenteritis

(4) Female genital tract—during estrus

(a) The uterus contains the most number of mast cells during proestrus and the least during estrus.

b. Parasitism—some parasites characteristically produce more eosinophilia than others, as there is a direct correlation between the amount of contact between the tissues of the host and the parasite, with a humoral substance produced by sensitized large lymphocyte exposure

(1) Filariasis (heartworms)—especially after destruction of the microfilaria

(2) Hookworms—moderate reaction

(3) Lungworms

(4) Strongyles

(5) *Spirocerca*

(6) *Echinococcus*

(7) Fascioliasis

(8) Trichinosis

(9) Fleas—flea-bite allergy or dermatitis

c. Allergies

(1) Allergic bronchitis or sinusitis—may be confirmed by demonstrating eosinophils in a smear of nasal or bronchial secretions

(2) Hay fever—eosinophils may be present in conjunctival discharges

(3) Gastrointestinal or food allergy

(4) Skin allergies—urticarial skin lesions and vesicles

(5) Anaphylactic reaction

(6) Angioneurotic edema

(7) Drying-off period in cows—mild allergic response to the milk protein retained in the mammary gland

d. Adrenocortical insufficiency—in some cases; initial screening can be accomplished by the Thorn test:

(1) Obtain a preinjection blood sample for an eosinophil count.

(2) Inject 10 to 25 units of ACTH intramuscularly.

(3) A decrease in eosinophils of at least 50% from the base-line value 4 hr after the injection, or a fall of at least 70% within 7 hr after the injection, indicates normal adrenocortical function.

e. Eosinophilic myositis

f. Eosinophilic panosteitis—infrequently

g. Decomposing body protein

(1) Chronic suppurative disease

(2) Malignancies

h. Hemopoietic disorders

(1) Eosinophilic leukemia

(2) After splenectomy—in about 1 mo

i. Neoplasms—especially those involving the ovary, bone, and serous membranes

j. Following radiation therapy—2 or 3 wk later

4. Eosinopenia

a. Systemic stress—in response to release of endogenous corticosteroids

(1) Stress of disease—either acute or chronic

(2) Inflammation—acute or chronic

(3) Intoxications

(4) Trauma

b. Hyperadrenocorticism

c. Administration of corticosteroids or ACTH

(1) Results in eosinopenia in 4 to 8 hr

(2) With one dose, eosinophils will reappear in the circulation within 24 hr.

(3) After prolonged corticosteroid therapy several days may be required for the eosinopenic condition to disappear.

C. Basophil

1. Kinetics

a. Basophils are produced in the bone marrow from the undifferentiated stem cell and have a life span of 10 to 12 days.

b. Mast cells are the connective tissue counterpart of basophils in the peripheral blood but differ by having a round nucleus, a stellate or round shape, and more numerous delicate granules.

c. The characteristic color of the granule is due to its content of sulfated acid mucopolysaccharides, which appears to vary in different species.

2. Functions

a. Basophilic granules are lysosomal structures, similar to the granules in the mast cell, and contain heparin in a bound form with histamine, serotonin, and hyaluronic acid, all of which are easily released.

(1) Injury to tissue releases histamine and serotonin to initiate the inflammatory response by causing increased permeability, capillary inflammatory response, and attraction of eosinophils.

(2) Heparin is a potent anticoagulant.

(3) Degranulation can occur with postprandial lipemia, possibly due to lipoprotein lipase releasing endogenous heparin to promote a clearing of the lipemia.

(a) Giving 2 mg/kg or 110 units/lb of heparin to a normal dog with dietary lipemia will clear the plasma in 15 min, but it is unlikely to clear the lipemia associated with diabetes mellitus or liver disease.

b. It is involved in cellular immune reactions.

(1) Differentiation and production of basophils can be initiated by antigenic stimulation.

(2) Basophils are implicated in the mechanism of immediate and delayed hypersensitivity.

(3) Antibodies attach to the basophil membrane and induce lysis by contact with an antigen.

3. Basophilia

a. Sometimes associated with an eosinophilia—heartworms and chronic respiratory disease, especially

b. Hyperadrenocorticism in the dog—with eosinopenia

(1) This is a contradiction to the basopenia that develops with stress.

c. Basophilic leukemia—rare; care should be taken not to confuse this with mast cell sarcoma

d. Hypothyroidism
e. Tissues that contain many mast cells
(1) Skin and subcutaneous tissue
(2) Lung
(3) Gastrointestinal tract
(4) Uterus
(5) Scrotum
(6) Serosal linings
(a) Heparin in the mast cells of the serosal linings prevents clotting of blood following chronic hemorrhage into body cavities.

D. Lymphocyte
1. Kinetics (Fig. 10.7)
a. In the embryo, stem cells from the bone marrow seed the thymus and the bursa equivalent, which is probably the bone marrow, producing two fundamentally different populations of conditioned cells:
(1) T or thymic-dependent lymphocytes—cells with the capacity to initiate cell-mediated immune (CMI) responses
(2) B or bursa-equivalent (bone marrow derived) lymphocytes—cells that can produce humoral antibodies and are precursors of plasma cells; independent of thymic activity
(a) Plasma cells—specifically modified cells that are derived from B lymphocytes and are the major cellular source of humoral antibodies (immunoglobulins)

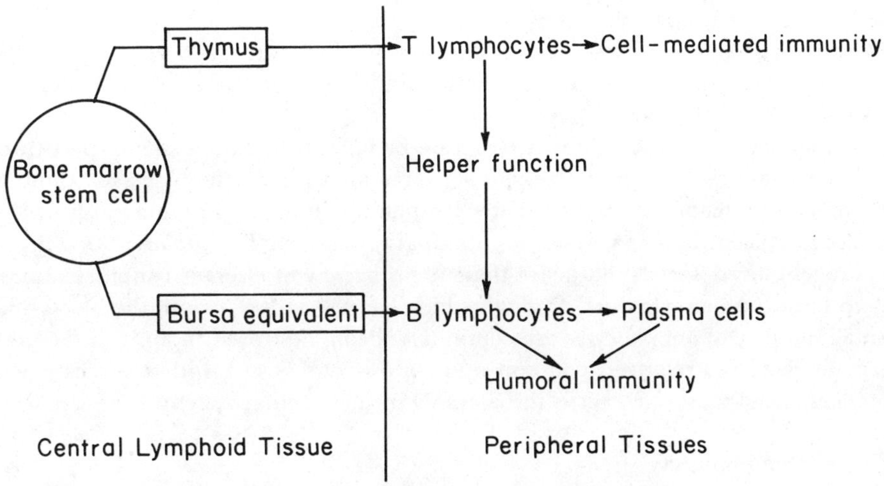

Fig. 10.7. Kinetics of the lymphocyte.

b. The conditioned cells migrate and colonize the lymph nodes and provide clones of lymphocytes with specific reactivity.
c. Circulating small lymphocytes represent two functional populations of lymphoid cells, although they cannot be differentiated by conventional or electron microscopy.
d. Locations of T and B lymphocytes

Location	T lymphocytes	B lymphocytes
Blood	+ + +	+
Bone marrow	+	+ + + + as precursors
Lymph node	+ + + deep cortex	+ germinal centers
Spleen	+ + +	+ +
Thoracic duct	+ + +	+
Thymus	+ + + +	Rare

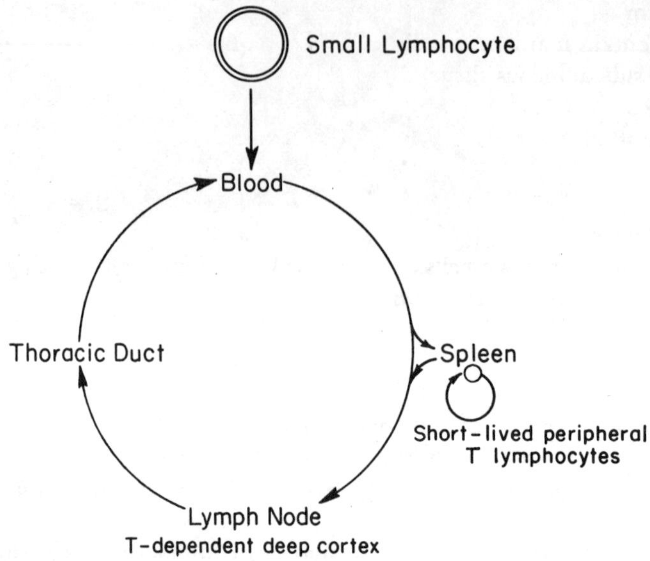

Fig. 10.8. Recirculation of lymphocytes.

e. The life spans of lymphocytes vary.
   (1) Long-lived lymphocytes—survive for years; predominate
   (2) Short-lived lymphocytes—live for hours, days, weeks, or at most a few months
f. Recirculation of lymphocytes (Fig. 10.8)
   (1) Lymphocytes have the ability to migrate between lymphatic tissue in part through their ability to enter and leave the blood freely. They circulate through the blood for about 2 hr, migrate through postcapillary venules, enter lymphatics, and reach peripheral lymphatic tissues (lymph nodes, spleen, Peyer's patches of intestinal wall, etc.). The majority of recirculating lymphocytes are long-lived T cells that leave these areas by way of efferent lymph channels that eventually join to form the thoracic duct, through which lymphocytes return to the blood and recirculate.
g. A small number of lymphocytes are continually being destroyed, mainly in the gut, and are replaced.
h. Normally there is a relatively constant number of lymphocytes, with a decrease as the animal ages.
   (1) These lymphocytes are distributed evenly in the vascular system.

2. Functions
   a. Cell-mediated immunity
      (1) Response of T cells to antigenic challenge (Fig. 10.9)

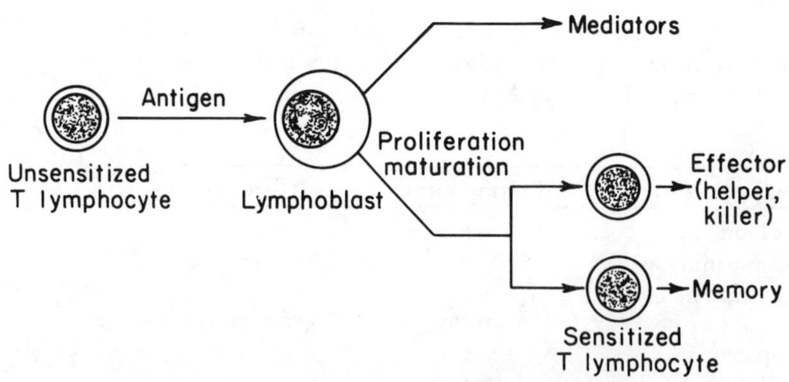

Fig. 10.9. Response of T cells to antigenic challenge.

(2) Rate of response—hours to days
(3) Examples:
(a) Delayed hypersensitivity
(b) Tuberculin-type
(c) Allograft rejection
(d) Contact dermatitis
(e) Tumor surveillance—possibly
(f) Graft host reactions
(g) Certain autoimmune reactions

b. Humoral immunity
(1) Response of B cells to antigenic challenge (Fig. 10.10)
(2) Rate of response—minutes to hours
(3) Examples:
(a) Bacterial opsonization and lysis
(b) Anaphylaxis
(c) Allergies—hay fever and asthma
(d) Virus and toxin neutralization
(e) Immune complex diseases
(f) Certain autoimmune reactions

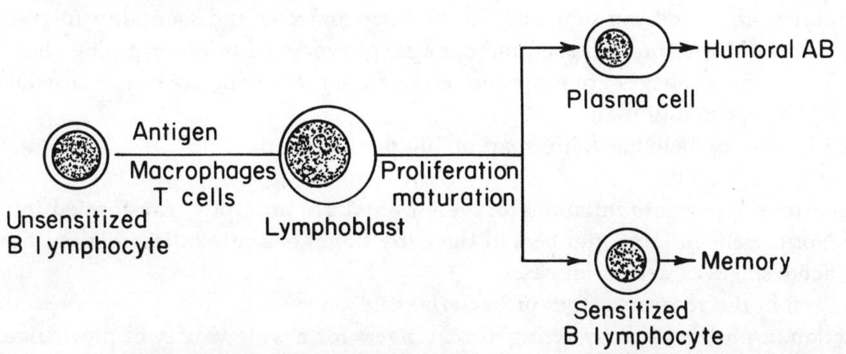

Fig. 10.10. Response of B cells to antigenic challenge.

3. Lymphocytosis—absolute number of lymphocytes is above the normal
a. Marked physiologic leukocytosis may increase lymph flow with dumping of an increased number of lymphocytes into the circulation.
(1) Frequently seen in the cat, where it should not be confused with lymphosarcoma, but may be observed in the dog and horse occasionally.
(2) More likely to occur in healthy animals than in those that are ill.
b. Normally seen as a result of immaturity in young cattle and cats.
(1) The number of lymphocytes decreases with age in all species.
c. Prolonged or abnormal antigenic stimulation—occasionally
(1) After vaccination—immunocytes may make an appearance
(2) Chronic infection
(3) Hypersensitivity
(4) Autoimmune disease
d. Hypoadrenocorticism
e. Lymphocytic leukemia
f. Lymphadenitis or lymphangitis—occasionally
g. Certain blood parasite infections—occasionally
(1) *Babesia*
(2) *Theileria*
(3) *Trypanosoma*
h. A relative lymphocytosis is the most common type—conditions that have a leukopenia and a neutropenia

4. Lymphopenia—<1000/microliter in the dogs and <1500/microliter in the cat
   a. Tissue redistribution of circulating cells—associated with:
      (1) Corticosteroids—effect is apparent in a few hours after administration, with a decrease up to 50%
      (2) Hyperadrenocorticism
      (3) Systemic stress—degree parallels the degree of lymphopenia
   b. Lysis of lymphocytes
      (1) Canine distemper—characteristic sign
      (2) Hog cholera
      (3) Bovine viral diarrhea
      (4) Infectious canine hepatitis—leukopenia is due to both lymphopenia and neutropenia
      (5) Corticosteroids—lysis of lymphocytes in all tissues and decline of lymphoid mitosis in lymph nodes
      (6) Radiation
      (7) Immunosuppressive drugs
   c. Extravasation of lymphocytes—reduces the available population of recirculating cells
      (1) Chylothorax
      (2) Chronic enteric disease

E. Monocyte
1. Kinetics
   a. Monocytes originate from stem cells in the bone marrow; and soon after migrating into the tissues, they can transform into a tissue macrophage (phagocytic histiocyte) in less than 24 hr.
      (1) Tissue macrophages are more numerous than the monocytes in the circulation, with a ratio of 400:1 reported in man.
      (2) The macrophage has a life span of 100 days or more.
2. Functions
   a. Monocytes migrate into inflammatory lesions and are promptly transformed into macrophages.
      (1) Not present in large numbers in the early stages of acute inflammation, but can appear in the acute stages of certain diseases
      (2) Seen in the recovery stages of bacterial infections
   b. Function in phagocytosis by acting as scavengers for a wide variety of particulate materials as well as bacteria
      (1) Have special enzyme systems, including nucleases, proteinases, and carbohydrases and are rich in lipases
      (2) Under severe conditions will phagocytize while in the bloodstream, as in intravascular hemolysis
   c. Interact with lymphocytes in immune reactions
3. Monocytosis—>1350/microliter in the dog and >850/microliter in the cat
   a. Corticosteroids or stress stimulate an increase in:
      (1) Dogs
      (2) Cats—occasionally
      (3) Cattle
   b. During the recovery or late phase of acute disease and in all chronic suppurative diseases
   c. Diseases with tissue debris where the monocytes can act as scavengers
      (1) Hemolytic anemia or hemorrhage into the tissues
      (2) Thrombocyte destruction
      (3) Exudate in pleural or peritoneal cavities
      (4) Pyometra
      (5) Retained placenta
   d. Granulomatous inflammatory response
      (1) Tuberculosis
      (2) Brucellosis
      (3) Systemic mycotic infections
      (4) Protozoan infection
   e. Monocytes are chemotactic to lipid-rich material—have high lipase activity
      (1) Migrate into milk in mammary glands that are involuting

B BLOOD PICTURE IN SPECIFIC CONDITIONS

I. DOG

ACTH (119)

1. Injection of 5 to 50 international units of ACTH in normal dogs, or in dogs in which no adrenocortical deficiency exists, results in a 75 to 99% decrease in circulating eosinophils within 7 hr.

Adrenocortical insufficiency (118)

1. There is a relative lymphocytosis and sometimes an absolute lymphocytosis.
2. A relative eosinophilia is not a consistent finding, but if it is present, the Thorn test can be used to determine if the eosinophilic insufficiency could be associated with adrenocortical insufficiency.
   a. Administration of ACTH fails to produce an eosinopenic response.
3. There may be an elevated PCV due to hemoconcentration, but after proper hydration a slight to marked anemia is sometimes seen.
   a. When present, the anemia is usually normocytic normochromic, with little evidence of bone marrow response.

Amyloidosis (144)

1. If the amyloidosis is generalized and chronic in nature, a nonregenerative anemia may be present.

Anesthesia, pentobarbital (75)

1. A leukopenia with a relative lymphocytosis reaches its maximum in 90 min, and then returns to normal.
2. Transient decreases in total erythrocytes, PCV, and hemoglobin values are noted.

Babesiasis (178)

1. Leukocytosis of varying degrees may be present, associated with a neutrophilia.
2. A progressive anemia develops, associated with a marked decrease in the number of erythrocytes per microliter and a low hemoglobin level.
   a. The anemia is of the regenerative type, with evidence of a bone marrow response seen in the blood smear.
3. *Babesia canis* can be demonstrated in most acute cases, but in the chronic form the organisms in the erythrocytes are scarce and often cannot be found.

Blastomycosis (139)

1. A neutrophilic leukocytosis with a marked shift to the left is reported.

Cardiac hemangiosarcoma (102)

1. Findings disclose anemia, leukocytosis due to neutrophilia, and shift to the left. Nucleated erythrocytes are frequently abundant, probably as a result of active hematopoiesis and hypoxia.

Chlorpromazine hydrochloride (86)

1. Hemodilution results from chlorpromazine administration.

Colitis, granulomatous (192)

1. The total leukocyte count will fall within the normal range in most dogs, but leukocytosis may occur in a severe case when secondary bacterial processes play a role.
2. A severe case rarely may lose enough blood to show a low PCV.

Copper deficiency (67, 194)

1. Normocytic normochromic anemia is produced.

Dermatosis, allergic (103)

1. In many types of allergic dermatoses, there is an increase in the number of eosinophils.

Diabetes mellitus (144)

1. Leukocytosis occurs as a result of tissue necrosis, stress, secondary infection, or pancreatitis.
2. The PCV is elevated.

Distemper (23, 146, 169)

1. The total leukocyte count will vary, depending upon the stage of the disease.
   a. In the early acute stage, there is a leukopenia.
   b. Leukocytosis is present in later stages in about 20% of the cases.
2. A shift to the left of neutrophils is associated with the leukocytosis and sometimes with the leukopenia.
3. Moderate anemia may be seen in the terminal stages.

Endocarditis, acute bacterial (144, 176)

1. The usual picture is one of a neutrophilic leukocytosis, but a leukopenia may occur in the presence of overwhelming septicemia.
2. There is a marked shift to the left, with very young forms such as myelocytes and even myeloblasts.
3. Thrombocytes are usually normal in number, sometimes with giant forms, but an occasional case may have a thrombocytopenia.

Endotoxicosis (*Escherichia coli*) (92)

1. There is a gradual increase in the PCV.
2. Leukocytes disappear within 5 min following endotoxin administration and gradually return during 5 hr postinjection.
3. Differential leukocyte counts reveal that the primary loss of circulating leukocytes is in the segmented neutrophils.

Eosinophilic myositis (205)

1. The percentage of eosinophils may vary from 20 to 60%.

Estrogen (46)

1. Large doses of natural or synthetic estrogens produce a gradual anemia and a profound leukocytosis, which is followed by a leukopenia.
2. During the period of leukocytosis, there is a neutrophilic shift to the left.
3. Thrombocytes are reduced in number.

Ethylene glycol poisoning (142)

1. Increased PCV, hemoglobin content, and total erythrocyte count are produced.
2. Neutrophilia, lymphopenia, and eosinopenia probably result from adrenocortical response to stress.

Haemobartonellosis (17)

1. A severe anemia develops with reduction in the total erythrocyte count, in hemoglobin, and in PCV.
2. The total leukocyte count will vary from normal to subnormal during the period when parasites can be demonstrated.
   a. The leukopenia appears to be associated with all cell types.
3. Parasitized erythrocytes contain long rods, chains of coccoid forms, and violin-bow forms but are not demonstrable once treatment has been initiated.

Heartworms (60)

1. Leukocytosis and eosinophilia are seen.

Hepatitis, infectious canine (ICH) (12, 13, 40, 72, 116, 184, 186)

1. A brief prefebrile leukocytosis precedes the leukopenia, which is characterized by a rapid decline in total leukocytes from the 3rd to the 5th postinoculation day.
   a. The average total leukocyte count is under 7000/microliter, with some reports that the leukopenia is usually about 2000.
   b. The reduction in the number of neutrophils is most marked, but other cell types are also depressed. Eosinophils disappear from the blood entirely at the point of maximum leukopenia.
2. During the period of recovery, usually after the 6th day, a leukocytosis develops, which is associated with a lymphocytosis and a marked increase in immature lymphocytes.
   a. The leukocytosis lasts 2 to 3 days.
3. The PCV may show a definite trend downward throughout the course of the disease, or it may be variable.
4. Thrombocytes are markedly reduced in number, but the prolonged coagulation time is more likely to be due to a prothrombin deficiency produced by the damaged liver or to disseminated intravascular coagulation.

Histoplasmosis (19)

1. There is a leukocytosis with an increase in immature neutrophils.
2. Anemia

Hydronephrosis (144)

1. When the kidney has a secondary bacterial infection, a leukocytosis may be detected.

Hyperadrenocorticism

1. Leukocytosis results from the release of cells from the bone marrow.
2. The differential leukocyte picture is characterized by a lymphopenia, eosinopenia, neutrophilia, and monocytosis.

Hypertrophic osteodystrophy (122)
1. During the febrile state, a leukocytosis with a shift to the left occurs.
2. A slight anemia may be seen in some cases.

Hypothermia (195)
1. In dogs cooled below 20°C, the total erythrocyte count and hemoglobin and PCV levels will increase. Leukocytes of all types nearly disappear, and thrombocytes disappear.
2. A slight anemia may be seen in some cases.

Lead poisoning (26, 211)
1. Lead poisoning produces a defect in erythrocyte maturation, and the striking finding is the absence of polychromasia and reticulocytes in the presence of numerous nucleated erythrocytes. There are numerous nucleated erythrocytes and erythrocytes with basophilic stippling in the absence of a severe anemia.

Leptospirosis (22, 126, 144)
1. Leukocytosis with a marked shift to the left is characteristic of the acute form, with the total leukocyte count as high as 35,000/microliter after the 5th day of infection. Leukocytosis may be absent in some subclinical cases, and occasionally a transient leukopenia may be seen early in the course of the disease at the time of febrile response.
2. In some cases, a decrease in hemoglobin of 1 to 2 g/dl and a commensurate PCV decrease are suggestive of hemolysis. The icterus in the hematocrit tube, however, is due to hepatocellular damage. Because of hemoconcentration, there may be an increase in the total erythrocyte count, hemoglobin, and PCV.

Metritis (hyperplastic endometritis) (98, 128)
1. The total leukocyte count is seldom over 25,000/microliter and is usually normal to moderately elevated. The elevation is due to a neutrophilic shift to the left.

Myositis, atrophic (202)
1. There is no eosinophilia.

Myositis, eosinophilic (202)
1. An eosinophilia is frequently but not invariably seen.

Nephritis, chronic interstitial (144, 171)
1. The total leukocyte count is generally above the mean normal value (20,000 to 30,000/microliter).
2. The differential picture is typical of the response to stress, with mature neutrophilia, lymphopenia, eosinopenia, and monocytes generally within upper normal limits.
3. When the chronic renal disease is progressive and irreversible, a nonregenerative anemia will develop that is normocytic normochromic.

Nephrosis (ischemic and chemical) (144)
1. When acute, a nonregenerative anemia does not develop.

Panosteitis (25)
1. Eosinophilia is an inconstant finding.

Parasitism, hookworms (24, 166)
1. A microcytic hypochromic anemia is produced.
2. When leukocytosis develops, it consists mostly of mature neutrophils.
3. Eosinophilia is variable and occurs after new infections or at the time parasites reach maturity.

Pneumonia (59)
1. Mild
   a. Slight anemia
   b. Marked leukocytosis with an absolute and relative neutrophilia
   c. Marked eosinopenia and lymphopenia
2. Severe
   a. Severe anemia
   b. Marked leukopenia with a relative neutrophilia and shift to the left
   c. Marked decrease in eosinophils and lymphocytes

Polycythemia vera (53)
1. There is an absolute increase in the number of erythrocytes, as well as increased hemoglobin and PCV values.

Pregnancy
1. An anemia develops between 7 and 9 wk after estrus and is probably of a normocytic normochromic type.

Primidone
1. Has been reported to cause a marked leukopenia and neutropenia after long-term treatment.

Prostatic abscess (149)
1. Leukocytosis

Pyelonephritis (144)
1. Leukocytosis will occur if a large quantity of renal tissue is actively infected, but it will not occur if only a small portion of renal parenchyma is involved.

Pyometra (21, 79, 98, 109, 144)
1. There is usually a marked leukocytosis (20,000 to 100,000 or more), with the average total leukocyte count being 50,000/microliter or over.
2. There is a marked neutrophilic shift to the left.
   a. The immature neutrophils often have a light blue staining cytoplasm with toxic granulation and may contain Döhle bodies.
3. The PCV is usually within normal limits, but occasionally there may be a nonregenerative anemia or a hemoconcentration.

Rabies (31)
1. The number of leukocytes increases on the appearance of clinical signs, reaching 15,000 to 19,000/microliter, and declines somewhat on the day of death.
2. Neutrophils exceed 90% from the time of appearance of clinical signs to death.

Renal cortical hypoplasia (144)
1. Profound nonregenerative anemia may occur in later stages.
2. The leukocytes are often affected by a stress response, producing a neutrophilic leukocytosis, lymphopenia, and eosinopenia.

Reserpine (2)
1. The PCV, total leukocyte count, and hemoglobin are less than normal, possibly due to a cytotoxic effect upon hematopoietic components.

Salmon disease (44)
1. The total erythrocyte count is normal or high normal due to hemoconcentration.
2. The total number of leukocytes varies from 15,000 to 28,000/microliter with a neutrophilic shift to the left.
   a. No eosinophils are present, and an absolute lymphopenia may occur.

Systemic lupus erythematosus (SLE) (144)
1. A regenerative hemolytic anemia is characterized by marked reticulocytosis, nucleated erythrocytes, and spherocytosis.
2. Thrombocytopenia is common.
3. Positive Coombs' test and LE cell demonstration are necessary to confirm.

Tetanus
1. There is a shift from an initial leukopenia to a moderate leukocytosis and a gradual return to the normal range.

Thallium poisoning (210)
1. There is commonly a leukocytosis due to neutrophilia, a shift to the left, lymphopenia, and eosinopenia.
2. Hemoconcentration is found in about half the cases prior to the administration of fluids.
3. Basophilic stippling is not seen in the erythrocytes, and anemia is uncommon.

Tracheobronchitis (kennel cough) (161)
1. A leukocytosis ranging from 16,000 to 26,000/microliter is usually seen.

Tranquilizers (42, 181)
1. The PCV is consistently reduced.
2. Total leukocyte counts are decreased by all the tranquilizers except chlorpromazine given intramuscularly.

Urinary tract infection (cystitis) (30, 131)
1. Erythrocyte counts are normal.
2. There may be a moderate leukocytosis with a slight shift to the left.

Vitamin B_6 deficiency (27)
1. Microcytic hypochromic anemia is seen.

II. CAT

Aspirin intoxication
1. Suppression of the erythropoietic centers can occur with long-term (35 days) doses of 5 g daily.

Chloramphenicol toxicity (171)
1. A marked decrease in the percentage of rubricytes, with vacuolization of the cytoplasm; occasional vacuolization of the nuclei of numerous early cells of the myeloid and erythroid cell series have been reported in the bone marrow. It is possible that cats already having some form of hematopoietic depression might be more susceptible to the toxic effects of chloramphenicol than normal cats. Aplastic anemia as reported in man has not been reported in cats.

Feline infectious anemia (haemobartonellosis) (66, 89)
1. Total erythrocyte counts, PCV, and hemoglobin levels are low.
2. A moderate leukocytosis is usually seen.
3. Parasitized erythrocytes contain coccal, ring, or rod forms of *Haemobartonella felis*.

Feline infectious peritonitis (FIP)
1. The total leukocyte count can range from a leukopenia to a marked leukocytosis (1700 to 52,000/microliter with a median around 13,000.
2. Generally there is a neutrophilia with a mild shift to the left. A marked lymphopenia is characteristic as well as an eosinopenia. Monocytes are in the normal range.
3. Anemia is present in 40% of the cases as a result of bone marrow depression, with the cell type being normocytic normochromic.

Feline panleukopenia (feline enteritis) (9, 18, 93, 104, 140)
1. A marked leukopenia (<8000) is seen, with an average total leukocyte count at the height of the disease reported as 1350 or 2000/microliter.
2. The leukopenia is due to a panleukopenia with a reduction of all cell types.

Griseofulvin intoxication
1. Occasionally cats, especially kittens, can develop a leukopenia (3000/microliter) and an anemia after 3 wk of treatment.

Respiratory disease complex
1. Feline picornavirus infection (FPI)
   a. An initial leukopenia will return to the normal or high normal range unless a leukocytosis is caused by secondary bacterial infection.
2. Feline pneumonitis (*Chlamydia*) (93, 115, 140)
   a. A normal to slightly increased total leukocyte count is seen.
3. Feline viral rhinotracheitis (FVR, herpes virus)
   a. The total leukocyte count is raised from 30,000 to 50,000/microliter.
4. Reovirus
   a. The total leukocyte count is normal.

Steatitis (yellow fat) (133)
1. A leukocytosis with a neutrophilia; varying degrees of eosinophilia may be seen.

Streptococcal infection
1. A neutrophilic leukocytosis is observed.

Thallium poisoning
1. Acute
   a. Leukopenia and anemia are typical of illnesses of short duration.
2. Chronic
   a. Longer illnesses are usually accompanied by a neutrophilic leukocytosis, a shift to the left, and moderate anemia.

Toxoplasmosis
1. Acute
   a. There is often a leukopenia, absolute neutropenia, absolute lymphopenia, and a marked degenerative shift to the left.
   b. Mild anemia
2. Chronic
   a. Anemia

Urethral obstruction

1. Hematologic values vary little from normal values.

III. HORSE

ACTH (6)

1. ACTH in adequate dosage will produce an eosinopenia.

Adenoviral infection in foals (113, 114)

1. A severe absolute lymphopenia is a consistent finding in adenovirus-infected foals. The finding of near normal numbers of lymphocytes in convalescent foals suggests that resistance is associated with lymphocytes.
2. In addition to lymphopenia, an irregular but progressive decrease in the number of neutrophils produces a progressively declining total leukocyte count.

Adrenalin (3)

1. Adrenalin in doses adequate to produce hyperglycemia will not cause an eosinopenia.

Arthritis, septic (joint-ill) in foals (193)

1. There is an increase above normal in relative numbers of segmented and nonsegmented neutrophils.

Butazolidin

1. After 3 wk of continuous treatment a slightly subnormal leukocyte count develops, which returns to the normal range in another 2 wk of continuous treatment.
2. Differential leukocyte counts show no significant deviations from normal.

Colitis ''X'' (162)

1. There is a marked leukopenia (less than 3000 to 4000/microliter).
2. Hemoconcentration

Contagious bronchopneumonia (199)

1. A neutrophilic leukocytosis is seen, with the degree of neutrophilia depending upon the severity of the infection.
2. An eosinopenia is typical.
3. There is no change in the erythrocyte picture.

Corticosteroids (6, 168)

1. Eosinopenia

Endotoxemia (*Aerobacter aerogenes*) (36)

1. There is a leukopenia followed by a leukocytosis. There is a dramatic fall of neutrophils, monocytes, and eosinophils within an hour; and although the lymphocytes do not fall as precipitously as neutrophils, there is a reduction of 50%. At the 5th hour, there is a return of neutrophils to the peripheral blood, due in part to band forms.
2. Initially, there is a marked elevation in PCV and plasma proteins, followed by a fall between the 3rd and 6th hours, probably produced by hemodilution. After the 6th hour, hemoconcentration again produces a rise in the PCV and plasma proteins.

Endotoxemia (*Escherichia coli*) (33, 34)

1. There is an initial neutropenia attributed largely to the sequestration of these cells within the pulmonary, hepatic, and splenic blood vessels. The sequestration and destruction of granulocytes is associated with fibrin thrombi in the pulmonary circulation after administration of the endotoxin.
2. In addition to the early neutropenia, there is a lymphopenia and hemoconcentration.

Equine infectious anemia (EIA) (54)

1. There is a fluctuating decrease and increase in the total number of erythrocytes.
2. A tendency to leukopenia and, later, a general trend to a relative or absolute lymphocytosis can be noted during the disease process.

Exercise, fright, or apprehension (8, 167, 170, 187)

1. There is a physiologic leukocytosis, with lymphocytes as well as neutrophils elevated above normal and monocytes and eosinophils remaining within the normal range.
2. A large reservoir of erythrocytes can be released to the circulation within minutes following excitement or strenuous exercise. The spleen is capable of supplying an erythrocyte volume equal to about one-third of the circulating erythrocyte mass.

Fistula of the withers (43)

1. A slight leukocytosis with a neutrophilia and shift to the left is seen.

Hematinics (100)

1. There is no significant change in either PCV or hemoglobin after 8 wk of treatment with ferrous sulfate, vitamin B_{12}, iron dextran, crude liver, or copper with iron.

Hepatic insufficiency, primary (68)

1. Hemoglobin and erythrocyte values are within normal limits, while the PCV is in the high normal range, as there is slight dehydration.
2. There is a leukocytosis and a shift to the left in most cases.

Histamine (3)

1. Histamine in doses that produce clinical signs also produces an eosinopenia.

Influenza (70)

1. The total leukocyte count is usually low, although not always frankly leukopenic. The decrease is due to a lymphopenia that lasts from several hours to 3 or 4 days. The neutrophils may be stable or show a tendency to increase.
2. There may be a moderate normocytic normochromic anemia with a tendency in some cases to a microcytic hypochromic anemia.

Insulin (3)

1. Eosinopenia

Intestinal infarction (acute surgical colonic infarction) (138)

1. The rapid decline in numbers of circulating leukocytes is directly related to the appearance of increased numbers of leukocytes in the peritoneal fluid, the invasion of the peritoneal fluid by enteric bacteria, and the increased production of peritoneal fluid.
2. The increase in PCV seems to be directly related to the rate of production of peritoneal fluid and probably reflects the loss of plasma fluid to peritoneal fluid.
3. The decrease in blood thrombocyte concentrations is probably due to the sequestration of thrombocytes in the infarcted intestine and in the form of microemboli scattered throughout other tissues.

Leptospirosis (80, 130)

1. Usually a leukocytosis is seen, with an increase in the proportion of mature and immature neutrophils.

Parasites

1. Ascarids (7)
   a. No demonstrable effect on the peripheral blood is noted with *Parascaris equorum* infections.
2. Strongyles (7, 55)
   a. Leukocytosis is a constant reaction.
   b. Eosinophils are relatively absent or present in small numbers in the acute case, whereas in the subacute reaction the percentage of eosinophils steadily increases.
   c. A normocytic normochromic anemia may be seen due to bone marrow hypoplasia.

Poll evil (91)

1. Leukocytosis with increasing neutrophilia and shift to the left is noted.

Promazine (152)

1. There are no significant changes in hemoglobin content, erythrocyte count, or blood cell volume.
2. There is a slight decrease in the leukocyte count with a relative increase in lymphocytes and a decrease in neutrophils.

Purpura hemorrhagica (91)

1. There is a well-marked leukocytosis due to neutrophilia.
2. Anemia is of the normocytic normochromic type.
3. The thrombocytes are usually reported to be normal in number.

Quittor (43)

1. A normal to slightly elevated total leukocyte count with a neutrophilic shift to the left may be seen.

Strangles (31, 91)

1. A leukocytosis with a marked shift to the left and neutrophilia are described.
2. Anemia is usually normocytic and may be due to streptococcal hemolysins or to bone marrow depression.

Tetanus (31)

1. A leukocytosis is present, but hemoglobin and erythrocytes are normal.

Viral arteritis (95)

1. Leukopenia is a constant finding, usually evident by the 2nd day after exposure and persisting up to 13 days.
2. Lymphopenia is more severe than neutropenia.

IV. CATTLE

Abomasal impaction (94)
1. The total leukocyte count and differential count may be normal or may reflect traumatic peritonitis or shock. (84)

Abomasum, left displacement (159)
1. Total and differential leukocyte counts, PCV, and hemoglobin usually lie within normal limits.

Abomasal lymphosarcoma (94)
1. The total leukocyte count may be normal or elevated.
2. The presence of an increased number of immature and abnormal lymphocytes has been reported to be pathognomonic.

Abomasal ulceration (94)
1. Anemia

ACTH (4, 83)
1. ACTH in adequate dosage will produce an eosinopenia within 2 to 4 hr.
   a. In the presence of normal adrenal glands, circulating eosinophils will decrease by 66 to 93% within 10 hr.

Adrenalin (4)
1. Adrenalin in doses of 5 mg/kg injected subcutaneously will not produce a significant eosinopenia. Occasionally (1 cow in 6), an eosinopenia is produced by 10 mg/kg.

Anaplasmosis (38)
1. At the time the disease is first clinically apparent, the total erythrocyte count will be approximately 4 million/microliter but will soon drop below 2 million/microliter in severe infections.
2. PCV and hemoglobin values will be reduced.
3. A leukocytosis and increase in immature forms is generally seen.

Aspergillosis (35)
1. A marked leukopenia and relative lymphocytosis is noted.

Bacillary hemoglobinuria (154)
1. Anemia is reflected by a low total erythrocyte count and hemoglobin level.
   a. At the time when the characteristic hemoglobinuria is first observed, from 30 to 50% of the erythrocytes may have been hemolyzed.
2. There may be a wide variation in the total leukocyte count, but in the majority of cases it will range from 10,000 to 16,000/microliter.

Bovine virus diarrhea (BVD) (151, 153, 207)
1. A leukopenia, with a total leukocyte count around 3000 and as low as 1500/microliter, occurs early in the course of infection prior to the onset of clinical signs and the febrile period. With the onset of clinical sign a leukocytosis may be present, followed by a severe leukopenia in some cases, so that a diphasic pattern may occur.
2. A relative lymphocytosis generally occurs following the febrile period.
3. The total erythrocyte count is essentially normal in the initial stages but may be 12 to 15 million/microlite near death.

Bracken poisoning (71)
1. A leukopenia with a reduction of segmented neutrophils is seen.
2. There is a reduction of thrombocytes.
3. In later stages there is a reduction in the total erythrocyte count.

Brisket (high mountain) disease (20, 165, 203)
1. The total erythrocyte count is variable and may be high, normal, or low.
2. Hemoglobin values are usually normal to elevated but occasionally are reduced.
3. Variations in the total leukocyte counts are seen, but they are usually high.
   a. High total leukocyte counts coinciding with temperature elevations are believed to indicate secondary infections.

4. Neutrophilia, eosinopenia, and lymphopenia are usually reported, but occasionally lymphocytosis and eosinophilia are seen.

Brucella vaccination (76)

1. By the 5th day following vaccination, when the serum agglutinins are becoming apparent, the total erythocyte count and hemoglobin content show significantly reduced values. This downward trend continues until the 12th day, then increases to normal by the 26th day.
2. There is a close correlation between the total leukocyte count and agglutinins. A gradual increase in the total leukocyte count occurs as agglutinins appear, and the count declines as agglutinins decline.
3. The increase in the total leukocyte count is due to a rise in neutrophils, but only an occasional animal will have an increase in band forms. The percentage of lymphocytes is inversely proportional to the number of neutrophils. The number of monocytes increases.

Brucellosis (15, 63)

1. A reduction in the total number of erythrocytes occurs following infection.
2. There is a significant drop in the total number of leukocytes per microliter.
3. Of the differential types, the mean percentages of neutrophils, monocytes, and basophils increase, while those of the lymphocytes and eosinophils decrease.

Cassia occidentalis (coffee senna) toxicosis (123)

1. There are no marked alterations in hematologic findings until the last 12 hr prior to death when hemoconcentration due to severe diarrhea produces an elevated PCV and hemoglobin concentration.

Corticosteroids (74, 171)

1. Administration of hydrocortisone analogs produces varying degrees of leukocytosis and neutrophilia.
2. 9 alpha-fluoroprednisolone produces leukocytosis, neutrophilia, monocytosis, eosinopenia, and lymphopenia, with a threefold to sixfold increase in mature neutrophils usually indicating a large pool of reserve neutrophils.
3. A mild eosinopenia is produced by synthetic corticosteroids.

Diarrhea, neonatal (48)

1. Changes in the PCV occur infrequently. In spite of the dehydration, it is possible that the plasma volume is maintained or that the erythrocytes are either destroyed as part of the catabolic response to diarrhea or moved out of the general circulation.

''Drying off' of lactation (171)

1. There is a leukocytosis with a definite increase in eosinophils.

Emphysema, pulmonary (132)

1. The blood and bone marrow findings are normal.

Indigestion, acute (85)

1. There is no leukocytosis, but in slightly over half the cases there will be a shift to the left with 6% or more nonsegmented neutrophils or the presence of an excess of neutrophils over lymphocytes, or both.

Indigestion, acute, with toxemia (173)

1. There is usually a leukocytosis produced by flushing of all available leukocyte types into the general circulation due to the increased heart rate (physiologic leukocytosis) and the effect of stress. With little cause for diapedesis, the neutrophils remain in the blood producing a significant neutrophilia and leukocytosis.
2. The degree of shift to the left is variable with half the cases having metamyelocytes released during the extreme stress conditions. The increased circulation of blood and lymph possibly maintains the lymphocyte, eosinophil, and basophil numbers at greater levels than would be anticipated with release of the corticosteroids of stress.

Infectious bovine rhinotracheitis (IBR)

1. There are conflicting reports, ranging from a leukopenia (156) to no change in the blood picture (73, 163) to a leukocytosis (191).

Insulin (4)

1. In doses of 1.25 units/kg, insulin has an inconsistent effect on the eosinophils.

Iron supplement for calves

1. Calves receiving an iron supplement, either orally or intramuscularly, will have a significant increase in hemoglobin levels and PCV values as compared to calves receiving no iron.

Johne's disease (5, 124, 157)

1. No definite changes in the total erythrocyte count, total leukocyte count, or hemoglobin level are seen.

2. A variable degree of neutrophilia and lymphopenia is observed, while a significant eosinopenia is a feature of infection.

Lead poisoning (37, 171)

1. In some cases, anemia will develop and is of the hemolytic type, due to abnormal structure, fragility, and permeability of the erythrocytic membrane.
2. Basophilic stippling may be present and apparently is of two types: one consisting of an accumulation of iron deposits unusable for hemoglobin formation, and the second of granules, presumably damaged mitochondria.
   a. Keep in mind that basophilic stippling is commonly seen in bovine erythrocytes when there is active erythrogenesis from a number of causes.

Malignant catarrhal fever (148)

1. There is a progressive leukopenia commencing at about the same time as generalized enlargement of the lymph nodes.
2. The leukopenia affects all cell types, but there is a relative monocytosis, with the appearance of large, primitive forms.

Mastitis, acute (172, 185)

1. Shortly after the onset of clinical signs of mastitis there is a leukopenia due to a depression of neutrophils and lymphocytes. Within a few hours or days, the total leukocyte count increases (but not to the point of leukocytosis) as a result of increased numbers of neutrophils, many of which are immature.
2. With the disappearance of clinical signs the leukocyte picture returns to normal.

Nitrate or nitrite long-term feeding (204)

1. Total hemoglobin and erythrocyte concentrations increase in proportion to blood methemoglobin levels.

Parasitism

1. Ascarids (77)
   a. Hemoglobin and PCV values remain within normal limits.
   b. A leukocytosis often follows infection and frequently parallels changes in eosinophil counts.
   c. Continual infection with *Ascaris suum* eggs results in circulating eosinophil levels that fluctuate and are dose dependent.
2. Coccidiosis (65)
   a. Hemoglobin and PCV values are lowered in severely affected calves that have hemorrhaged into the intestinal tract.
3. Hookworms and nodular worms (51)
   a. Anemia
   b. Neutrophilic leukocytosis
4. Lungworms (*Dictyocaulus viviparus*) (160, 164, 197)
   a. Marked eosinophilia develops.
   b. No significant reduction in the PCV is produced.
5. Stomach worms (*Ostertagia ostertagi*) (117)
   a. Little alteration occurs in the hemoglobin, PCV, or total leukocyte values.
   b. Occasionally an eosinophilia is produced.

Parturition (62, 129, 183)

1. At parturition, the total leukocyte count is increased, due mainly to an increase in neutrophils, but lymphocytes and monocytes are also increased. Eosinophils are depressed.
2. The total leukocyte count may fall or continue to be increased by the first day after calving. The decline in total leukocytes is due to a reduction in both neutrophils and lymphocytes.
3. The erythrocytes show a slight decrease in the latter half of gestation, with a marked decrease noted 36 hr after parturition and then a rapid return to the normal picture.

Porphyrinuria, congenital (174, 196)

1. Cattle with high levels of uroporphyrin may have a hemolytic anemia, even in the absence of sunlight exposure. The anemia has been classified as macrocytic normochromic. A marked anisocytosis, metarubricytes, and basophilic stippling are present.
2. Hemoglobin is consistently low.
3. There is a leukocytosis, with a neutrophilia and a shift to the left commensurate with the infected skin lesions. Percentages of monocytoid lymphocytes and eosinophils are increased when the skin lesions are present.

Pregnancy (125, 171)

1. There is a slight increase in the total leukocyte count up to and including the 3rd month, after which it slowly falls. The increase is usually less than 1000/microliter. A second leukocytosis is noted during the 2 wk immediately prior to parturition.
2. The leukocytosis is mainly due to an increase in neutrophils, although the lymphocytes increase up to the 3rd month, followed by a continuous decrease throughout the rest of gestation.
3. The erythrocytes show a slight decrease in the latter half of gestation. A marked decrease is noted 36 hr after parturition, with a rapid return to the normal picture.

Psittacosis-lymphogranuloma group infection (182)

1. There is a leukopenia at the 3rd and 4th day, but a return to the original leukocyte values occurs by the 7th day in cows. However, 1-week-old calves have a leukocytosis during the 3rd and 4th days followed by a return to normal after 7 to 9 days.

Retained fetal membranes (127, 183)

1. The total leukocyte count may be normal or depressed.
2. The number of neutrophils decreases, but there is an increase in the number of immature forms. There may be a monocytosis.
3. The number of erythrocytes and hemoglobin values remain normal.

Rift Valley fever (57)

1. A leukopenia is produced.

Rinderpest (121)

1. Leukopenia is usually apparent on the day before or the day of the initial temperature rise. Within the first 2 days of fever, the total leukocyte count may drop to 4000/microliter or under. In convalescence, the total leukocyte count returns to normal about 5 wk after the last signs of illness.
2. Two or 3 days after the initial leukopenia, a marked shift to the left is seen, with the appearance of immature neutrophils.

Shipping fever (16, 87)

1. As soon as the typical signs of shipping fever are apparent, there is an increase in total erythrocytes, total leukocytes, band neutrophils, and metamyelocytes.
2. The numbers of segmented neutrophils, lymphocytes, monocytes, and eosinophils decrease.

Traumatic pericarditis (10)

1. The total leukocyte count is usually increased early in the course of the disease but later may drop rapidly.
2. A neutrophilia with a marked shift to the left is characteristic.

Traumatic reticulitis (10, 29, 39, 99, 120)

1. About half of the chronic cases will have a total leukocyte count in the normal range, but it is more likely to be elevated if complicated by other conditions.
2. A consistent finding is the appearance of immature forms of neutrophils, even though a neutrophilia is present in only two-thirds of the cases.
3. High eosinophil counts are occasionally seen in some chronic cases.

Trichloroethylene-extracted soybean oil meal poisoning (32)

1. Aplastic anemia with normocytic normochromic erythrocytes is noted, with a progressive drop in the PCV and hemoglobin reduced to 5 to 9 g/dl of blood.
2. There is a leukopenia with a neutropenia and relative lymphocytosis.
3. Thrombocytopenia completes the picture of pancytopenia.

Winter dysentery (158)

1. A leukopenia has not been seen.

V. SHEEP

Ammonia intoxication (101)

1. A slight drop occurs in the total leukocyte count.
2. Increases are produced in the total erythrocyte count, hemoglobin concentration, and PCV. There are no changes in the erythrocyte indices (MCV, MCHC, and MCH).

Bluetongue (110)

1. A leukopenia develops, the lowest counts coinciding with the height of the fever 6 to 7 days after infection.

a. The leukocyte count falls to 4000 to 5000/microliter, with a neutropenia, lymphopenia, and eosinopenia
2. The PCV drops as much as 15%.

Copper poisoning, chronic (147)
1. Hemoglobin and PCV values are low.
2. A neutrophilic leukocytosis is usually seen.

Enterotoxemia (*Clostridium perfringens* type A) (88)
1. A hemolytic anemia is present.
2. Agranulocytosis is seen.

Epinephrine (209)
1. A 2-mg dose will produce an 80% decrease in eosinophils in 6 hr.

Insulin (209)
1. 25 units of insulin will cause a 92% decrease in eosinophils by the 6th hour.

Ketosis, starvation (28)
1. A severe hemoconcentration is characterized by increased PCV and hemoglobin values.

Listeriosis (143)
1. A neutrophilic leukocytosis with a shift to the left and suppression of lymphocytes is found.

Locoweed poisoning (90)
1. Erythrocyte, leukocyte, hemoglobin, and PCV values are all within normal limits.

Mastitis, acute (155)
1. The total erythrocyte count falls during infection, but returns to normal on recovery.
2. A neutrophilic leukocytosis develops during the infection.

Muscular dystrophy (141)
1. Low total erythrocyte count and hemoglobin values are seen.

Nitrogen mustard (apholate) (208)
1. A significant leukopenia occurs, with the absolute numbers of lymphocytes and neutrophils markedly decreased. Eosinophils and monocytes are sometimes decreased.
2. No appreciable changes are found in erythrocyte numbers, hemoglobin content, or PCV.
3. Thrombocytopenia develops.

Parasitism (61, 201)

Haemonchus contortus
1. Because *H. contortus* is a bloodsucking parasite, an anemia is produced that is characterized by a marked reduction in hemoglobin concentration and PCV that is similar to that produced by periodic bleeding.

Trichostrongyloidosis (excluding *H. contortus*)
1. There is a severe anemia resulting from toxic depression of erythropoiesis, with the total erythrocyte count sometimes declining to as low as 2 or 3 million.
2. Total leukocyte counts are normal or may be elevated.

Pingue (*Hymenoxys richardsonii*) poisoning (1)
1. An increase in band neutrophils occurs, while there is a significant drop in the number of lymphocytes.
2. The PCV increases.

Pregnancy (155)
1. The total erythrocyte count and hemoglobin values show a tendency to decrease late in gestation.
2. A neutrophilic leukocytosis is seen during the last month of pregnancy.
3. A slight eosinophilia is seen throughout the period and drops rapidly at parturition.
4. Monocytes and basophils are constant.
5. The lymphocytes decrease in proportion to the increase in neutrophils.

Radiation (69)
1. Lambs that receive 30 R of total body radiation show a significant decrease in total leukocytes and lymphocytes.
2. No significant changes occur in neutrophilic, PCV, and hemoglobin values.

Rift Valley fever (58)
1. There is a leukopenia of short duration that tends to be more severe in young lambs than in adult sheep. The lowest leukocyte counts are evident when there is the maximum amount of fever and virus in the blood.
2. Changes are not detectable in the PCV.

VI. PIG

ACTH and adrenocortical extract (112)

1. A marked increase in the total leukocyte count, with a lymphopenia and neutrophilia, is seen within 2 hr following administration of adrenocorticotropic hormone and adrenocortical extract.

African swine fever (52)

1. There is a leukopenia associated with a significant increase in the percentage of neutrophils, especially the juvenile forms, and a decrease in the percentage of lymphocytes.
2. The total erythrocyte count; hemoglobin value; PCV; and percentages of eosinophils, basophils, and monocytes remain normal.

Agalactia, postpartum (135, 136)

1. Circulating eosinophils tend to be depleted, indicating that the postpartum agalactia is associated with an increase in adrenocortical function.
2. A transient decrease in total leukocyte counts and segmented and nonsegmented neutrophils occurs at 1 to 24 hr after parturition.

Atrophic rhinitis (78)

1. There is no change in the total erythrocyte, total leukocyte, or differential counts.

Aujeszky's disease (179)

1. The total leukocyte count is usually well below 10,000/microliter.

Clay pigeon target (coal tar) poisoning (49, 97)

1. 24 to 48 hours before death, there is a marked decrease in hemoglobin and PCV.
2. Values for total leukocyte and differential cell counts remain within normal limits.

Copper deficiency (200)

1. A leukopenia is usually present.
2. A microcytic hypochromic anemia develops.

Endotoxicosis (*Escherichia coli*) (50, 134)

1. There is a marked leukopenia noted within minutes, followed in 24 hr by an increase above normal levels in the number of leukocytes and in the percentage of band and metamyelocyte cells.

Esophagogastric ulcers (47)

1. Progressive microcytic anemia after a transient hemoconcentration is a characteristic hematologic pattern. As the anemia progresses, hemoglobin values as low as 3.3 g/dl, total erythrocyte counts as low as 1,580,000/microliter, and PCV as low as 12% are observed.
2. Lymphocytosis and neutropenia are often observed in chronic cases.

Ethylene glycol poisoning (145)

1. A neutrophilic leukocytosis and a marked increase in band neutrophils develops along with an eosinopenia.

Exercise

1. The total leukocyte count increases with an increase in neutrophils.

Folic acid deficiency (206)

1. A severe macrocytic anemia develops.
2. Leukopenia
3. Some thrombocytopenia

Gestation and lactation (189)

1. The PCV and hemoglobin concentration decrease during both gestation and lactation.

Hog cholera (swine fever) (56, 41, 106, 179, 188, 190)

1. The total leukocyte count will fall below 9000/microliter within 2 to 6 days after exposure.
   a. The count may be less than 4000, but commonly does not fall below 5000/microliter.
   b. Usually a total leukocyte count of 9000 or less in pigs 8 wk of age or older is considered diagnostic of hog cholera.

Iron deficiency (200)

1. Hemoglobin levels decrease as low as 2 to 3 g in 3 to 4 wk, and the anemia is a microcytic hypochromic type.

Lead toxicosis (107)

1. The effect on the number of circulating erythrocytes and the hemoglobin is not pronounced. The greater decrease of hemoglobin than erythrocytes suggests that the toxic action of lead affects synthesis of pyrrole groups essential for hemoglobin production.

2. Basophilic stippling of erythrocytes is observed only after the pigs become moribund.

Leptospirosis (64)

1. A neutrophilic leukocytosis develops between the 4th to 8th days after exposure.
2. Many of the neutrophils are immature forms.

Listeriosis (175)

1. An increased number of monocytes are present.

Lysine deficiency (11)

1. A normocytic normochromic anemia develops.

Moldy corn poisoning (180)

1. In acute cases, large hemorrhages result in anemia.
2. In chronic cases, anemia may be due to hemolysis.

Parasitism

Ascarids (198)

1. Eosinophil counts increase by the 4th day postinfection and continue to increase until the 12th to the 16th day, after which the counts decrease to preinfective levels by the 20th to the 28th day.
2. A mild anemia develops that is noticeable 32 days after infection.

Trichuris (150)

1. Anemia develops from the hemorrhagic enteritis and the bloodsucking habits of the parasites.

Parturition (111)

1. At parturition there is a well-marked lymphopenia and neutrophilia.
   a. The blood cell reaction is usually apparent 6 to 30 hr before parturition, but in exceptional cases it may be evident as early as 9 days before farrowing or may be delayed until after farrowing has started.

Pasteurellosis (96)

1. Total leukocyte counts of 20,000/microliter or more are usually found.

Pneumonia and/or influenza (179)

1. A slight leukopenia is noted in influenza, but not nearly to the same degree as seen with hog cholera.
2. Most cases of pneumonia show leukocyte counts of 15,000/microliter or above.

Protein deficiency (200)

1. Anemia
2. Leukopenia and decrease in lymphocytes are seen.

Pyridoxine (vitamin B_6) deficiency (200)

1. A severe microcytic hypochromic anemia is seen.

Riboflavin (vitamin B_2) deficiency (200)

1. Normocytic anemia

Rift Valley fever (57)

1. A leukopenia is seen.

Rinderpest (81)

1. The leukopenia that develops is due to the neutrophils and lymphocytes being decreased in relatively the same proportion. There is no shift to the left. The remainder of the hematologic values show no significant changes.

Salmonellosis (106, 179)

1. The average total leukocyte count is 30,000/microliter with a range from 16,000 to 56,000/microliter.

Salt poisoning (45)

1. PCV and total leukocyte counts remain essentially normal.

Septicemia, streptococcal (14)

1. The total leukocyte counts are 20,000/microliter or more.

Swine erysipelas (177, 179)

1. The total leukocyte count is above 15,000/microliter producing a mononuclear leukocytosis with a neutropenia.

Transmissible gastroenteritis (105)

1. For most pigs the total leukocyte count is within normal limits, but in some a leukopenia of moderate degree develops during the febrile period. During recovery there tends to be a leukocytosis.

Vitamin E deficiency (137, 200)

1. The total leukocyte count is increased, and the number of neutrophils is increased at the expense of the lymphocytes.
2. Low hemoglobin and PCV values are exhibited, while the mean corpuscular hemoglobin concentration is within normal limits.

Yellow fat disease (108)

1. There is a hypochromic anemia.

11 PROTEIN

I. General considerations

A. Protein production

1. The liver produces all the albumin and most of the globulins; a small amount of gamma globulin is produced by reticuloendothelial tissue.
   a. The production of albumin is subject to a mechanism regulating colloidal osmotic pressure and is secondary to alterations in globulin concentration. (3)
2. The liver synthesizes lipoproteins; glycoproteins; mucoproteins; fibrinogen; prothrombin; and clotting factors VII, VIII, IX, and X.

B. Abnormalities in plasma proteins are not indicative of a specific disease but of a condition that alters the tissues responsible for the balance between protein synthesis and catabolism or mechanical loss. (13)

1. Many diseases and conditions produce similar alterations in plasma protein fractions, but changes can be of diagnostic value in demonstrating that a pathological process is occurring and may contribute to a diagnosis, especially when they are related to history, clinical signs, laboratory tests, and other test results. (13)

C. For interpretation of the total plasma protein concentration, it may be necessary to know the amounts of albumin and/or globulin as well, since a decrease in one fraction may be masked by an increase in the other.

D. Progressive alterations in plasma proteins by analysis of serial samples usually provide more worthwhile information than individual blood samples, but this may not always be practical. (13)

II. Methods of analysis

A. Total serum or plasma protein

1. Goldberg refractometer (TS Meter, American Optical, or Japanese models)
   a. Hold the instrument in a horizontal position.
   b. Loading procedures
      (1) With the cover plate in position on the measuring prism, place a drop of serum or plasma on the exposed portion as close to the plate as possible so that the liquid will be drawn into the space between the prisms by capillary action.
      (2) An alternate procedure is to swing the cover plate over the body of the instrument to expose both the prism and the cover plate and place the serum sample on the measuring prism. Close the cover plate over the measuring prism without delay to reduce evaporation.
   c. To hold the instrument for reading, press the plastic cover gently but firmly to spread a minimal volume of sample into a thin, even layer over the prism. Expose it to a bright light.
   d. Obtain the optimum contrast between the light and dark boundary by having the instrument properly tilted with respect to the light source.
   e. Bring the scale seen in the eyepiece into sharp focus by rotation of the eyepiece.
   f. Make the reading on the appropriate scale at the point where the dividing line between bright and dark fields crosses the scale.
   g. It may be necessary to use a conversion table to obtain serum or plasma protein in g/dl if the model of refractometer does not have a direct reading for serum protein.

(1) Various scales are available on different models, but the most useful clinical combination is the one that reads total serum protein in grams and reads urine specific gravity directly.
(2) Other scales (such as refractive index or total solids) can usually have the results converted to total protein by means of a conversion chart.

h. This method is simple and quick and compares favorably with the biuret chemical method.

i. Limitations to reliable results
(1) Cloudy serum, lipemic serum, or serum with free hemoglobin will increase the refractive index to give an erroneously high value. (40)
(a) Increased amounts of bilirubin in the serum will not increase the reading. (40)
(2) With a refractometer not compensated for temperature:
(a) Serum samples read shortly after removal from low temperatures, such as the refrigerator, will give inaccurate results. Simply allow the serum to warm to room temperature to correct this problem, or use a temperature correction chart.
(b) Heat from the hand holding the refractometer for a prolonged period, while reading a number of samples, can alter the reading. Place the refractometer on the table and allow it to cool at brief intervals, and this problem will not occur.
(3) With some species there may be a difference in reading a fresh sample and the same sample after several hours have elapsed. It is also important to cap the tube to avoid evaporation, for this will surely increase the reading.
(4) Avoid Bromsulphalein (BSP) dye. (2)

2. Biuret method—colorimetric
3. Copper sulfate specific gravity method (1)
a. A graded series of copper sulfate solutions of known specific gravity is prepared. Accurate preparation is critical.
b. From approximately 1 cm, a small drop of serum or whole blood is allowed to drop into each of the solutions where it immediately becomes encapsulated in copper proteinate.
c. In 15 to 20 sec the mass rises or sinks in the copper sulfate solution unless it is the same specific gravity. Each dilution has a different specific gravity that indicates the amount of protein in grams for the blood that is tested.
d. The error is reported to be less than ± 0.2 g.

B. Serum protein fractions
1. Chemical—for measurement of albumin
a. Salt separation
b. HABA dye binding—2-(4′-hydroxyazobenzene)-benzoic acid
(1) Used in many automated clinical chemistry instruments, such as the SMA/12 (Technicon) and blood analyzer systems (such as the Ames/BMI).
(2) It consistently produces lower albumin values than the chemical or electrophoretic methods since sera of different species have different dye-binding activities.
c. Bromcresol green—produces better results than HABA dye
2. Seroflocculation or turbidity tests
a. Normally, albumin inhibits the precipitation of globulins by one of a variety of reagents available in the various tests; but with a low albumin or increased globulin concentration (low A/G ratio) precipitation occurs.
b. Examples of these tests and their reagents

Test	Reagent
Cephalin-cholesterol	Cephalin-cholesterol
Thymol turbidity	Thymol
Takata-Ara	Mercuric chloride
Formol-gel	Formaldehyde
Zinc sulfate	Zinc sulfate

c. Usually unreliable in animals since the tests are standardized to the human A/G ratio, which is not the same as in animals, so false-positive reactions can occur. (9)

d. Since immunoglobulins appear in the serum of newborn animals only after they have received colostrum, the use of a turbidity test is reported to be reliable for detection if colostrum has been given.
   (1) In calves, 36% sodium sulfite will detect immunoglobulins 2 to 19 hours after nursing. (44)
   (2) The estimation of immunoglobulins in neonatal calf serum can be determined with the zinc sulfate turbidity test. (30)

3. Electrophoresis (2)
   a. Paper or cellulose acetate electrophoresis allows fractionation and semiquantitation of proteins into 5 components, while with immunoelectrophoresis 30 or more components of serum protein can be separated.
      (1) Albumin
      (2) Alpha-1 globulin
         (a) Lipoprotein
         (b) Antitrypsin
         (c) Glycoprotein
         (d) GC-1-globulin
      (3) Alpha-2 globulin
         (a) Lipoprotein
         (b) Macroglobulin
         (c) Haptoglobin
         (d) Ceruloplasmin
      (4) Beta globulin
         (a) Lipoprotein
         (b) Transferrin
         (c) Hemopexin
         (d) 1-C-globulin
      (5) Gamma globulin
   b. Limitations
      (1) Only when the qualitative pattern is normal is there a valid quantitation of protein fractions in grams per deciliter of blood. With abnormal proteins or alterations in the albumin or globulin concentrations, quantitation is misleading due to alterations in the staining properties of individual abnormal or normal protein fractions.
      (2) Protein fractions expressed as percentages are useless unless the total serum protein value is also known.

4. Immunoglobulins—found in both the beta and gamma fractions
   a. Types
      (1) IgG
      (2) IgA
      (3) IgM
      (4) IgD
      (5) IgE
   b. Abnormalities
      (1) Deficiency
      (2) Increased levels
         (a) Polyclonal—broad band of diffuse hyperglobulinemia
            [1] Immune system is persistently stimulated due to protracted infection
         (b) Monoclonal—spikelike electrophoretic pattern
            [1] Composed of a paraprotein (M component), which is the product of a single clone of cells
            [2] Examples—multiple myeloma, lymphosarcoma, macroglobulinemia, L-chain disease

III. Interpretation

A. Normal values

Species	No.	Age	Total serum protein (g/dl)	Albumin g/dl	Albumin %	Reference
Dog		Birth	4.08			(38)
		2 days	4.18			(38)
		1 wk	3.32			(38)
		6-7 wk	4.9-5.6 (5.2)			(43)
		8-9 wk	5.0-7.0 (5.6)			(43)
		10-12 wk	5.5-6.5 (6.2)			(43)
		4-6 mo	6.3-7.0 (6.7)			(43)
		1-1½ yr	6.5-7.7 (7.1)			(43)
		2-3½ yr	6.9-7.8 (7.5)			(43)
		<1 yr	6-6.5			(23)
		Mature	6.8-7.2			(23)
		Advancing age	7.0-7.5			(23)
	15	2-7 yr	6.64		53.8	(21)
		Adult	5.3-7.3 (6.3)	3.1-4.0 (3.56)		(27)
	20	Adult	6.3 ± 0.4	3.36 ± 0.33	53.5	(4)
Cat			6-7.5			(39)
			6.9	2.7-3.2 (3.0)		(33)
Horse		Adult	6-8			(39)
	70	Adult	7.3		33.5	(21)
	30		7.1 ± 0.38	3.1 ± 0.34		(22)
	10	Adult	7.29	2.87 ± 0.49	39.6	(18)
Cattle		Newborn	4.0-5.3 (4.7)			(43)
		2-7 days	4.7-5.3 (4.9)			(43)
		1-24 days	5-7.6 (6.1)			(24)
	15	Newborn	4.2-5.3 (4.9)			(10)
	9	22 days	5.5-7.0 (6.5)			(10)
		½-12 mo	7.9			(47)
		15-30 mo	6.97 ± 0.53	3.20		(6)
		>2 yr	7.16		43.1	(21)
		Adult	7.85		42	(8)
		Adult	9.20	3.39		(35)
		Adult	6.1-8.1 (7.11)	2.7-3.9 (3.31)		(36)
		5-9 yr	7.56 ± 0.5	3.44		(37)
		Adult	6-8			(39)

A. Normal values (*continued*)

Species	No.	Age	Total serum protein (g/dl)	Albumin g/dl	Albumin %	Reference
Sheep	10	2-3 mo	5.46		56.8	(21)
	27	122 days	5.81 ± 0.54	2.96		(26)
		Adult	5.83		14	(8)
			6-7.5			(39)
Goat	10	3-6 mo	5.7		63	(21)
		Adult	6-7.5			(39)
	15	7-9 mo	6.25 ± 0.35	3.95 ± 0.26		(16)
Pig		Birth	2.22			(39)
	47	Birth	2.22		16.7	(31)
	17	Birth	2.3-4.2 (2.98)	0.39-0.94 (0.59)		(46)
	26	6 hr	3.67		9.5	(31)
	18	12 hr	5.67		8.0	(31)
	36	24 hr	5.20		8.9	(31)
	40	1 wk	4.8-8.0 (6.31)	0.90-2.37 (1.81)		(46)
	47	1 wk	5.07		15.0	(31)
		1-5 wk	4.75			(39)
	34	2 wk	4.78		44.3	(31)
	94	3 wk	4.75		47.6	(31)
	40	8 wk	4.4-7.6 (5.66)	1.94-3.45 (2.49)		(46)
		2-3 mo	5.5			(39)
	84	9 wk	5.41		40.9	(31)
	36	3 mo	5.68		45.3	(31)
	10	3-4 mo	7.77		34.2	(21)
		4-6 mo	6.8			(39)
	79	5½-6½ mo	7.4 ± 0.6	3.4		(25)
	76	6 mo	6.80		48.6	(31)
	11	1 yr	7.51		52.7	(31)
		1 yr or over	7.5-7.97			(39)
		Adult	7.07		42	(14)
Man		Adult	6.0-8.0	4.0-5.0 (3.8)	52	(2)
Monkey (rhesus)	5		6.7 ± 0.2	3.9 ± 0.15		(17)
Rabbit	24	>4 mo	5.9		62	(21)
			7.20 ± 0.11	4.11		(20)
Guinea pig	8		5.68 ± 0.09	2.28		(20)
Rat	8		6.71 ± 0.15	1.94		(20)
Mouse	5		3.99	3.38		(15)
Chicken	15	>3 mo	4.08		35.5	(21)
Turkey	29	Adult	4.40		66.5	(29)
Duck	10	1 day	4.43 ± 0.57	2.41 ± 0.35		(32)

B. Alterations in total serum or plasma protein
 1. Increased
  a. Polycythemia
   (1) Relative polycythemia—the total plasma protein in hemoconcentration increases in proportion to the water lost
    (a) With severe dehydration, the total protein will increase to 9 g or more. (41)
    (b) Lactating cows may have plasma protein as high as 8 g and occasionally 8.5 g as a result of water loss in milk secretion and heat control (40)
    (c) When anemia is present along with dehydration, the low to normal PCV can be misleading and can mask the dehydration unless the plasma protein concentration is checked and observed to be increased. (41)
   (2) Transient polycythemia—the result of splenic contraction due to epinephrine release will increase the PCV by 20 to 25% within minutes, but the plasma protein level in the dog will be only slightly increased and will be about 0.6 g in the horse (11, 41, 43)
  b. Increased gamma globulin production
   (1) Response to antigens can increase total protein up to 8.5 g and can be differentiated from hemoconcentration by electrophoresis. (41)
    (a) Infectious and suppurative diseases
    (b) Many chronic diseases—tuberculosis in mammals (13)
   (2) Aging—generally an increase in total serum protein and globulin and a decrease in albumin concentration (13)
 2. Decreased
  a. Inadequate production
   (1) Age—lowest in the newborn of all species (12)
    (a) In the newborn dog and during the first 2 wk, globulin is greater than albumin concentration, but after the 2nd week the A/G ratio increases significantly above 1 and remains above 1 throughout life. Total plasma protein concentration is stabilized at 6 mo in the dog. (38)
    (b) In the pig, rapid changes in total serum protein and in the electrophoretic pattern occur in the first 24 hr of life as a result of colostral absorption of gamma globulin. Rapid changes also occur in the subsequent 3-wk period because of the catabolism of serum gamma globulin, the immediate anabolism of serum albumin, and the absence of significant production of gamma globulin. (31)
   (2) Malnutrition (23)
    (a) Low protein or nitrogen diet—decreases concentration of albumin
    (b) Anorexia or cachexia—total protein is reduced, especially if there is no associated dehydration and the A/G ratio is reduced
    (c) Inadequate digestion and/or absorption—protracted diarrhea, chronic pancreatitis, fibrosis, malabsorption
   (3) Hepatopathy—especially when chronic, results in reduced albumin production
    (a) Fibrosis
    (b) Lipidosis
    (c) Neoplasia
   (4) Neoplasia—when lymphoid tissue and liver are involved
   (5) Pregnancy and lactation—failure to meet increased needs (23)
    (a) Sheep—albumin is decreased during the first half of pregnancy, while globulin is decreased during the second half of gestation due to globulin-rich colostrum
    (b) Cattle—a 10 to 30% decrease due to drop in globulin
  b. Loss of protein from the body
   (1) Acute blood loss (42)
    (a) The measurement of low total plasma protein will detect dilution of the plasma protein by extravascular fluid movement in response to the reduction in total blood volume. The fluid shifts begin within minutes and continue for several hours, and there is a gradual return of the plasma protein concentration toward normal as recovery takes place.

(b) Especially in the horse, demonstration of blood loss during the 12-hr period after hemorrhage by the PCV or hemoglobin level is unreliable due to the large number of erythrocytes released into the circulation from the vast splenic reservoir, thus masking the actual reduction in erythrocytes. (42)

(2) Chronic blood or protein loss

(a) Gastrointestinal loss of serum protein via exudation or leakage into the lumen of the gut—exudative or protein-losing enteropathy (23, 45)

(b) Parasitism—decrease in total protein and albumin and increase in concentration of gamma globulins (13)

(c) Renal disease—glomerular damage allows albumin and smaller amounts of globulin to pass into the urine and, when severe, will result in hypoalbuminemia and low total plasma protein (34)

c. Loss of blood or protein into body cavities (43)

C. Alterations in protein fractions

1. Albumin decreased (hypoalbuminemia)—most striking change (13)

a. Inhibition of synthesis

(1) Malnutrition

(a) Lack of proper amino acids

(b) Lack of enzymes and impaired digestion

(c) Impaired absorption—diarrhea, malabsorption

(2) Liver disease that is diffuse and usually chronic in nature

(a) Fibrosis (cirrhosis)

(b) Malignancies—diffuse

(c) Necrosis

(d) Inflammations

b. Increased protein catabolism from stress conditions

(1) Fever

(2) Infection

(3) Trauma

(4) Pregnancy—during first half of pregnancy in sheep

c. Leakage of albumin through damaged vessels and tissue

(1) Glomerular lesions—nephrosis, glomerulonephritis, amyloidosis

(2) Protein-losing enteropathy—in addition to the normal catabolism of albumin that occurs in the intestinal tract, increased losses are associated with chronic enteric diseases as the result of changes that alter permeability or obstruct intestinal lymphatic drainage (45)

(a) Johne's disease (35)

(b) Acute enteritis in calves (45)

(c) Ulcerative colitis (23)

(d) Parasitism

(e) Abomasal disorders in cattle (45)

(f) Intestinal neoplasia

(g) Lymphangiectasia

d. Secondary to increases in globulin concentration since colloid osmotic pressure is maintained within normal limits by a regulatory mechanism (3)

e. Edema, ascites, and hydrothorax may be produced by a decrease in colloidal pressure associated mainly with albumin levels that are lowered to between 1 and 2 g/dl and less with globulin molecules that are fewer in quantity because they are heavier. (34)

2. Globulins increased

a. Alpha globulins (4, 5)

(1) Acute inflammatory processes, especially in the dog and pig

(2) Acute and chronic renal disease

(3) Destruction of tissue

(4) Neoplastic conditions

(5) Fever

b. Beta globulins (4, 5)

(1) Hepatic disease

- (2) Abnormal lipid metabolism—diabetes mellitus, hypothyroidism
  - (a) Beta globulins contain the majority of lipoproteins that bind free and esterified cholesterol and phospholipids in serum.
- (3) Heavy helminth infection in the horse
- (4) Chronic skin disease in the dog
- (5) Eosinophilic myositis in the dog

c. Gamma globulins (4, 5)
- (1) Reflect the response of the reticuloendothelial system to antigens
  - (a) Correlation between the concentration of gamma globulins and antibody titers; more pronounced in chronic inflammations—tuberculosis, brucellosis (13)
- (2) Magnitude of the increase during infectious disease depends upon (13):
  - (a) Its severity
  - (b) Inherent host response
- (3) While absent or very low at birth, there is a rapid increase in gamma globulins in the newborn animal. However, within 1 to 2 days after birth, intact protein cannot be absorbed through the intestinal wall. (31)
- (4) While changes occur after bacterial, fungal, and parasitic infections, there is little or no change in the plasma protein picture in most viral infections even though high antibody titers may be produced. (13)
  - (a) No changes occur in foot-and-mouth disease in cattle (7, 37), vesicular stomatitis in cattle, or in Newcastle disease or infectious bronchitis in the chicken.
  - (b) Changes occur in equine infectious anemia; albumin is reduced.
- (5) Cirrhosis of the liver (4, 5)

d. Alpha and gamma globulins increased (4, 5)
- (1) Transition stage between acute and subacute or chronic inflammation
- (2) Various infectious diseases
- (3) Polyarthritis
- (4) Chronic arthritis in the dog

e. Beta and gamma globulins increased
- (1) Hepatitis and other liver damage in the dog and cattle (4, 5)
- (2) Hyperplastic endometritis and pyometra in the dog (4, 5)
- (3) In many, principally responsible for increased serum protein with age (28) and after intake of colostrum (31)

f. Alpha, beta, and gamma globulins increased (4, 5)
- (1) Complicated diseases
- (2) Malignant tumors
- (3) Impaired liver function (2)

g. Albumin:globulin ratio (A/G ratio)
- (1) Normal species variation
  - (a) Albumin predominates over globulin—dog, sheep, goat, man
  - (b) Relative amounts of albumin and globulin are nearly equal or globulin tends to be in excess of albumin—horse, cattle, pig
- (2) The ratio is usually altered by a decrease in albumin and/or an increase in globulins.
  - (a) Liver diseases—especially when chronic and generalized
  - (b) Bacterial infections—especially when chronic, e.g., tuberculosis, Johne's disease, brucellosis, erysipelas, arthritis (13)
  - (c) Parasitic diseases—*Haemonchus, Trichostrongylus, Ostertagia,* trypanosomiasis, babesiasis, fascioliasis (13)
  - (d) Viral infections—blockage in protein synthesis and passage into interstitial spaces because of increased permeability of the vascular system, e.g., canine distemper, infectious canine hepatitis, equine infectious anemia
  - (e) Fungal infection—candidiasis in the goat (13)
  - (f) Burns—reduced or normal A/G ratio as more albumin than globulin is lost into the burned area; following fluid loss the total serum protein is increased but falls following rehydration
  - (g) Young animals—in the newborn dog and during the first 2 wk, globulin is greater than albumin concentration (12)

12 FIBRINOGEN

I. General considerations

A. Fibrinogen is a soluble plasma protein produced in the microsomes of hepatic parenchymal cells and is stored in the cell until required. (2, 7)
   1. Fibrinogen has a turnover time estimated to be 50 hr.
   2. The half-life of canine fibrinogen has been found to be somewhere between 2.3 and 2.7 days. (9)

B. Among the various species, differences appear in the fibrinopeptides A and B released from the action on fibrinogen by thrombin. (9)

C. Fibrinogen is not normally found in serum, as consumption during the clotting of normal blood is usually complete.

D. Location of fibrinogen in the body
   1. Blood plasma—three times as much fibinogen is found in plasma as in lymph (9)
   2. Lymph
   3. Connective tissue
   4. Interstitial spaces

E. Action of fibrinogen
   1. Coagulation
      a. Fibrinogen is converted to fibrin by action of thrombin or thrombin-like enzymes.
      b. Adequate fibrinogen is present for hemostasis if a good clot is formed when blood is drawn into a tube. (3)
      c. Clotting is impaired with fibrinogen concentration below 60 mg/dl. (3)
   2. Fibrinogen provides defense against injury by migration into extravascular spaces to confine or localize invasive disease processes. (14)
   3. Peptides released from fibrinogen act on smooth muscle and might aid in regulating capillary-fed blood circulation. (13)
   4. In many species the erythrocyte sedimentation rate (ESR) is accelerated by increase in the fibrinogen level.
      a. It would appear that fibrinogen determination would be quicker and more specific than the ESR, especially in animals with a very slow ESR.

F. Heating plasma to 56°C precipitates fibrinogen but not albumin or globulin (8).

II. Methods of fibrinogen measurement—although several methods give similar results when normal blood samples are tested, pathologic specimens often produce wide variations (3)

A. Chemical methods—thrombin is added to plasma, producing a fibrin clot that may be washed, dried, and weighed, or the tyrosine or nitrogen content may be determined
   1. Time consuming
   2. In the presence of large amounts of heparin and a normal amount of fibrinogen, this method will indicate an absence of fibrinogen because no clot will be produced on the addition of the thrombin.

B. Turbidometric—fibrinogen in the plasma is precipitated by ammonium sulfate and the resulting turbidity is measured photometrically

C. Immunologic (Fi) test—antifibrinogen is complexed with latex particles and mixed with diluted blood. At plasma fibrinogen levels of 100 mg/dl or less, agglutination is not demonstrated.
   1. Rapid and requires little experience, but not especially quantitative
   2. Does not differentiate between breakdown products of fibrinogen or fibrin and fibrinogen

D. Thrombin time—measures the amount of functional fibrinogen in the plasma (5)

E. Heating the plasma to 56°C in a microhematocrit capillary tube to precipitate the fibrinogen—simple and a fairly reliable measure of fibrinogen with the Millar method (3, 5, 8, 12, 15)

1. Schalm method (15, 16, 17)
   a. Collect blood in EDTA to fill two microhematocrit tubes or other suitable tubes for plasma collection and centrifuge at a moderate speed for 10 min to clear the plasma.
   b. Place a drop of plasma from one of the tubes on the prism of the refractometer to determine the total plasma protein in grams per deciliter.
   c. Suspend the other capillary tube in a beaker of water, in a water bath, or under a stream of hot tap water that is 56° to 58°C for 3 min.
      (1) A plain capillary tube filled with plasma can be substituted for the capillary tube with whole blood that has been centrifuged.
      (2) Immerse in such a way that the entire column is surrounded by the warm water.
   d. Centrifuge the capillary tube to spin down the precipitated fibrinogen.
   e. Measure the protein concentration in the fibrinogen-free plasma, again using the refractometer. The difference between the two plasma protein readings is the fibrinogen concentration in milligrams per deciliter.
      (1) For example, a difference of 0.5 g between the two protein readings would indicate a fibrinogen concentration of 500 mg/dl.
   f. This method results in low readings when compared to the Ratnoff-Menzie assay used as a reference standard (5).
2. Millar method (5, 14)
   a. Blood is collected in EDTA and whole blood is drawn into a microhematocrit tube and sealed at one end.
   b. Spin for 5 min in a microhematocrit centrifuge.
   c. Place the tube in a water bath at 56°C (±1°C) for 3 min, making sure the plasma column is completely under the surface of the water.
   d. The precipitated fibrinogen is packed on top of the buffy coat by centrifugation, this time for 3 min.
   e. The length of the column of the packed precipitate (AB) is measured in relation to that of the original column of plasma (AC). (See Fig. 12.1.)
      (1) Reading of the column is facilitated by using a microscope with an ocular micrometer, and readings are made to the nearest 0.1 mm.

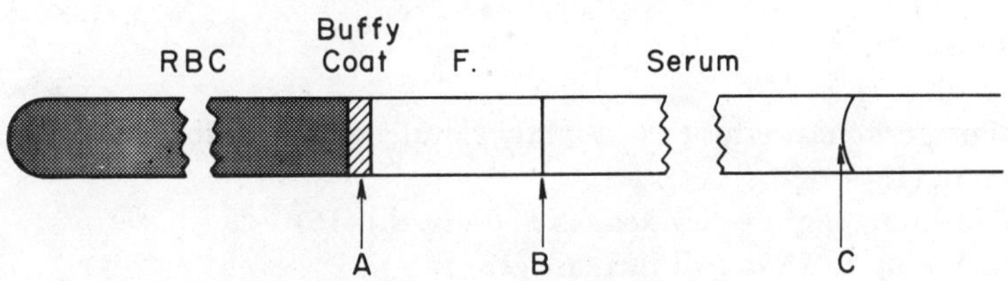

Fig. 12.1. Reading the plasma column in the Millar method.

   f. The amount of fibrinogen in the plasma is calculated by:

      (AB/AC) x 100 = ml/dl

   g. To convert ml/dl to mg/dl, multiply by 100:

      (ml/dl) x 100 = mg/dl

   h. This method compares favorably with the Ratnoff-Menzie assay (5).

III. Plasma protein: fibrinogen ratio (PP:F) (15)

A. When hemoconcentration occurs, it leads to a concentration of blood constituents and does not allow a direct interpretation of the extent of fibrinogen increase.

Total protein – fibrinogen = remainder ÷ fibrinogen = PP:5
PP:F less than 15:1 = an absolute increase in fibrinogen
PP:F less than 10:1 = marked increase in fibrinogen

IV. Interpretation

A. Normal ranges of fibrinogen
1. Cattle—450 to 750 mg/dl, with 800 mg/dl considered as abnormal (13, 15, 17)
2. Horse—200 to 400 mg/dl, with 500 mg/dl considered as abnormal (15, 16, 17)
3. Dog—200 to 400 mg/dl, with 500 mg/dl considered as abnormal (13, 16)
4. Cat—200 to 400 mg/dl (17)
5. Man—200 to 400 mg/dl (13)

B. Increased fibrinogen levels
1. General causes
a. Inflammation—bacterial, chemical, traumatic, or neoplastic
(1) Acute inflammation—reaches peak and then declines
(a) Favorable response—fibrinogen level rapidly returns to normal
(b) Unfavorable responses—fibrinogen level remains high, or plasma fibrinogen fails to increase during acute inflammatory stages
(2) Chronic inflammation—remains high as long as the disease is present and active
b. Tissue destruction—increases within 24 hr of tissue injury
2. Specific conditions
a. Dog
(1) Distemper—varies from 200 to 800 mg/dl (16)
(2) Leptospirosis—increase in fibrinogen and some reduction in fibrinolytic activity (6)
(3) Wound infections (13)
(4) Bone fractures
(5) Traumatic injuries
(6) Surgery (13)
(7) Peritonitis (13)
(8) Pneumonia (13)
(9) Pleural or peritoneal effusions—slightly elevated; rate of fibrinogen utilization may exceed liver production (15)
(10) Pyometra—only slightly elevated (to 600 mg/dl) (16)
(11) Pregnancy—up to 25 mg/dl increase (13)
(12) Pyelonephritis (16)
(13) Chronic interstitial nephritis (16)
(14) Malignancies—may exceed 1000 mg/dl in some forms (16)
b. Cat—does not elevate fibrinogen as readily in response to disease as other species (17)
(1) Feline infectious peritonitis (FIP)—200 to 700 mg/dl with an average of 400 mg/dl, but less than half with PP:F ratio $<15:1$
(2) Steatitis (17)
(3) Otitis interna (17)
(4) Urethral obstruction (17)

c. Cattle—elevation of fibrinogen is a more sensitive indicator of an inflammatory process than the total leukocyte count (17), as cattle have a greater capacity to produce fibrinogen in response to different stimuli than other species (13)

(1) Peritonitis—including traumatic reticuloperitonitis (13)
(a) 70% are over 1000 mg/dl
(b) 50% are over 1300 mg/dl
(c) 10% are over 2000 mg/dl
(2) Pericariditis
(3) Endocarditis
(4) Pneumonia—average 1300 mg/dl (13)
(5) Enteritis
(6) Nephritis
(7) Pyelonephritis
(8) Mastitis
(9) Liver damage—multiple abscesses, fatty degeneration
(10) Acute indigestion and rumen impaction (17)
(11) Septicemia and/or septic arthritis in calves (17)
(12) Following abortion
(13) *Brucella abortus* vaccination—moderate increase (13)
(14) Bracken poisoning (13)
d. Horse (16)
(1) Peritonitis
(2) Pleuritis
(3) Fractures
(4) Inflammation of guttural pouch
(5) Abscesses
(6) Salmonellosis

C. Decreased fibrinogen levels (hypofibrinogenemia, fibrinogenopenia)
1. General causes
a. Blood samples that contain a clot
b. Liver disease—especially severe or advanced cases
c. Terminal states
d. Rapid removal of fibrinogen from the circulation due to increased destruction by fibrinolysin or following release of thromboplastin into the circulation (13)
(1) Fibrinous exudation into serous cavities
(2) Obstetrical accidents or complications
(3) Shock
(4) Complications of major abdominal or pulmonary surgery
(a) The bovine lung has little fibrinolytic activity. (13)
(5) Extensive neoplasia—especially of bladder, pancreas, or prostate (13)
e. Nutritional disorders—occasionally
2. Specific conditions
a. Congenital fibrinogenopenia—rare, but described in man and calves (4)
b. Virus diarrhea in cattle—can be high, low end of normal, or subnormal (13)
(1) Lack of fibrinogen response may be due to inadequate stimulus to production
c. Streptococcal infections of the horse and dog—if fibrinolysin appears in the plasma (15)
d. Granulocytic leukemia in the dog—the low fibrinogen level is helpful in differentiating the leukocytosis from an inflammatory response (15)
e. Disseminated intravascular coagulation (consumptive coagulopathy)
(1) Administration of incompatible blood transfusion (9, 10)

D. No alterations in fibrinogen levels
1. General causes
a. Hemorrhage or repeated bleeding (13)
b. Transfusion of blood or Locke's solution (13)
c. Age (13, 15)

d. Change in type or amount of ration (13)
e. Sex
f. Exercise
g. Treatment with coumarin-based drugs (9)

2. Specific causes
   a. Dog
      (1) Lymphosarcoma—infiltrating cells in the liver interfere with fibrinogen production (16)
      (2) Splenectomy
   b. Cat (17)
      (1) Panleukopenia—averages 400 mg/dl
      (2) Feline infectious anemia—100 to 300 mg/dl
      (3) Lymphosarcoma—200 to 400 mg/dl
      (4) Myeloproliferative disorders—100 to 300/dl
      (5) Pyelonephritis—100 to 600 mg/dl (average 400 mg/dl) but with hemoconcentration
   c. Cattle (17)
      (1) Acetonemia
      (2) Anaplasmosis
      (3) Simple indigestion
      (4) Foot-and-mouth disease vaccination (13)

13 ERYTHROCYTE AND ITS DISORDERS

A PRODUCTION, LIFE SPAN, DESTRUCTION

I. Erythrocyte maturation (Fig. 13.1)

A. Stem cells (hemocytoblasts), with the stimulation of erythropoietin, differentiate into rubriblasts.
B. Normally, with four mitotic divisions, the rubriblast matures to the reticulocyte by a continual process of differentiation in approximately 72 hr. The reticulocyte matures to the erythrocyte in the ensuing 48 hr.

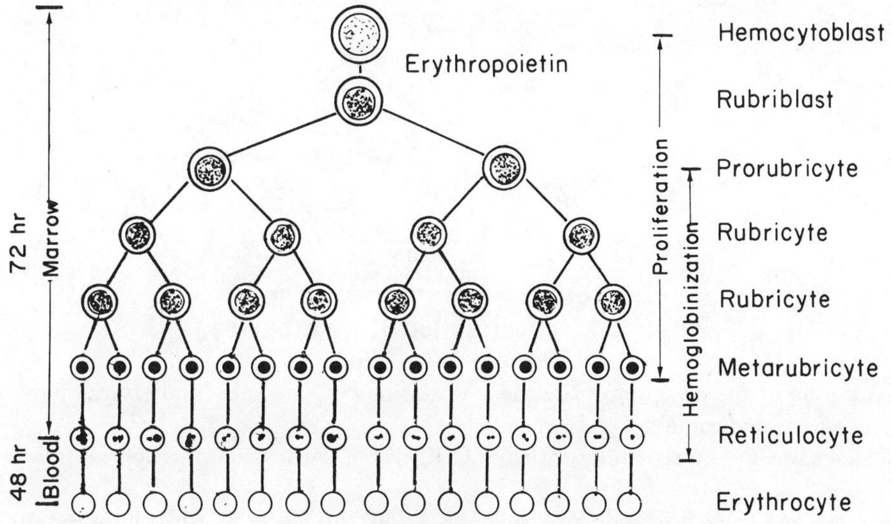

Fig. 13.1. Maturation of erythrocytes.

II. Life span of the erythrocyte

A. In the circulation the life span of the erythrocyte varies with the species of animal. The following average life spans in days have been established by isotope labeling with either ^{59}Fe or ^{14}C:

Species	Mean life span (days)
Cattle (adult)	160
Cattle (3 mo)	55
Horse	140-150
Sheep	70-153
Goat	125
Dog	110-122
Cat	68
Pig	63
Rabbit	68
Chicken	20

B. Reticulocytes and polychromatophilic erythrocytes are seen in normal blood of species with a short life span, while none are seen in animal species with prolonged erythrocyte life spans where the reticulocytes mature in the bone marrow.
   1. No reticulocytes are seen in normal healthy animals.
      a. Horse
      b. Cattle
      c. Sheep
      d. Goat
   2. Animals with a shorter life span for erythrocytes have normal numbers of reticulocytes
      a. Dog and cat—0.5 to 1%
      b. Pig—up to 2%
      c. Rabbit, rat, mouse, guinea pig—2 to 4%

III. Destruction of the erythrocytes (Fig. 13.2)

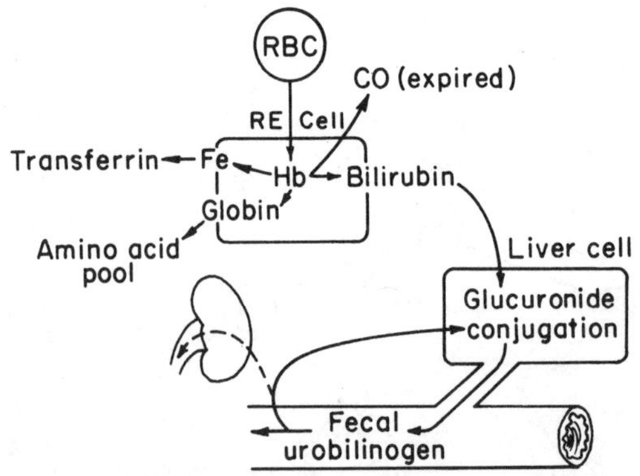

Fig. 13.2. Destruction of erythrocytes.

A. At the expiration of the erythrocyte life span, the aging cell becomes smaller and denser as the concentration of glycolytic enzymes diminishes.
B. Direct phagocytosis by the reticuloendothelial (RE) tissues is the usual method of destruction of the aging cells.
   1. Erythrocytes and their fragments are processed by all the RE cells, with the spleen as the most sensitive tissue for filtration of cells.

C. Hemoglobin is disassembled in a matter of minutes after the phagocytosis is initiated.
   1. Iron is made available for reuse by the bone marrow.
   2. Amino acids return to the protein pool of the body.
   3. The protoporphyrin ring is broken with release of the carbon through the lungs as carbon monoxide.
   4. The rest of the pyrrole molecule is transported to the liver as free bilirubin.
   5. Free bilirubin is conjugated in the liver to glucuronide and is excreted through the common bile duct to the intestine, where it is converted to urobilinogen by bacterial action.

IV. Requirements for normal erythropoiesis (Fig. 13.3)

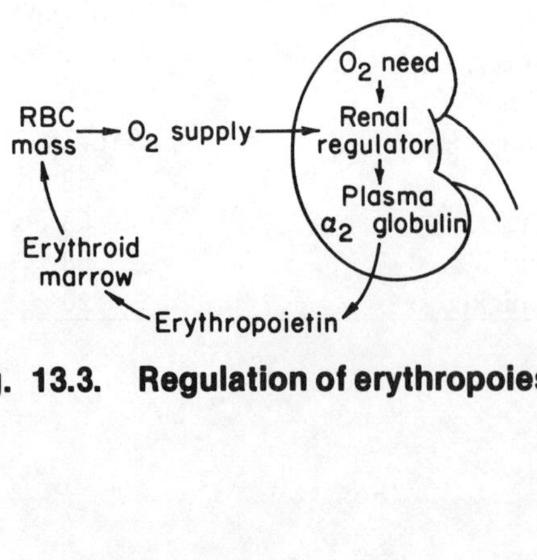

Fig. 13.3. Regulation of erythropoiesis.

A. Functional bone marrow
B. Erythropoietin
  1. Within the kidney is a sensing mechanism that equates oxygen supply with tissue oxygen requirements to maintain hemoglobin concentration within narrow limits.
  2. This regulating device generates a renal erythropoietic factor that produces erythropoietin by acting on an alpha-2 globulin substrate of the plasma.
  3. An increased output of erythropoietin is found in anemia and other forms of hypoxia.
  4. A decrease in erythropoietin output is associated with:
    a. Hyperoxia
    b. Hypertransfusion
    c. Reduction in tissue oxygen requirement
  5. Results of erythropoietin stimulation
    a. Increase in the number of developing cells
    b. Increase in the rate of maturation due to shortening of the mitotic cycle
    c. Increase in cell release from the bone marrow
      (1) Reflected in the blood smear by reticulocytes or polychromatophilic erythrocytes
        (a) Since the cells remain enlarged, there will be an increased mean corpuscular volume and mean corpuscular hemoglobin, but a slightly decreased mean corpuscular hemoglobin concentration, so that the degree of bone marrow stimulation will be reflected in the erythrocyte indices.
    d. Increase in hemoglobin synthesis within the individual cell

C. Iron supply
  1. An inadequate supply of iron limits erythrocyte production.

B RECOGNITION AND SIGNIFICANCE OF IMMATURE AND ABNORMAL ERYTHROCYTES

I. Signs of increased erythrocyte production

A. Anisocytosis—variation in the size of cells, especially erythrocytes
  1. Commonly seen in most anemias
    a. Large erythrocytes among the normal ones represent newly released cells from the bone marrow and increased erythrocyte production.

B. Macrocytes—immature erythrocytes
  1. Reticulocytes large and often macrocytic
  2. Indicates active bone marrow
  3. Occasionally indicates a defect in maturation of the cell
    a. Megaloblastic anemia—B_{12} and folic acid deficiencies

C. Nucleated erythrocytes
D. Reticulocytes—any nonnucleated cells of the erythrocytic series containing RNA that, when supravitally stained with new methylene blue or brilliant cresyl blue, will have discernible granules or a diffuse network of fibrils
E. Polychromasia—erythrocytes that show a faint, bluish tint due to an admixture of the characteristic colors of hemoglobin and basophilic erythrocytic cytoplasm
  1. Increased erythrocyte production and increased young erythrocytes
  2. If stained with new methylene blue, many cells would be reticulocytes.

F. Howell-Jolly bodies—nuclear remnants in young erythrocytes
   1. Feline and equine erythrocytes normally have Howell-Jolly bodies up to 1% of their erythrocytes.
   2. Indicate increased erythrocyte production
      a. Following acute blood loss or destruction
      b. In regenerative anemias
   3. A poorly functioning spleen may not be capable of removing nuclear remnants.
      a. Sluggish "pitting" function of spleen
      b. Follows splenectomy

G. Basophilic stippling—erythrocyte that shows blue-staining basophilic granules scattered throughout
   1. Seen with Romanowsky stains, but not with supravital stains
   2. Represents abnormal aggregates of RNA fraction altered so as to stain with Romanowsky stains such as Wright's
   3. Seen in anemias of almost all types
      a. Abundant in poisoning by heavy metals, especially lead
      b. Indicates defective erythropoiesis
      c. Increases with intense erythrogenesis in cattle and sheep

II. Other erythrocyte abnormalities

A. Acanthocytes ("burr" or "spur" cells)—erythrocytes with spinelike or sharp points
   1. Damage to the membrane of the erythrocyte
      a. Faulty technique and use of hypertonic fluids
   2. Autoimmune disease
      a. Autoimmune hemolytic anemia
      b. Thrombocytopenic purpura
   3. Severe disease
      a. Kidney—uremia
      b. Spleen—hemangiosarcoma
      c. Liver—occasionally
   4. Pyruvate kinase deficiency
   5. Abetalipoproteinemia

B. Basophilic stippling (punctate basophilia)
   1. Indicates defective erythropoiesis
   2. Seen in almost all types of anemias
      a. Abundant in poisoning by heavy metals, especially lead

C. Bowl or cup-shaped erythrocytes (wet film) or punched out centers (stained smear)
   1. The bowl shape assumed while the cell passes through a capillary is retained when it enters the larger vessels, rather than reverting to the normal biconcave form.
      a. Primary defective cellular formation
         (1) Distortion results from inadequate stromal framework allowing permanent distortion of cells as they travel through small capillaries to the peripheral circulation.
         (2) Acute disease—common to all animals
         (3) Chronic disease—frequently seen in the dog
   2. Artifacts in making the blood smear
      a. The use of "precleaned" slides may produce this type of artifact.

D. Distemper inclusion bodies—light blue stain of varying size, usually associated with young erythrocytes (macrocytes and polychromatophilic cells)
   1. Usually larger than Howell-Jolly bodies
   2. Rarely found in cases of canine distemper

E. Erythrocyte refractile (ER) bodies
  1. Morphology
    a. Unstained wet mounts—highly refractile bodies near the periphery or sometimes protruding
    b. Wright's stain—small circular pale areas at the edge of erythrocytes
    c. New methylene blue stain—blue black, called Heinz bodies
  2. Especially common in cat blood—as many as 10% in normal cat blood
  3. Toxic change thought to be altered hemoglobin
  4. Increase in number and size in a variety of chronic toxic diseases

F. Heinz bodies (ER bodies)—intraerythrocytic mass of denatured globin, irregular in shape, and appearing as a refractile granule when slightly out of focus
  1. Seen to best advantage with new methylene blue or methyl violet stains
    a. Not seen with Romanowsky dyes except as a pale area
  2. May be one or more in a cell and sometimes in plasma outside the erythrocyte
  3. Size varies
    a. Dog—1 to 2 microns in diameter
    b. Cat—larger, often ⅓ to ½ of erythrocyte diameter
  4. Represent areas of denatured hemoglobin and damaged erythrocytic stroma
  5. Hemolytic anemias associated with toxic drugs
    a. Phenothiazine and its derivatives
    b. Urinary antiseptics containing methylene blue—cat
    c. Phenylhydrazine
    d. Sodium nitrate
    e. Naphthalene (moth balls)
    f. Glucose-6-phosphate dehydrogenase deficiency—results in oxidative damage from a number of drugs with resulting Heinz body production in man

G. Hypochromasia—significant decrease in the density of the characteristic hemoglobin color for the stained or unstained erythrocyte
  1. Metabolic or toxic interference with hemoglobination
  2. Deficiency
    a. Iron—usually; includes chronic blood loss
    b. Copper
    c. Pyridoxine—necessary for utilization of iron in hemoglobin synthesis
    d. Riboflavin—dog
    e. Pyruvate kinase—Basenji breed of dog

H. Leptocytes—thin erythrocytes of decreased volume in relation to their diameter, often characterized by abnormality of shape
  1. Patterns of leptocytes
    a. Target cell
    b. Folded cell—raised fold traverses the center of the cell
  2. Best seen in thicker areas of the blood smear
  3. Associated with:
    a. Bone marrow depression anemia
    b. Aging change
    c. Chronic infections—suggested when there is an absence of erythrogenesis
    d. Inherited or acquired metabolic interference with erythrocyte metabolism
    e. Certain splenic diseases or splenectomy
    f. Hyperlipemia and hypercholesterolemia
    g. Biliary obstruction
  4. In the erythrocyte sedimentation rate the leptocytes tend to fall more slowly and show little tendency to participate in rouleaux formation.
    a. Lead to a minus value in the corrected ESR
  5. Accumulate in the lower portion of the buffy coat, resulting in a pink to red color

I. Microcytes—erythrocytes that are smaller than normal
  1. Seen in iron deficiency anemia—cells are hypochromic
    a. There is a maturation arrest in the rubricytic stage, and as a consequence the cells have an additional mitotic division, resulting in microcytic cells.
      (1) The bone marrow may be hyperplastic with many rubricytes and metarubricytes, but no stainable iron.
  2. Erythrocytes become smaller as they age but retain normal hemoglobin and stain deeply acidophilic.

J. Ovalocytes—elliptical erythrocytes
  1. Normal
    a. Few in a normal blood smear
    b. Camellidae family—alpaca, llama, camel, vicuna
  2. Macrocytic anemia—increased number
  3. Hereditary elliptocytosis—man
    a. Inherited as simple dominant
    b. Usually harmless

K. Poikilocytes—erythrocytes with an abnormal shape
  1. Usually abundant in most anemias
    a. Often reflects fragmented, aged erythrocytes before removal by the spleen
    b. Hemolytic anemia
  2. Microvascular pathology
    a. Uremia
    b. Vascular neoplasia
    c. Vasculitis
    d. Thrombosis
    e. Heartworm disease—sometimes

L. Rouleaux formation—arrangement of erythrocytes in a roll or column with flat surfaces facing, in which they appear as figures resembling stacks of coins
  1. Normal
    a. Marked—horse
    b. Moderate—cat, pig
    c. Slight—dog
    d. Absent—cattle, sheep
  2. Signs of defective erythropoiesis with interference at the developmental stage in the bone marrow
    a. Nutritional deficiency
      (1) Vitamin B complex
      (2) Protein
      (3) Iron
    b. Metabolic interference
      (1) Endogenous agents
      (2) Exogenous agents

M. Schistocytes—irregularly shaped fragments of erythrocytes
  1. Aging change
  2. Hemolytic anemias
  3. Microvascular pathology
    a. Thromboses of small vessels
    b. Splenic neoplasms

N. Siderocytes—erythrocytes containing nonhemoglobin iron granules that stain blue with the Prussian blue reaction
  1. In smears with Romanowsky dyes these iron granules are occasionally seen and appear as basophilic rods known as Pappenheimer bodies.

2. Abundant in hemolytic anemias
3. Seen after splenectomy

O. Spherocytes—spheroid erythrocytes of decreased diameter in relation to volume and having the microscopic appearance of hyperchromatic microcytes
1. Hemolytic anemias
   a. Autoimmune hemolytic anemia
   b. Hemolytic disease in the newborn—puppies
2. Hypersplenism—spleen is responsible for removing spherocytes from the circulation
3. Hyposplenism—occasionally
   a. When the erythrocyte is retained in the spleen for a long period, it may become permeable to sodium ions and take spherical form.
4. Bacterial toxins—occasionally

P. Stomatocytes—erythrocytes with a shape deformity in which there is a linear rather than a central area of pallor
1. Inherited hemolytic anemia
   a. Man
   b. Alaskan Malamute breed of dog

Q. Target cells—erythrocytes with a central rounded area of pigmented material, surrounded by a clear zone without pigment, and a dense ring of cytoplasm about the periphery of the erythrocyte
1. A form of leptocyte
2. Intense erythropoiesis in the dog
   a. Are reticulocytes and differ from those target cells seen in bone marrow depression anemia; seen with polychromasia
3. Bone marrow depression—seen without polychromasia
   a. Kidney disease—end stage
   b. Splenic disease or removal of spleen
   c. Liver disease—commonly seen
4. Artifacts in blood film—conditions favoring hypertonicity of plasma
   a. Slow drying of smears

R. Crenation—shrinkage of cells with the formation of irregular margins and a number of prickly points
1. Not an intrinsic abnormality of the erythrocyte but associated with improper technique
   a. Dehydration effect associated with slow drying or extreme temperatures
   b. Poor smearing technique
      (1) Dirty glassware

C ANEMIA

I. General considerations

A. Anemia is a decrease below normal in the number of erythrocytes per microliter, the hemoglobin value, and the packed cell volume (PCV).

B. Anemia is not a diagnosis but a sign of underlying disease.
   1. The objective of the laboratory is to determine the type of anemia as an aid in discovering the cause. A search for the underlying cause is essential, so that it can be remedied or removed and can serve as a guide for proper therapy.

II. Erythrocyte indices

A. Erythrocyte indices define the size and hemoglobin content of the erythrocyte from values obtained for the erythrocyte count, the hemoglobin concentration, and PCV.

1. Mean corpuscular volume (MCV)

a. The MCV expresses the average volume of the individual erythrocyte and is calculated from the formula:

$$\text{MCV} = \frac{\text{PCV x 10}}{\text{erythrocyte count (millions/microliter)}}$$

and the result expresses the mean volume of the erythrocyte in femtoliters (fl).

b. Example—erythrocytes 6.5 million/microliter and PCV 43%

$$\text{MCV} = \frac{43 \text{ x } 10}{6.5} = 66.2 \text{ fl}$$

c. Interpretation

(1) Normal MCV—normocytic

(a) Acute hemorrhage

(b) Hemolysis

(c) Lack of blood formation

(2) Increased MCV—macrocytic

(a) Increased activity of the bone marrow in some conditions usually associated with normocytic anemia such as acute hemorrhage and hemolysis

(b) Some deficiencies of hematopoietic factors

(3) Decreased MCV—microcytic

(a) Iron deficiency

(b) Copper deficiency in some animals

(c) Some deficiencies of hematopoietic factors

2. Mean corpuscular hemoglobin concentration (MCHC)

a. The MCHC is the concentration of hemoglobin in the average erythrocyte, or the ratio of weight of hemoglobin to the volume in which it is contained, and is calculated from the formula:

$$\text{MCHC} = \frac{\text{hemoglobin (g/dl) x 100}}{\text{PCV}}$$

and the result is expressed in grams per deciliter (g/dl).

b. Example—hemoglobin 14 g/dl of blood and PCV 45%

$$\text{MCHC} = \frac{14 \text{ x } 100}{45} = 31 \text{ g/dl}$$

c. Interpretation

(1) Normal MCHC—normochromic

(a) In many types of anemia an increase or decrease in the average size of the cell is accompanied by a corresponding increase or decrease in the average hemoglobin content, so that the MCHC remains within the normal range.

(2) Decreased MCHC—hypochromic

(a) In the true hypochromic anemia the reduction in hemoglobin is relatively greater than the average decrease in erythrocyte volume.

(3) Increased MCHC

(a) There are no conditions in which the MCHC is increased above the normal range, since the erythrocyte cannot be supersaturated with hemoglobin.

(b) In so-called hyperchromic anemia there is an increase in the weight of hemoglobin in the average erythrocyte, but the concentration of hemoglobin per unit volume is not increased.

3. Mean corpuscular hemoglobin (MCH)

a. The MCH is the amount of hemoglobin, by weight, in the average erythrocyte and is calculated from the formula:

$$MCH = \frac{\text{hemoglobin (g/dl) x 10}}{\text{erythrocyte count (millions/microliter)}}$$

and the result is expressed in picograms (pg).

b. Example—hemoglobin 13.5 g/dl of blood and erythrocytes 6.5 million/microliter

$$MCH = \frac{13.5 \times 10}{6.5} = 20.8 \text{ pg}$$

c. Interpretation

(1) The MCHC is a more valuable measurement than MCH because in anemias in which the MCH is not altered proportionately with MCV the lack of correlation is indicated by a change in the MCHC.

B. Normal values for erythrocyte indices

Species	MCV (fl)	MCHC (g/dl)	MCH (pg)
Horse, Thoroughbred	42(37-50)	33(31-35)	13.3
Horse, draft	44(39-52)	33(31-35)	15.2-18.6
Cattle	50(40-60)	30(26-34)	14.4-18.6
Sheep	32(23-48)	32(29-35)	9.0-13.0
Goat	20(18-24)	32(30-35)	5.0-7.4
Pig	63(50-68)	32(30-34)	16.6-22.0
Dog	70(60-77)	33(31-34)	19.0-23.0
Cat	45(40-55)	33(31-35)	13.0-17.0
Man	87(82-92)	34(32-36)	29(27-31)

C. Morphologic classification of anemia

Classification	MCHC normal	MCHC decreased
MCV normal	Normocytic Normochromic	Normocytic Hypochromic
MCV increased	Macrocytic Normochromic	Macrocytic Hypochromic
MCV decreased	Microcytic Normochromic	Microcytic Hypochromic

D. Differential diagnosis in anemia (See chart.)

Differential Diagnosis in Anemia

Necessary Examinations

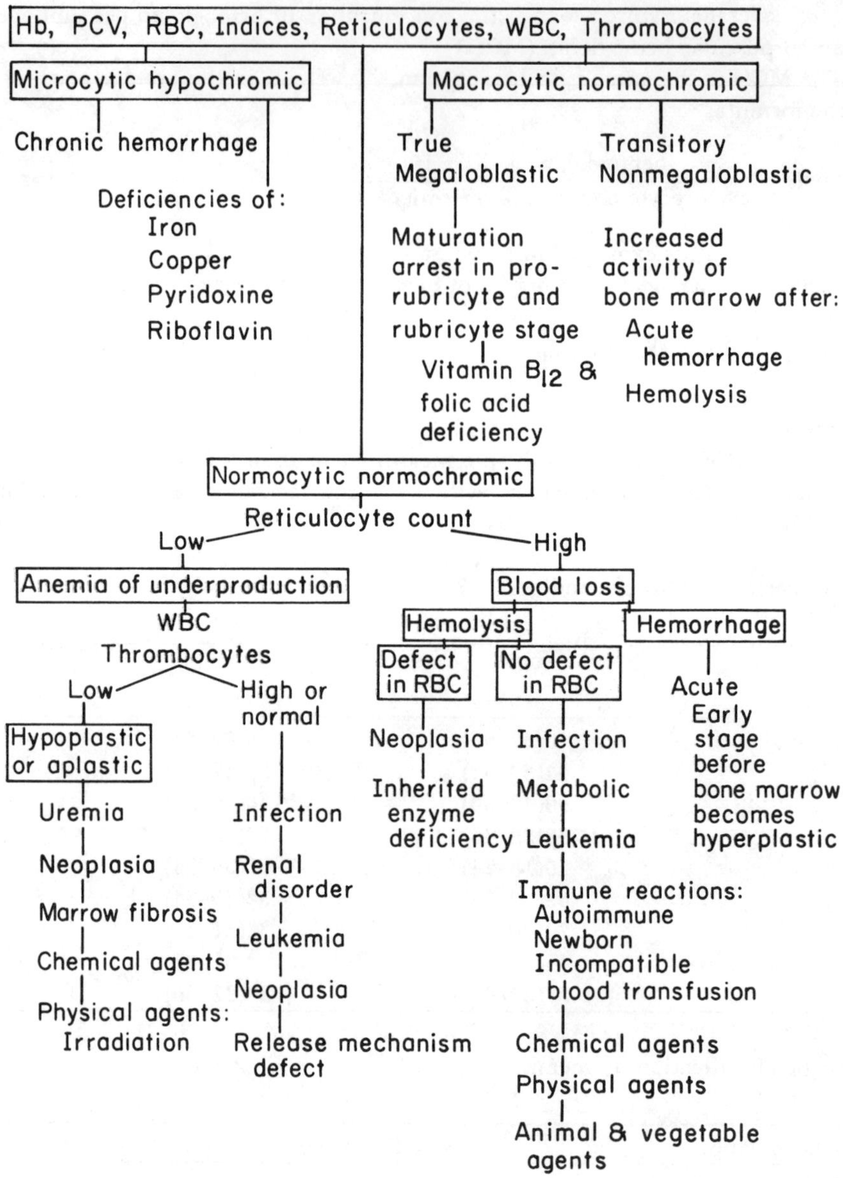

III. Clinical evaluation—establishment of the correct diagnosis of the underlying cause of the anemia begins with an adequate history and a physical examination that cannot be too thorough

A. History
1. Time of onset of clinical signs
a. Abrupt onset—suggests acute hemorrhage or hemolysis
b. Gradual—suggests chronic hemorrhage or bone marrow depression
2. Evidence of blood loss
a. Hematuria
b. Melena
c. Hemoptysis
d. Blood in vomitus

3. Performance status—weakness and fatigue after exertion
4. Existence of an underlying condition—renal disease, leukemia
   a. Weight loss
5. Exposure to drugs
6. Exposure to toxic chemicals in environment—lead

B. Physical examination
1. Fever—common manifestation of infection, leukemia, hemorrhage, or hemolysis
2. Character of mucous membranes, eye, and skin
   a. Pale
   b. Icteric—liver disease
   c. Pale and icteric—hemolysis
   d. Cyanotic
   e. Petechia or ecchymoses—platelet or vascular defect
3. Palpation
   a. Internal masses
   b. Splenomegaly
   c. Hepatomegaly
   d. Lymphadenopathy
4. Signs of underlying disease
5. External wounds—evidence of being hit by car, bullets

IV. Laboratory evaluation

A. Initial laboratory tests to evaluate the anemic patient
1. PCV and color of supernatant plasma
2. Hemoglobin
3. Total erythrocyte count—if either PCV or hemoglobin is low
4. Examination of blood smear for immature and abnormal erythrocytes
5. Erythrocyte indices—MCV, MCHC, MCH
6. Total plasma protein
7. Reticulocyte count
8. Total leukocyte count and differential
9. Platelets
10. Bone marrow evaluation

B. Subsequent laboratory tests that may be necessary
1. Coombs' test
2. Lupus erythematosus preparation
3. Serum iron
4. Total iron binding capacity
5. Stain for iron in bone marrow
6. Total and indirect bilirubin
7. Urine bilirubin
8. Erythrocyte fragility
9. Erythrocyte enzymes—pyruvic kinase
10. Erythrocyte survival

V. Classification of anemia according to cause

A. Acute hemorrhage—relatively large amount of blood lost extravascularly in a brief period; regenerative type of anemia; normocytic normochromic, later pseudomacrocytic
1. Trauma—accidental or surgical
   a. Internal
   b. External

2. Disease process with damage to vascular wall, allowing blood to escape
   a. Rupture of large vessel—mesenteric, etc.
   b. Rupture of friable neoplasm—splenic hemangiosarcoma
3. Coagulation defect
   a. Disseminated intravascular coagulation
   b. Warfarin
   c. Sweet clover

B. Increased erythrocyte destruction—regenerative anemia; normochromic later pseudomacrocytic; icterus in acute hemolysis
   1. Extrinsic abnormalities
      a. Infection
         (1) Bacterial
            (a) Leptospira—in cattle, occasionally in the dog
            (b) *Clostridium hemolyticum*—bacillary hemoglobinuria
            (c) *Clostridium perfringens* (type A)—lambs
            (d) *Staphylococcus* and *Streptococcus* toxins
         (2) Viral
            (a) Equine infectious anemia
         (3) Blood parasites
            (a) *Anaplasma*—probably due to several causes (hemolytic, autoimmune, bone marrow depression)
            (b) *Haemobartonella*—dog, cat (feline infectious anemia)
            (c) *Eperythrozoa*—swine
            (d) *Babesia* or *Piroplasma*
            (e) Trypanosomes
            (f) Malaria
      b. Antibody-mediated destruction
         (1) Isoimmune agents
            (a) Hemolytic disease of the newborn—foal, puppy, pig
            (b) Transfusions
            (c) Vaccines
         (2) Autoimmune agents
            (a) Autoimmune hemolytic anemia
            (b) Lupus erythematosus
            (c) Leukemias
            (d) Anaplasmosis
      c. Chemical agents
         (1) Phenothiazine and derivatives
         (2) Methylene blue
         (3) Copper
         (4) Lead
         (5) Coal tar derivatives
         (6) Naphthalene (moth balls)
         (7) Saponin
      d. Animal and vegetable agents
         (1) Snake venom
         (2) Poisonous plants
            (a) Wild onion
            (b) Broom
            (c) Ranunculus
            (d) Frosted turnips
            (e) Oak shoots
      e. Mechanical disruption
         (1) Microangiopathic hemolytic disease

(2) Vascular prothesis
(3) Burns
f. Physical agents
(1) Heat
(2) Ultraviolet radiation
g. Reticuloendothelial sequestration
(1) Hypersplenism
(2) Acute infection
2. Intrinsic erythrocyte abnormality
a. Erythrocyte enzyme
(1) Pyruvate kinase deficiency—Basenji breed of dog
b. Cell shape abnormalities
(1) Acanthocytosis
c. Hemoglobinopathy
(1) Sickle cells—deer, goats
d. Heme and porphyrins
(1) Erythropoietic porphyria
(2) Hepatic porphyria

C. Decreased erythrocyte production
1. Disturbance of stem cell proliferation and differentiation—nonregenerative type of anemia; normocytic normochromic, colorless plasma
a. Aplastic anemia—disorders associated with pancytopenia; bone marrow replaced by fat
(1) Chemical toxins—chloramphenicol, primidone, phenylbutazone, sulfas
(2) Radiation
(3) Unknown agents
b. Chronic renal failure—impaired erythropoietin production
(1) Often mixed with shortened life span of erythrocytes due to metabolic or mechanical environment, hemolysis, or hemorrhage from ulcerated gastrointestinal tract
c. Endocrine disorders—certain hormones are essential for the production of erythrocytes and hemoglobin synthesis
(1) Thyroid
(a) Administration of thyroxin, dessicated thyroid, and triiodothyronine increases the rate of erythrocyte production and is related to the release of renal erythropoietin.
(b) Anemia is normocytic normochromic, with reticulocyte reduction.
(2) Gonads
(a) Androgens stimulate erythrocyte production by increasing production of erythropoietin or enhancing erythropoietin effect on the bone marrow, or both.
(b) Estrogens suppress erythrocytes by suppressing erythropoietin production or inhibition of erythropoietin at the stem cell level.
(3) Adrenal
(a) ACTH and adrenocortical hormones stimulate release of renal erythropoietin.
(b) Hypoadrenocorticism (Addison's disease) may produce a mild normocytic normochromic anemia.
(4) Pituitary
(a) Growth hormone stimulates erythrocyte production.
2. Disturbance of differentiated cell proliferation and maturation
a. Impairment of DNA synthesis (megaloblastic anemia)—macrocytic normochromic
(1) Vitamin B_{12} and folic acid deficiency—rare in animals
(a) Maturation arrest in prorubricyte and rubricyte stage
b. Hemoglobin synthesis—microcytic hypochromic anemia
(1) Iron deficiency
(2) Chronic blood loss
(a) Gastrointestinal lesions—ulcers, enteritis

(b) Bleeding from neoplasms into tissues or body cavities
(c) Parasitism
Internal—hookworms, coccidia, stomach worms, whipworms, liver flukes, nodular worms
External—lice, fleas, ticks
(d) Genitourinary tract bleeding
(e) Coagulation defects

3. Multiple or unknown mechanism
  a. Anemia of chronic disorders—common; moderate normocytic normochromic anemia
    (1) Associated with:
      (a) Chronic inflammation
      (b) Chronic infection
      (c) Neoplasia—disseminated or necrotizing
    (2) Characterized by:
      (a) Relative bone marrow failure
      (b) Decrease in serum iron
      (c) Decrease in total iron binding capacity
      (d) Increase in iron stores in RE cells of bone marrow
  b. Nutritional deficiency anemia other than B_{12} or folic acid
    (1) Starvation
    (2) Protein deficiency—reduces erythropoietin production and produces a maturation block at the rubricyte level
    (3) Vitamin C deficiency—monkey
    (4) Vitamin B (pyridoxine) deficiency
    (5) Pantothenic acid deficiency—moderate normocytic anemia in swine
    (6) Niacin deficiency—niacin required for erythrocyte respiration
      (a) Normocytic anemia in swine
      (b) Macrocytic anemia in the dog
    (7) Vitamin E deficiency—mild macrocytic anemia in the monkey
    (8) Copper deficiency
      (a) Copper is the cofactor for numerous enzyme systems.
      (b) A deficiency decreases absorption of iron, release of iron from body stores, and utilization of iron in hemoglobin synthesis.
      (c) A deficiency decreases the life span of erythrocytes.
      (d) Macrocytic hypochromic anemia in swine
    (9) Cobalt deficiency
      (a) Cobalt is an essential constituent of B_{12} and is incorporated into this vitamin in the ruminant.
      (b) Macrocytic anemia in ruminants
  c. Anemia of neoplasia
  d. Anemia with marrow infiltration—bone marrow is invaded or replaced; competition between these cells for nutritional factors; usually signs of regeneration, although the number of erythroid precursors is reduced; myelophthisic
    (1) Tumor cells
    (2) Leukemic cells
    (3) Granulomas
    (4) Disseminated fungal infections

VI. Correlation of causes of anemia with laboratory findings

A. Regenerative anemias—acute hemorrhage or hemolysis; normal active bone marrow with active erythrogenesis to compensate for erythrocyte loss in the anemia
  1. Acute hemorrhage—response varies with amount of blood loss, duration, and site of hemorrhage
    a. Immediately following loss of erythrocytes and plasma
      (1) Blood volume alone is decreased.
      (2) Splenic contraction and bone marrow releases mature erythrocytes to mask loss of cells from vessels; normocytic normochromic cells.

b. First few hours
   (1) Most of the fluid volume is replaced to produce a dilution of the plasma and plasma protein concentration; total of WBC and platelets increases.
c. First 12 hours
   (1) PCV, hemoglobin, and total erythrocyte counts may be misleading due to dilutional effect.
   (2) Recovery is denoted by gradual increase in plasma protein to normal.
d. Up to 72 hours
   (1) An occasional metarubricyte and reticulocyte is released from bone marrow.
e. 72 hours (3rd day)
   (1) It requires 2 to 4 days for a significant number of new cells to enter circulation in response to hemorrhage when the number of cells from the reserve stores are not sufficient to prevent hypoxia and stimulation by resulting erythropoietin release.
f. 5th to 6th day
   (1) Peak response to a single bleeding episode occurs between the 5th and 6th day; pseudomacrocytosis.
      (a) Reticulocytes—increased
      (b) Metarubricytes
      (c) Howell-Jolly bodies
      (d) Polychromasia
      (e) Basophilic stippling—sometimes
      (f) Poikilocytes—possible
      (g) Anisocytosis—due to reticulocytosis
g. 1 to 3 weeks
   (1) PCV increases by the 4th day and gradually increases to normal at 1 to 3 wk.
h. Seldom enough blood loss to produce an iron deficiency
   (1) Must be massive loss, since iron is available in storage and diet
i. Internal blood loss
   (1) Into body cavities—peritoneal, pleural
      (a) Blood is absorbed by lymphatics as an autotransfusion—2/3 in 24 hr and the remainder in 2 to 3 days, provided the source of hemorrhage has been corrected
   (2) Blood loss into body tissue
      (a) If there is a large accumulation of blood, it must be broken down; pigment breakdown may result in an icteric condition, which is possible to confuse with hemolysis.
j. The degree of regenerative response in the blood smear will vary with the species.
   (1) Dog—good response
   (2) Cat—none
   (3) Horse—none; diphasic sedimentation rate provides a clue to response
   (4) Calves—reticulocytes appear only after severe and sudden blood loss, and disappear early in the recovery phase, even though macrocytosis persists

2. Hemolysis
   a. Regenerative signs are marked and commensurate with the degree of anemia.
      (1) Reticulocytosis is marked.
         (a) Reticulocytosis that is sustained for more than a few days is usually evidence of hemolytic anemia; the more severe the anemia, the higher the reticulocyte count.
      (2) Nucleated erythrocytes may be seen.
      (3) Associated with the reticulocytosis will be macrocytosis, which is responsible for anisocytosis, as well as polychromasia.
   b. Icteric plasma should be seen in acute hemolytic crisis but may be present or absent in chronic hemolytic anemia.
   c. Neutrophilic leukocytosis is often present within hours.
   d. Erythrocyte abnormalities often depend upon the cause of the hemolysis.
      (1) Autoimmune hemolytic anemia
         (a) Autoagglutination and rouleaux formation
         (b) Spherocytes—may be present, but may also be seen occasionally in any type of hemolysis
         (c) Positive Coombs' test

(d) Thrombocytopenia—common
(2) Blood parasites—on the surface of the erythrocyte
(a) Shorten the erythrocyte life span
(3) Microangiopathic anemia
(a) Schistocytes
(4) Drug toxicity
(a) Heinz bodies
(5) Basophilic stippling may be seen.
(a) Intense erythrogenesis in cattle
(b) Lead poisoning—nucleated erythrocytes without reticulocytes (due to maturation arrest); poikilocytes
e. Erythrophagocytosis is seen occasionally, especially in the bone marrow.
f. Target cells may be seen during intense erythrocyte production.
g. The Van den Bergh test (serum bilirubin) will have increased amounts of free bilirubin (indirect-reacting bilirubin).
h. Urobilinogen is increased in urine and feces.

B. Nonregenerative anemias
1. Lack of erythropoietin stimulation or defective bone marrow
a. Normocytic normochromic erythrocytes
b. Pale to colorless plasma
c. Leptocytes—target cells and folded cells common
d. Poikilocytes
e. Leukocyte and platelet counts variable and dependent upon the cause
f. Anemia of chronic disorders
(1) Serum iron and total iron binding capacity (TIBC) are decreased, but iron can be demonstrated in the RE cells in the bone marrow by using special stains.

C. Signs of defective proliferation or maturation of erythrocytes
1. Microcytic hypochromic erythrocytes in nutritional iron deficiency or chronic blood loss
a. The reticulocytes and nucleated erythrocytes are numerous.
b. Anisocytosis, polychromasia, and Howell-Jolly bodies are commonly seen.
c. Fragmented cells are seen occasionally.

D SPECIAL ANEMIAS

I. Autoimmune hemolytic anemia

A. Occurrence
1. Age
a. Most of the canine cases occur between the ages of 2 and 8 yr.
b. Next in frequency are the cases that are over 8 yr.
c. Occasional cases occur in younger animals.
2. Sex
a. Three times more frequently in female than in male dogs
3. Species
a. Dog—most often
b. Cat—undoubtedly occurs, but is difficult to diagnose

(1) To establish the fact that the cat is actually producing an autoantibody against its own erythrocytes, it is necessary to take the coated antibody erythrocytes from the patient, destroy the erythrocytes, and have the antibody react with another cat's erythrocytes in a test tube.
(a) It has not been possible to do this with cat erythrocytes and establish the autoantibody nature of the disease.
(2) A positive Coombs' test can occur when upper respiratory virus of the coryza patient is absorbed on the erythrocyte membrane and produces a membrane change, but this is not an autoantibody.
c. Horse
d. Cattle—infected with *Anaplasma marginale*
(1) An autoantibody is a gamma globulin that reacts with the erythrocytic membranes of infected calves.
(2) Demonstrated by:
(a) A single precipitin band in immunoelectrophoresis (IE) tests
(b) Passive hemagglutination (PHA)
e. Mouse
f. Man

B. Clinical signs
1. Sudden onset
2. Fever
a. Initially in half of the cases
b. Does not persist longer than 1 to 2 days
3. Weakness—extreme
4. Pallor—in all cases
5. Icterus
a. In half of the cases
b. Degree dependent upon the number of spherocytes and their hemolysis
c. Usually not pronounced
6. Splenomegaly—in half of the cases
7. Hepatomegaly—less commonly
8. Lymphadenopathy
a. Popliteal, mandibular, and prescapular lymph nodes are slightly enlarged in half of the cases.
9. Thrombocytopenic purpura
a. Present in one-third of the cases
b. Clinical signs of thrombocytopenic purpura
(1) Hemorrhages in skin, mucous membranes, nose, eye
(2) Melena
(3) Hematuria
(4) Epistaxis
10. Anorexia
11. Depression
12. Dyspnea
13. Dark urine—sometimes
14. Recurrence common

C. Laboratory findings in the dog
1. Coombs' test—positive
a. Demonstrates the presence of globulin intimately associated with the erythrocytic membrane
b. Must use rabbit anti-canine globulin serum
c. Usually positive in recurrent crisis
(1) In almost all cases, becomes positive when a relapse is imminent
d. Becomes negative as the patient recovers
e. False negative after corticosteroid therapy is initiated
2. Packed cell volume
a. Usually between 5 to 20% and not over 30%

b. Icteric plasma
3. Marked thrombocytopenia—in 75% of affected dogs
   a. Fewer than 100,000/microliter
4. Morphologic changes in the erythrocytes
   a. Spherocytosis—spherocytes are small in size, dark staining, and lack a central pallor
      (1) Present early, but easily hemolyzed and removed by the spleen
      (2) Not a constant finding
   b. Macrocytic erythrocytes
   c. Polychromasia

Antibody + RBC → Membrane change → Spherocyte / Increased susceptibility to phagocytosis → Premature hemolysis

5. Reticulocytosis
   a. Marked
   b. Better measure of intensity of bone marrow response than the number of nucleated erythrocytes
6. Spontaneous agglutination of erythrocytes
   a. In early stages of 25% of the cases
7. Leukocytes
   a. Total leukocyte count—20,000 to 40,000/microliter
   b. Neutrophilia with shift to the left
   c. Monocytosis
8. Urine
   a. Proteinuria
   b. Normal specific gravity
   c. Bilirubinuria
   d. Urobilinogen increased
9. Blood urea nitrogen—may be elevated in early stage
10. Increased erythrocyte fragility

D. Direct Coombs' test on canine erythrocytes
1. Procedure
   a. Obtain 3 to 5 ml of fresh blood from the patient.
      (1) Collect in EDTA or allow to clot and take an appropriate number of cells from the clot.
      (2) Sample should be received in the laboratory within one hour of collection.
   b. Centrifuge for 5 min to concentrate the cells if sample is in EDTA.
      (1) Discard the supernatant plasma.
   c. Add two drops of concentrated erythrocytes to 5 ml of isotonic saline and mix. Centrifuge at 1500 rpm to pack the cells. Discard the supernatant. Repeat two times.
   d. Prepare a 2 to 3% suspension of the erythrocytes in saline.
   e. Add two drops of the erythrocyte suspension to two drops of Coombs' serum in a small test tube.
   f. Mix well, incubate for 15 to 30 min at 37°C.
   g. Centrifuge for approximately 1 min at 1000 rpm.
   h. Flick the tube to allow the erythrocytes to swirl and resuspend. Watch for a tendency to agglutinate.
   i. Grade macroscopic reactions as follows:
      (1) Negative—cells swirl up, no macroscopic agglutination
      (2) 3+ reaction—small to large groups; check microscopically
      (3) 4+ reaction—the whole button comes off the bottom of the tube
   j. Grade microscopic reactions as follows:
      (1) Trace—erythrocytes in groups of 3 or less; should be repeated
      (2) 1+—small groups of 4 to 8 erthrocytes
      (3) 2+—larger groups of about 10 erythrocytes
      (4) 3+—large groups incorporating most of the erythrocytes

(5) 4+ —button does not break up

k. A control tube containing washed erythrocytes from a normal dog and saline must always be run in parallel with the test sample.

2. Absorption of commercial anti-canine globulin serum—to remove nonspecific agglutinins and avoid false positive reactions
   a. Inactivate Coombs' antiserum at 57°C in water bath for 30 min to inactivate the complement.
   b. Collect fresh, normal dog whole blood in ACD solution and wash the erythrocytes five times in isotonic saline.
   c. The inactivated rabbit antiserum (Coombs' serum) is added to 25 to 50% of its volume of packed, normal, washed canine cells.
      (1) Incubate 1 hr at 37°C in a water bath with occasional mixing.
      (2) Allow to stand overnight in the cold (4°C).
   d. Centrifuge and remove serum.
   e. Test for nonspecific agglutinins
      (1) Two drops of a 2% suspension of normal canine erythrocytes (washed three times) and two drops of absorbed antiserum (Coombs' serum) are incubated at 4°C, room temperature, and 37°C for 30 min and observed for gross and microscopic agglutination.
      (2) Repeat absorption if agglutination is noted at this step.

E. Treatment

1. Interfere with production of antibodies or inhibit antigen-antibody reaction
   a. High levels of glucocorticoids—prednisolone or prednisone (1 mg/lb of body weight per day to start)
      (1) Give in 2 to 3 divided doses.
      (2) Maintenance levels of 2.5 to 5 mg daily is eventually achieved by a gradual reduction in the dose as improvement is evident.
   b. Testosterone can be used with corticosteroid therapy to offset the catabolic effect.
2. Blood transfusions
   a. Usually contraindicated
      (1) Animals appear better for a short period, become jaundiced in about 12 hr, and are dead in 18 hr.
      (2) Rapid hemolysis, shock, and death often occur.
   b. Reserve for emergency case as a last resort when the animal is not responding and hemoglobin or PCV are extremely low.
   c. Use only fresh, compatible blood.
   d. Administer corticosteroid before transfusion to reduce the likelihood of a reaction.
3. Splenectomy
   a. Suggested if the condition recurs on declining dose of corticosteroids or after adequate maintenance dosage
      (1) Leukemoid reaction, declining at about a week, may occur after the splenectomy.
   b. Usually contraindicated, as the spleen represents only a fraction of the reticuloendothelial system, and antibody production is not diminished
4. Supportive therapy
   a. Antibiotics to avoid infection when large doses of corticoids are used
   b. Fluid therapy—for dehydration
5. Plasma transfusion—to limit hemorrhaging from marked thrombocytopenia
   a. Must use fresh blood, as the life span of the platelets is limited.
   b. Centrifuge whole blood at 1500 rpm for 15 min or allow erythrocytes to settle naturally. Use platelet-rich plasma.

II. Systemic lupus erythematosus (SLE) is an autoimmune, progressive nonorgan-specific disorder, characterized as a collagen-vascular disease in which a variety of tissues and organs are affected.

A. Types of autoimmune disease

1. Organ-specific diseases
   a. Autoimmune hemolytic anemia

b. Idiopathic thrombocytopenic purpura
c. Lymphocytic thyroiditis
d. Glomerulonephritis
2. Nonorgan-specific diseases
a. Systemic lupus erythematosus
b. Connective tissue disorders
(1) Rheumatoid arthritis
(2) Polyarteritis nodosa
3. Mixed or transitory
a. Granulomatous colitis
b. Myasthenia gravis
c. Active chronic hepatitis

B. Collagen-vascular diseases associated with antinuclear antibodies
1. Systemic lupus erythematosus
2. Rheumatoid arthritis
3. Polymyositis
4. Polyarteritis nodosa

C. Mechanisms in the production of the SLE lesions
1. Localization in vascular structures of preformed complexes formed from:
a. Antigen (DNA)
b. Antibody (anti-DNA)
c. Complement
2. Cytotoxic mechanisms—involve the formation of specific antitissue antibodies that damage the respective organs

D. Occurrence
1. Species
a. Dog
b. Cat
c. Mouse—New Zealand black (NZB)
d. Man
2. Sex—more common in young adult female dogs and women

E. Diagnosis of SLE in the dog
1. Presence of LE cells
2. One (according to Lewis), two (according to Schultz), or more of the following disorders occurring simultaneously or sequentially:
a. Autoimmune hemolytic anemia (positive Coombs' test)
b. Thrombocytopenic purpura
c. Symmetrical (rheumatoid) arthritis
d. Glomerulonephritis (membranous)

F. Conditions that occasionally occur with canine SLE
1. Skin
a. Dermatitis
b. Photosensitivity
2. Musculoskeletal manifestations
a. Generalized polymyositis
b. Arthritis
c. Arthralgia
3. Blood
a. Polyclonal gammopathy
b. Leukopenia

4. Thyroiditis
5. Pleurisy
6. Hepatitis
7. Central nervous system
   a. Seizures
   b. Apparent psychoses
8. Heart
   a. Pericarditis
   b. Valvular lesions

G. Laboratory findings in SLE
1. Demonstration of the LE cell—most reliable test in the dog
   a. Principle
      (1) The serum or plasma of patients with SLE may contain an IgG antibody to the nucleoprotein of the leukocytic nuclei.
         (a) This *in vitro* test involves subjecting the leukocytes to some trauma.
      (2) This antibody, the LE factor, causes the depolymerization of the deoxyribonucleic acid (DNA) of the nuclear chromatin of the injured leukocytes. After swelling of the nucleus, the cell ruptures, releasing a homogeneous, pink-staining mass.
      (3) When adequate IgG antideoxyribonucleoprotein (DNP) is present with complement, the altered nuclear material may be engulfed by phagocytes.
         (a) The phagocyte is usually a neutrophil, but occasionally it can be one of the other leukocytes such as a monocyte, eosinophil, basophil, lymphocyte, or plasma cell.
   b. Method
      (1) Clot method—the most consistent results are usually obtained with this method
         (a) Allow 7 to 10 ml of blood to clot and incubate at room temperature or 37°C for 2 hr.
         (b) Gently press the clot through a fine-mesh wire screen (Scientific Products) into a Petri dish or beaker.
            [1] One advantage of this method is that the fibrin remains on the screen.
         (c) Fill a Wintrobe hematocrit tube with the mashed clot and centrifuge at 2000 rpm for 15 min.
         (d) Discard the supernatant serum and prepare films from the buffy coat on either microscope slides or coverglasses.
         (e) Stain with any routine blood stain such as Wright's or Wright-Giemsa.
            [1] The LE cell mass is more prominent with new methylene blue stain than with an alcohol-fixed smear.
         (f) Scan several slides with the high power objective for suspicious cells and verify by using the oil immersion objective.
      (2) Rotary method
         (a) 5 ml of blood is placed in a heparinized tube with 5 glass beads. Rotate the tube for 30 min at room temperature.
            [1] The LE factor is inhibited by heparin in concentrations higher than 0.75 mg/10 ml.
            [2] The LE factor is inhibited by EDTA, so this anticoagulant should be avoided.
         (b) Centrifuge the blood and prepare blood films from the buffy coat.
         (c) Examine as described in the clot method.
      (3) Capillary method—recommended only when a limited amount of blood is available.
         (a) Collect blood in four or more heparinized capillary tubes and seal the red end.
         (b) Centrifuge for 5 min in a microhematocrit centrifuge.
         (c) Insert the stylet from a 20-gauge, 3-in. hypodermic needle into the capillary tube and mix the plasma and buffy coat by rotating the stylet 15 times.
            [1] The tip of the stylet should be slightly bent.
         (d) Incubate the capillary tubes at room temperature for 2 hr or at 37°C for 30 min.
            [1] Prolongation of the incubation times will not increase the yield of LE cells.
         (e) Centrifuge again as in step 2.
         (f) Break the tubes about 2 mm below the buffy coat, as the 2-mm erythrocyte layer helps to prevent loss of the buffy coat.

(g) Place the buffy coat on a glass microscope slide, avoiding an excess of plasma being delivered to the slide.
(h) Place a second slide on top of the buffy coat and make the smear by compressing gently and pulling slides away from each other at parallel planes.
(i) Stain with any conventional blood stain.

c. Interpretation
(1) LE cell
(a) Usually a neutrophil with its nucleus displaced to the cell border by a large, round mass of ingested nuclear material
[1] The color of the mass is usually magenta, lavender, or pink.
[2] The mass has lost the nuclear chromatin and appears as a uniform, homogeneous structure.
(b) Rosettes are groups of polymorphonuclear leukocytes surrounding a homogeneous nuclear mass.
[1] Highly suspicious as the LE factor but not acceptable as a positive LE test.
(c) The presence of LE cells with the simultaneous occurrence of one or more of the following disorders constitutes a diagnosis of SLE.
[1] Autoimmune hemolytic anemia—must be Coombs'-positive
[2] Thrombocytopenic purpura
[3] Rheumatoid arthritis
[4] Membranous glomerulonephritis
(2) The LE cell must be differentiated from:
(a) Tart cell—nucleophagocytosis with a monocyte phagocytizing a cell nucleus
[1] The ingested mass retains its nuclear chromatin network.
[2] The outer rim of the mass may show increased staining.
(b) Erythrophagocytosis—commonly present in autoimmune hemolytic anemia
(c) Phagocytosis of platelets
(d) Coalesced eosinophilic granules in canine blood can produce large red masses, but the nucleus will not be displaced to the cell border.

2. Antinuclear antibody (ANA) tests
a. Agglutination of coated latex particles
(1) Detects and quantitates antinucleoprotein serum factors associated with SLE
(2) Available as a commercial kit
(a) Lederle Diagnostics Systemic Lupus Erythematosus (SLE) Latex Test Kit (Lederle Laboratories)
b. Indirect immunofluorescence

3. Serum electrophoresis
a. Polyclonal type of hyperglobulinemia
(1) Increase in beta and gamma globulins

4. If autoimmune hemolytic anemia is present:
a. Blood
(1) Anemia
(2) Coombs' test positive—direct and indirect
(3) Reticulocytosis
(4) Spherocytosis
(5) Leukocytosis
b. Urine
(1) Bilirubinuria
(2) Urobilinogen—increased

5. If thrombocytopenic purpura is present:
a. Platelet count below 50,000
b. Bleeding time prolonged
c. Bone marrow—abundant megakaryocytes
d. Antiplatelet antibody present

6. If glomerulonephritis is present:
a. Proteinuria—persistent and marked
b. Nephrotic syndrome—if prolonged

(1) Proteinuria
(2) Hypoproteinemia
(3) Hypercholesterolemia
(4) Edema
c. Progressive renal failure
d. Renal biopsy—membranous glomerulonephritis
(1) Thickening of capillaries in the basement membrane
(2) Affected capillary walls have "wire loop" appearance.
(3) Not all glomeruli are equally affected.
7. If rheumatoid arthritis is present:
a. Rheumatoid factor positive
(1) Canine or feline IgG or globulin fraction reacted with latex particles.
(a) Commercially available
(b) Human reagent not suitable
b. Synovial fluid
(1) Moderate inflammatory change
(2) LE cells may be in smears.

III. Pyruvate kinase deficiency anemia

A. Occurrence
1. Basenji breed of dog
a. Simple autosomal recessive mode of inheritance
(1) Affected anemic parents—puppies are always anemic
(2) Carrier parents—puppies could be normal, anemic, or carriers
2. Man—congenital nonspherocytic hemolytic anemia

B. Erythrocyte metabolism (Fig. 13.4)
1. Energy production in the mature erythrocyte is mainly glycolytic, with 90% occurring through the Embden-Meyerhof pathway, as each mole of glucose goes to lactic acid with the net production of two moles of adenosine triphosphate (ATP).
a. Since mitochrondria are lacking in the mature erythrocyte, there is a lack of oxidative phosphorylation and only vestiges of Krebs cycle activity.
2. ATP is required for the energy-needing reactions in the erythrocyte.
a. Active cation transport across the erythrocytic membrane
(1) Sodium out of the cell
(2) Phosphorus into the cell
b. Maintains membrane deformability
c. Preserves the biconcave shape of the erythrocyte
3. Pyruvate kinase (PK)
a. PK catalyzes the phosphorylation of adenosine diphosphate (ADP) to ATP by phosphoenolpyruvate with the formation of pyruvate.
b. Pyruvate then reduces any NADH present to NAD with the formation of lactate.
c. PK deficiency, and subsequently an ATP deficiency, results in:
(1) Loss of integrity of the erythrocytic membrane
(2) Shortened erythrocytic life span
d. Leukocytes normally contain about 300 times as much PK as the erythrocytes and must be removed during assay, for in PK deficiency it is the erythrocytes that lack PK.

C. Clinical signs in the dog
1. Anemia usually develops by 2 to 7 mo of age.
2. Lethargy and decreased activity
a. Tires easily when exercised
3. Anemia is progressive—pale mucous membranes
4. Sensitive to cold

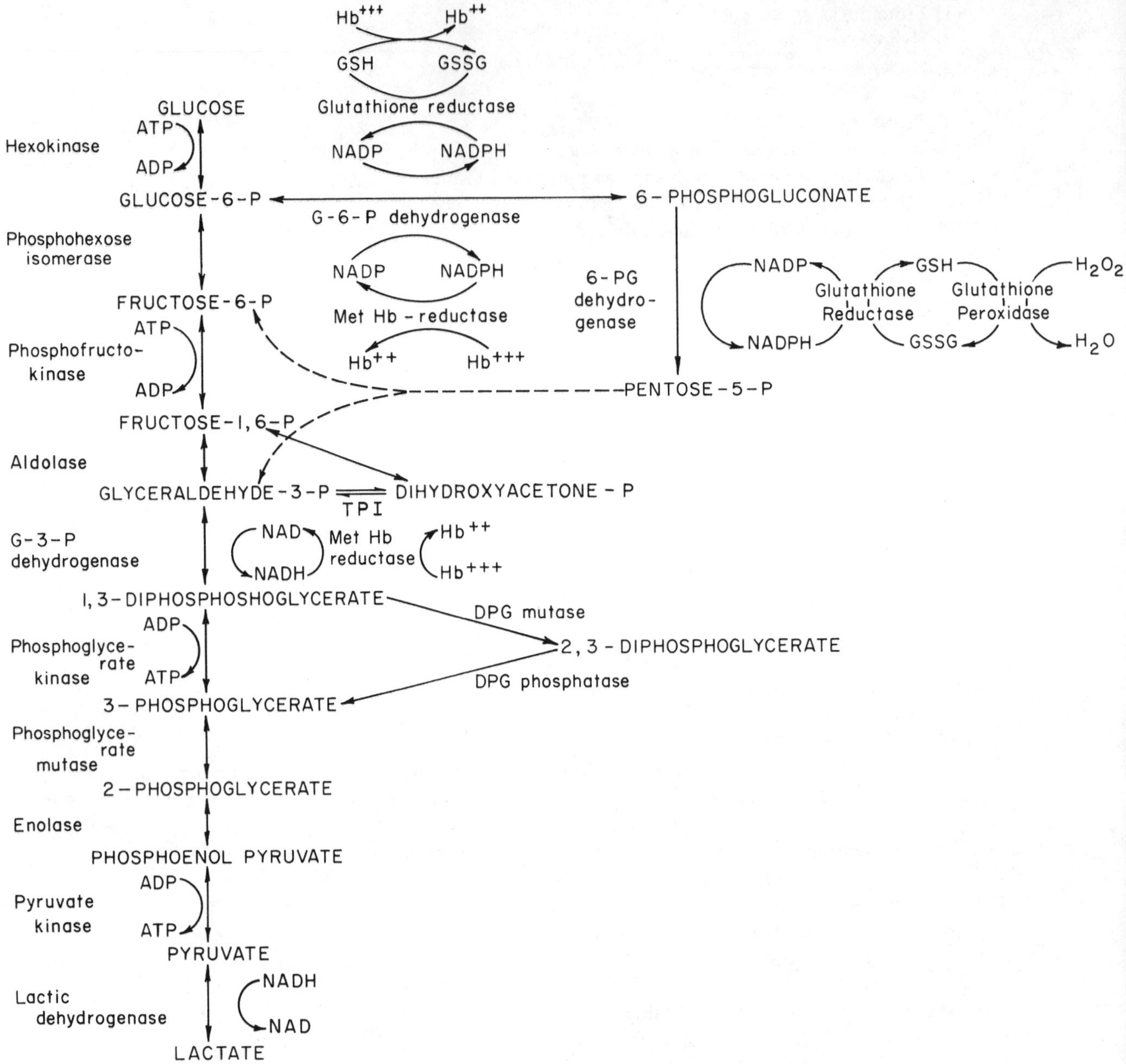

Fig. 13.4. Erythrocyte metabolism.

5. Splenomegaly—due to reticuloendothelial hyperplasia
6. Die before 2 or 3 yr of age unless repeated blood transfusions are given

D. Laboratory findings
1. Unresponsive anemia
2. PCV—15 to 30%, but as low as 5% at time of death
3. Hemoglobin—5 to 9 g
    a. No abnormalities on hemoglobin electrophoretic studies
4. Tremendous erythropoietic response to the anemia
    a. Polychromasia
    b. Metarubricytes
    c. Leptocytes
    d. Reticulocytes—tremendous; 40 to 60%

5. Macrocytic hypochromic
   a. Macrocytes are abundant, as the cells are in an immature stage.
   b. Hypochromic, because hemoglobin synthesis is incomplete in the young cell
      (1) Normally 70% of hemoglobin synthesis occurs in the reticulocyte.

IV. Anemia of chronic disorders

A. Synonyms
1. Simple chronic anemia
2. Anemia of chronic infection
3. Sideropenic anemia with reticuloendothelial siderosis

B. Etiology
1. This is a commonly encountered anemia and almost always can be expected as a complication with one of the following:
   a. Chronic inflammatory disease
      (1) Conditions regularly associated with anemia
         (a) Collagen diseases, especially rheumatoid arthritis
         (b) Ulcerative colitis
   b. Chronic infection
      (1) Almost all chronic suppurative infections will be complicated by anemia.
      (2) A sustained infection of 1 to 2 mo is required to produce the anemia.
         (a) At that point the anemia is stabilized by a balance between erythrocyte production and destruction.
   c. Necrotizing or disseminated neoplastic disease
      (1) Lymphosarcoma
      (2) Reticulum cell sarcoma
      (3) Carcinomas—especially those that are disseminated

C. Pathogenesis
1. Life span of the erythrocyte slightly to moderately decreased
2. Disturbance of iron metabolism
   a. Iron deposited in reticuloendothelial cells is not properly released to circulating transferrin and is poorly reutilized.
      (1) There is impairment of plasma transferrin iron transport to the bone marrow.
      (2) Serum iron is decreased.
      (3) Tissue iron stores are adequate or increased, as iron accumulates as ferritin in the tissues and reticuloendothelial system.
         (a) Transferrin has been shown to be sequestered around inflammatory foci.
3. Relative bone marrow failure
   a. Constitutes a major cause of the anemia, since the moderately shortened erythrocytic life span could easily be compensated for by a normal bone marrow
   b. The low serum iron impairs:
      (1) Proliferation of erythroid cells, as iron is a necessary component of several erythrocytic enzymes needed for rapid cell turnover in the bone marrow
      (2) Hemoglobin synthesis
   c. There can be failure to secrete adequate amounts of erythropoietin, as well as failure, sometimes, of the marrow to respond to erythropoietin.

D. Laboratory findings
1. The anemia is mild to moderate in intensity
   a. If the anemia is severe, additional problems contributing to the anemia should be investigated:
      (1) Blood loss from hemorrhage
      (2) Hemolysis
      (3) Renal disease

(4) Deficiency of protein
(5) Deficiency of iron
(6) Deficiency of vitamins

2. Erythrocytic indices
   a. Microcytic and hypochromic in many of the cases
   b. Normocytic and normochromic can be seen.
3. Reticulocytes are normal or slightly increased—nonregenerative anemia
4. Total leukocyte and platelet counts will depend upon the underlying disorder.
5. Serum iron is decreased.
   a. Occurs rapidly and precedes development of the anemia
   b. Essential for the diagnosis of anemia of chronic disorder
   c. Serum iron is the iron bound to transferrin, measured in micrograms/deciliter.
6. Total iron binding capacity (TIBC) is moderately decreased.
   a. TIBC is the total amount of transferrin measured as the total amount of iron it can bind, measured in micrograms/deciliter.
   b. Develops much more slowly, probably due to the longer half-life of transferrin than iron
7. Bone marrow
   a. Cellular pattern will be fairly normal.
   b. Alteration in iron content is the most important change.
      (1) Sideroblasts are decreased.
      (2) Reticuloendothelial iron is normal to increased.

E. Differential diagnosis
1. Chronic blood loss or iron malabsorption
   a. Reticuloendothelial iron is decreased.
   b. TIBC is increased.
   c. A diagnostic aid is to administer iron and reevaluate.
2. Renal impairment—bone marrow failure and shortened erythrocytic life span
   a. Blood urea nitrogen and creatinine are increased.
   b. Serum iron is normal or high.
3. Drug-induced bone marrow depression or drug-induced hemolysis
   a. Serum iron tends to be high.
4. Replacement of bone marrow by metastatic neoplastic tissue
   a. Serum iron is normal or increased.
   b. Bone marrow aspiration will detect abnormal cells.

F. Treatment
1. Should be to reduce or remove the underlying cause
2. Iron therapy will have little effect, as it will probably be sequestered in the reticuloendothelial system.
3. Transfusion is seldom necessary, as the anemia is rarely symptomatic.

8 POLYCYTHEMIA

Polycythemia is an increase above the normal in the number of erythrocytes in the circulating blood and is usually accompanied by a corresponding increase in the amount of hemoglobin and packed erythrocyte volume.

I. Relative polycythemia—the total erythrocyte mass is normal, but because the plasma volume is decreased the number of erythrocytes per unit volume of blood is increased; plasma protein concentration is increased

A. Dehydration—hemoconcentration as a result of a decrease in the volume of plasma without appreciable change in the total mass of erythrocytes

1. Loss of body fluids
   a. Vomiting
   b. Diarrhea
   c. Excessive sweating
2. Water deprivation or reduced fluid intake

B. Shift of body fluids from the plasma to the interstitial tissue
1. Shock—increasing hemoconcentration could act as a warning signal of ensuing circulatory failure
   a. Surgical shock
   b. Abdominal shock, especially in the horse—rapid onset of plasma pooling in and around the involved tissue
      (1) Intestinal torsion, intussusception, or volvulus
   c. Anaphylactic shock—increased vascular permeability with hemoconcentration
2. Burns—marked hemoconcentration as the fluid portion of the blood leaks into the tissues
3. Increased hydrostatic pressure in capillaries and veins
   a. Acute circulatory failure
   b. Increased catecholamines

C. Stress polycythemia (Gaisbock's syndrome)—chronic relative polycythemia seen mostly in the white human male and believed to be secondary to an abnormally low plasma volume
1. Most affected is the middle-aged male with a strong tendency toward obesity, hypertension, elevations of serum cholesterol and uric acid, thromboembolic disease, and arteriosclerosis.

II. Transient polycythemia—redistribution of erythrocytes within the vascular bed

A. The spleen acts as a reservoir for erythrocytes in the dog, cat, horse, and sheep and under the influence of epinephrine will contract to force the erythrocytes into the circulation; the plasma protein concentration is not affected; accompanying the erythrocyte increase is an increase in leukocytes, but without immature forms.
1. Exercise
   a. It has been suggested that the magnitude of increase in erythrocyte level in the horse stimulated by excitement or epinephrine injection is a more accurate measure of racing performance potential than the concentration of hemoglobin in the resting horse.
2. Excitement and fear
   a. Some breeds or individual dogs that become apprehensive when being examined may have abnormally increased levels of erythrocytes, PCV, and hemoglobin.
      (1) German Shepherds, Boxers, Beagles, Dachshunds, Poodles, and Chihuahuas most often exhibit a transient polycythemia.

III. Absolute polycythemia—increase in the total erythrocyte mass due to an increase in the production of erythrocytes

A. Primary
1. Polycythemia vera
   a. One of the myeloproliferative disorders, of unknown cause, characterized by an absolute increase in circulating erythrocyte mass, frequently a leukocytosis, and thrombocytosis and splenomegaly
   b. Occurrence
      (1) Dog
      (2) Cat
      (3) Cattle
      (4) Man
   c. Clinical signs—related directly or indirectly to increased erythrocyte mass and hyperviscosity of blood
      (1) Markedly reddened mucous membranes
      (2) Splenomegaly—consistently in man, variable in animals
      (3) Absence of dehydration

(4) Polydipsia and polyuria—the increased blood viscosity may activate compensatory mechanisms of the body

(5) Hemorrhagic episodes—epistaxis, hematuria, hematemesis

(a) May result from venous and capillary distention required to accommodate the increased blood volume

(b) Thrombosis may be associated with decreased velocity of blood flow, as thrombocytosis is not usually seen except in man.

(6) Neurologic or neuromuscular disorders—tissue hypoxia is the result of lowered velocity of blood flow and capillary distention

(a) Blindness

(b) Posterior weakness

(c) Circling

(d) Seizures

d. Hematologic findings

(1) Erythrocyte mass, total blood volume, and PCV increased

(2) Leukocytosis

(a) Usually seen in man

(b) Variable in animals

(3) Thrombocytosis—usually seen in man but not in animals

(4) Bone marrow—hyperplasia of the cellular elements, principally of the erythroid series

(5) Arterial oxygen saturation normal

(6) Erythrocyte half-life usually normal but shortened in the cat

(7) Accelerated plasma iron turnover rate with rapid uptake of radioactive iron by the bone marrow

(8) Erythropoietin level reduced or normal

2. Familial polycythemia—characterized by marked absolute elevation in circulating erythrocyte volume, but without leukocytosis or thrombocytosis

a. Occurrence

(1) Man

(2) Cattle—14 Jersey calves

b. Clinical signs

(1) Weakness

(2) Congestion of nasal mucosa and conjunctivae

(3) Skin, reddish cyanotic appearance

(4) Sometimes comatose or convulsions

(5) Intermittently blind

c. Hematologic findings

(1) PCV of at least 70%, hemoglobin greater than 20 g/dl

(2) Normal arterial oxygen saturation

(3) Plasma iron turnover rate increased

B. Secondary—increased stimulation of erythrocyte production characterized by an absolute erythrocytosis

1. Hypoxia—erythropoietin released in response to tissue hypoxia; arterial oxygen saturation decreased

a. High altitude acclimatization—air with low partial pressure of oxygen (PO_2)

b. Chronic pulmonary disease—most frequent cause

c. Alveolar hypoventilation—as a result of depressed respiratory center function

d. Heart disease

(1) Congenital—usually

(a) Right to left shunt

(b) Pulmonic stenosis

(c) Patent ductus arteriosus

(2) Acquired—erythrocytosis seldom occurs

e. Hemoglobinopathies—result in defective oxygen transport

(1) Methemoglobinemia

(2) Sulfhemoglobinemia

f. Physiologic in the newborn of some species during the neonatal period

(1) May be due to low oxygen content while *in utero* or when the fetal hemoglobin in the erythrocyte is being replaced by adult hemoglobin

(2) Varies with species—not usually seen in the puppy, kitten, calf, lamb, or kid

g. Cobalt toxicity—produces local hypoxia

2. Inappropriate erythropoietin or erythropoietinlike production—oxygen saturation normal; pyelogram or angiogram useful

a. Renal tumor

b. Renal vascular impairment

c. Renal cyst and hydronephrosis

d. Release of erythropoietinlike substance

(1) Cerebellar hemangioma

(2) Uterine myoma

(3) Hepatoma

IV. Differential features of polycythemia

			Secondary	
Feature	Relative	Polycythemia vera	Hypoxia	Renal disease
Red cell volume	Normal	Increased	Increased	Increased
Plasma volume	Decreased	Usually normal	Normal to decreased	Variable
Leukocyte count	Increased	Man—increased Animals—variable	Normal	Usually normal
Arterial oxygen saturation	Normal	Normal	Decreased	Normal
Erythropoietin level	Normal	Decreased to normal	Increased	Increased

14 LEUKOCYTE AND ITS DISORDERS

A ABNORMAL LEUKOCYTES

Basket cell: A degenerative cell that has ruptured and in which the cell nucleus appears as a pale-staining smear without prescribed form or shape; also called a smudged cell.

Charcot-Leyden crystal: Crystal found in secretions from sites where eosinophils are present in abundance, e.g., bronchial secretions in an asthmatic patient or stools associated with intestinal parasitism; derived from disintegration products of eosinophilic leukocytes.

Chediak-Higashi syndrome: Giant eosinophilic granules in the neutrophils that have been shown to be abnormal lysosomes. Described in four species: man, cattle, mink, and mice.

Döhle bodies: Small (1 to 2 microns) round or oval, gray-blue bodies in the cytoplasm of neutrophils; derived from incomplete utilization of ribonucleic acid in maturation of the cytoplasm. Seen in patients showing the toxic effect of systemic disease. Most commonly seen in the cat, occasionally in the dog and other animals.

Erythrophagocytosis: Erythrocytes engulfed by phagocytic cells such as monocytes; commonly seen in autoimmune hemolytic anemia and blood parasitism such as hemobartonellosis.

Giant neutrophils: Defective neutrophil maturation; may be due to delay in cytoplasmic maturation with failure of the cell to divide at the proper time while the nucleus continues its maturation. Seen in some severe inflammatory diseases in the cat, such as the recovery phase of panleukopenia, and occasionally in extreme leukocytosis.

Hypersegmented neutrophil: A segmented neutrophil with more than the normal number of lobes in the nucleus, usually more than 4. Indicates retention of the neutrophil in the circulation beyond its normal life span. May be seen in a variety of conditions. Corticosteroids of stress prevent diapedesis of cells, and cells continue to age within the circulation; may be seen in chronic diseases, as an artifact in old blood containing anticoagulants, in vitamin B_{12} and folic acid deficiencies, in myeloproliferative disease, and in autoimmune hemolytic anemia.

Immunocyte (reactive lymphocyte, virocyte): Lymphocyte with dark blue cytoplasm and a mature nucleus; indicates an immune response, as the cells are transformed from lymphocytes by an antigen to synthesize immune globulins.

Lupus erythematosus (LE) cell: A neutrophil (usually) that is distended by an intracytoplasmic, homogeneous, red-purple body, with the lobes of its nucleus compressed at the periphery of the mass.

Mast cell: Connective tissue cell in which the basophilic granules normally stain metachromatically. The cytoplasmic granules are usually large, may vary from large to minute rounded bodies, and tend to be uniform in size in a given cell. The granules seldom overlie the round, oval, or occasionally indented nucleus.

Pelger-Hüet anomaly: A rare, hereditary condition associated with a myeloproliferative disorder where neutrophils lack the usual nuclear segmentation: cytoplasm of the neutrophils and eosinophils appears mature, while the nuclei are nonsegmented and deeply stained due to greater than normal condensation of chromatin. Occurs in dog, man, and rabbits.

Plasma cell (plasmacyte): The nucleus has eccentric location of a round or oval nucleus that has extremely coarse chromatin. The chromatin stains deeply and is arranged similar to the spokes of a wheel. The cytoplasm is abundant, dark blue, and characterized by a perinuclear area of lighter staining. Vacuoles are often present. The cytoplasm contains gamma globulin and is shed into the lymph as antibodies.

Normally present in lymph nodes, connective tissue, and bone marrow. Not normally seen in peripheral blood, but may appear occasionally.

Pyknotic nuclei: Nuclear material becomes clumped and compressed. Degeneration of the nucleus occurs in the nucleus of the metarubricyte, which appears as a homogeneous dark blue structure, and in leukocytes kept too long in anticoagulant.

Tart cell: Nucleophagocytosis is produced by the phagocytosis of a nucleus (usually a lymphocyte) by a monocyte. The ingested nucleus usually retains some characteristic nuclear structure. It may be found in many conditions. Their significance is not entirely known. It is important to differentiate from the LE cell.

Toxic granulation: Neutrophils contain darker purple and coarser granules than normal. At times the cytoplasm is basophilic and vacuolated. Seen in severe infections and other toxic states that interfere with normal cytoplasmic maturation and thus inhibit the normal transformation of granules. Can be mimicked by overstaining.

Toxic neutrophil: Contains toxic granules, small to medium-sized vacuoles, and/or basophilic cytoplasm. Seen in severe infections, toxemia, and acidotic patients.

B LEUKEMIAS, LYMPHOMAS, AND MYELOPROLIFERATIVE DISORDERS

I. Terms

A. Leukemia—generalized, neoplastic, malignant proliferation of one of the leukocytic tissues (bone marrow, lymphoid tissue, reticuloendothelial system, and plasma cell system). The term is generally applied if the neoplastic cells are present at some time in the circulating blood.

1. Leukemia is not an intrinsic blood disease, for the blood is merely a moving stream interposed between the abnormal blood-forming tissues and the tissues in which the proliferating cells settle.

a. The blood findings may be inconsistent in reflecting the status of the proliferating tissue in the form of abnormal counts or cell types.

B. Lymphosarcoma—neoplasia of the lymphoid system

1. A variety of different terms have been applied to what is substantially a single disease: leukosis; lymphatic, lymphogenous, or lymphoid leukemia; malignant lymphoma; or Hodgkin's disease.

a. Some investigators restrict the term to lymphoid neoplasms that are unicentric in origin and spread by metastasis and invasiveness.

C. Malignant lymphoma—lymphoid malignancy characterized by multicentric origin and enlargement of many or all of the lymph nodes of the body

1. When the term multicentric is applied to an end stage seen at necropsy, it may be difficult to prove simultaneous origin in more than one anatomical site.

D. Reticulum cell sarcoma—neoplastic proliferation of reticulum cells of lymph nodes or other reticuloendothelial tissues resulting in tumor formation and infiltration of various tissues

E. Lymphoma—in the broadest sense, lymphoma is used to designate both solid tumors (lymphosarcoma) or leukemias of the lymphatic system

F. Reticuloendotheliosis—myeloproliferative disorder of the cat characterized by immature, undifferentiated (reticuloendothelial) cells in the blood and bone marrow, which are probably early erythroid precursor cells

G. Mast cell leukemia—a malignant proliferation of connective tissue cells rather than hematopoietic cells. In its systemic form, neoplastic mast cells are in the blood and bone marrow and have been misinterpreted as basophilic leukemia in some cases.

H. Granulocytic leukemia—malignant proliferation of neutrophils, eosinophils, and/or basophils
 1. Other terms by which granulocytic leukemia is known are myelogenous, myeloid, or myelocytic.

II. Classification of leukemia

Leukocyte count and stage of maturity	Cell type
Leukemic	Granulocytic
Subleukemic	Neutrophilic—usually
Aleukemic	Eosinophilic
	Basophilic
	Lymphocytic
	Lymphoblastic
	Lymphocytic
	Monocytic—related to reticulum cell sarcoma
	Plasmocytic—multiple myeloma
	Erythrocytic
	Stem cell—too primitive to identify

A. According to total leukocyte count and stage of cell maturity
 1. Leukemic—high leukocyte counts
 2. Subleukemic—normal leukocyte counts, but with abnormal differential counts showing primitive cells
 3. Aleukemic—normal total leukocyte counts and no abnormal or immature cells in the blood smear; usually seen during period of remission or treatment of one of the other types, or diagnosed by bone marrow aspiration

B. According to the type of proliferating cell observed in the blood smear, bone marrow, or lymphoid tissue
 1. Granulocytic—cell type derived from myeloid tissue
  a. Eosinophilic and basophilic can be included with granulocytic leukemia
 2. Lymphocytic—the blood picture may represent a generalized proliferation of leukocytic tissue characterized by a blood dyscrasia with secondary changes in the lymphoid tissue, or the blood picture may represent invasion of the blood by localized tumor cells (lymphosarcoma)
 3. Monocytic leukemia—associated with reticulum cell sarcoma
 4. Plasmocytic leukemia—the proliferating plasma cell is associated with multiple myeloma
 5. Stem cell leukemia—the proliferating cell is too primitive to be identified

C. According to duration of process—acute or chronic
 1. Although these terms are used in human leukemias, corresponding types cannot be transposed to the conditions described in animals.

III. Diagnosis of lymphoid malignancies

A. Diagnosis of feline lymphosarcoma
 1. History and physical examination
  a. General clinical signs—anemia, lethargy, weight loss, anorexia
  b. Alimentary form—vomiting, diarrhea, constipation
   (1) Enlarged mesenteric lymph nodes, intestine, spleen, and liver and enlarged irregular kidneys
  c. Anterior mediastinal form—dyspnea, coughing, choking, cyanosis
   (1) Noncompressible thorax with large anterior mediastinal mass
   (2) Pleural effusion
  d. Multicentric
   (1) Liver infiltrated—icterus, hepatomegaly

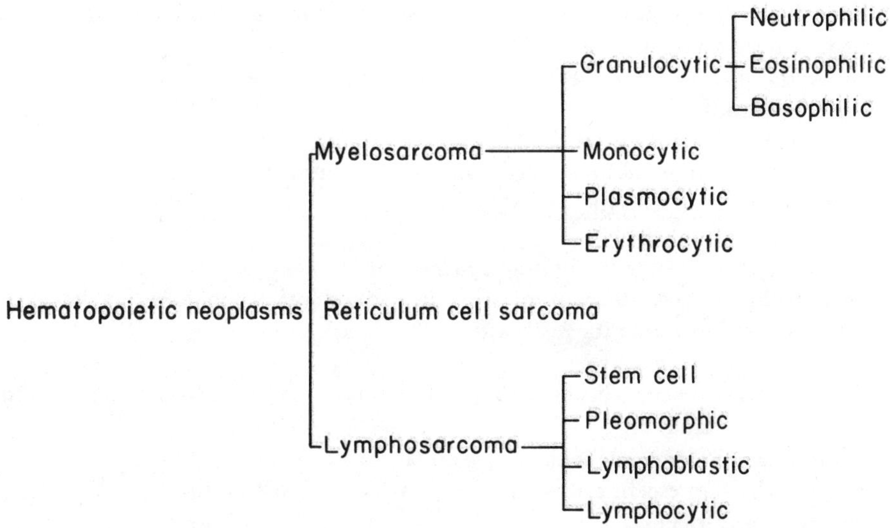

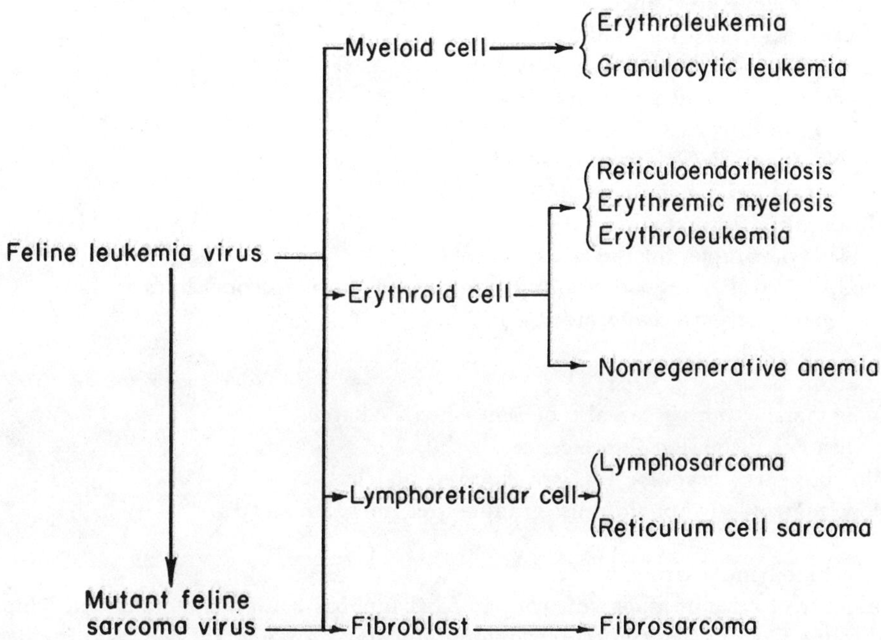

(2) Kidney infiltrated—uremia, large and irregular kidney
(3) Spleen infiltrated—splenomegaly
(4) Peripheral lymph nodes—involved only 10 to 20% of time

2. Hematology
   a. Anemia—the most consistent feature and seen in at least 50% of the cases
      (1) Normocytic normochromic and may be nonregenerative
      (2) Nucleated erythrocytes may vary from zero to more than 100—usually metarubricytes
      (3) PCV usually 10 to 20%
   b. Leukocytic picture
      (1) Absolute leukocytosis—30% of the cases
      (2) Leukopenia—10% of the cases (most likely to occur when sarcomatous masses are forming)
      (3) Absolute lymphocytopenia—40% of the cases
      (4) Leukemia—25 to 40% of the cases, as it is influenced by the stage of the disease; may have only a few immature lymphoid cells, which are more likely to appear in the peripheral blood in the terminal stages

(5) Absolute lymphocytosis of more than 14,000/microliter is a basic indication for a tentative diagnosis of lymphosarcoma.

c. Thrombocytes may be decreased in number and may vary in size.

3. Bone marrow aspiration

a. More than 15% lymphocytes in the bone marrow suggests a tentative diagnosis of lymphosarcoma.

(1) If the marrow is hypoplastic, a high lymphocyte count may indicate only that there is depression of the erythroid and leukocytic precursors.

4. Cytology

a. Pleural effusions—examine for immature forms of lymphocytes

b. Peritoneal lavage—inject 10 to 20 ml of sterile saline solution, massage the visceral organs gently, aspirate fluid, and examine for neoplastic cells.

5. Lymph node aspiration or biopsy

a. A normal lymph node contains 5 to 25% lymphoblasts, so blasts in excess of this maximum could suggest lymphosarcoma.

6. Immunofluorescent test for feline leukemia virus (FeLV)

a. Specificity of the fluorescent antibody detection of the FeLV group

(1) Diseases caused by FeLV

(a) Lymphosarcoma—90%

(b) Nonregenerative anemia—40%

(2) Diseases associated with FeLV

(a) Myeloproliferative disease—95%

(b) Feline infectious peritonitis—50%

(3) FeLV in healthy cats

(a) No known FeLV exposure—0.1%

(b) Known FeLV exposure—35%

(4) Multicentric fibrosarcoma—100%

b. Submission of samples for the test

(1) Send three unfixed, good quality blood smears on microscope slides to:
National Veterinary Laboratory, Inc.
P.O. Box 239
Franklin Lakes, N.J. 07417

(2) Bone marrow smears can also be sent when available.

c. Cells with FeLV showing fluorescence

(1) Blood smears—granulocytes, lymphocytes, platelets

(2) Bone marrow—lymphoid cells, granulocytes, megakaryocytes

B. Diagnosis of canine lymphosarcoma

1. In the majority of cases of malignant lymphoma (lymphosarcoma), the malignant lymphoid cells are confined to the fixed tissues and there is seldom invasion of malignant cells into the peripheral blood.

a. The blood picture in this aleukemic type may vary from leukopenia to a marked leukocytosis.

(1) The mean total leukocyte count is in the high normal range with a mild left shift and a moderate monocytosis.

(a) The mean lymphocyte values are within the normal range; in 20% of the cases there can be a lymphocytosis, while a frank lymphopenia is seen in 25% of the cases.

(2) Occasional neoplastic lymphocytes may appear sporadically in about 50% of the cases and are usually detected only after thorough examination.

(a) These cells may be classified as atypical if a nucleolus or nucleolar ring is present.

(b) Other morphologic features of atypical lymphocytes may include an irregular shape, deep blue and/or granular cytoplasm, and a diffuse nuclear pattern.

b. Lymphocytic leukemic leukemia is seen in 3 to 6% of canine cases of lymphosarcoma, and counts may be in excess of 75,000/microliter.

(1) Almost all the cells will be of lymphoid origin, with the cell maturity varying from lymphoblasts to mature cells.

(a) The mature lymphocytes are frequently atypical in appearance and easily smudged.

2. A thrombocytopenia is not a constant feature, being seen in about 10% of the cases, but hemorrhages are rare.
3. About 50% of the dogs will have protein values lower than corresponding normal dogs in the same age bracket, with the low values ranging from 4.5 to 6.5 g/dl. Decreased synthesis by lymphoreticular tissue is believed to be responsible.
4. Anemia is a feature in one-third of the canine lymphosarcoma cases and is mild in severity.
5. Bone marrow examination seldom yields evidence of neoplastic invasion.
6. Aspiration or biopsy and an impression smear of a lymph node with lymphadenopathy is the most helpful diagnostic procedure.
   a. Most or all the cells will be the large lymphoblastic type.
7. High serum calcium level due to pseudohyperparathyroidism may be present.

IV. Myeloproliferative disorders—include a complex of diseases characterized by unrestrained, purposeless proliferation and incomplete differentiation of a primitive mesenchymal cell of the bone marrow, which may involve one or more of the cell lines in defective maturation, either singly, in combination, or sequentially

A. Cat
1. Stages of progression
   a. Reticuloendotheliosis—proliferation of immature, undifferentiated cells in the blood and bone marrow with no evidence of a progressive maturation toward any cell type that would justify naming the cells. Results of electron microscopy study of cells in this disorder indicate that the proliferating primitive cells have surface specializations (coated vesicles) characteristic of erythroid cells.
   b. Erythremic myelosis—differentiation is present to a sufficient degree to suggest a cell line in the erythrocytic series, but without histologic evidence of neoplasia
   c. Erythroleukemia—a combination of proliferating erythremic and granulocytic primitive cells
   d. Granulocytic leukemia—abnormal proliferation of granulocytes
   e. Myelofibrosis—as a terminal event, the abnormal proliferation of the cells in the bone marrow may involve the fibroblast and the supporting connective tissue cell, leading to myelofibrosis

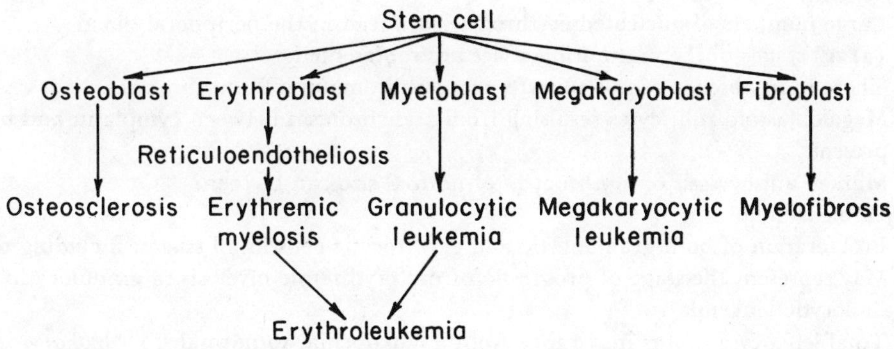

2. Etiology
   a. A C-type virus, similar to the feline leukemia virus, has been demonstrated in the bone marrow of some cats with reticuloendotheliosis, erythremic myelosis, and erythroleukemia
3. Clinical signs
   a. Rapid weight loss
   b. Anorexia
   c. Pallor
   d. Icterus—occasionally; from massive liver involvement; slight to profound
   e. Duration of the conditions usually unknown
      (1) May vary from a few days to several weeks
      (2) A rare case may have a long period of remission before relapse.
   f. Temperature may vary from normal to 106°F.
   g. Splenomegaly—moderate to severe; consistently seen

h. Hepatomegaly—consistently seen
i. Lymphadenopathy—mild; occasionally seen
j. Increased respiratory and heart rates
k. Listless

4. Blood picture
   a. Reticuloendotheliosis
      (1) Total leukocyte count ranges from leukopenia to a marked leukocytosis with an average of 22,000/microliter.
      (2) Profound, unresponsive anemia—average about 10% PCV
      (3) The proliferating, abnormal, undifferentiated cells constitute up to 55% (average 20 to 23%) of the circulating nucleated cells.
         (a) Size—12 to 16 microns
         (b) Shape—round to ovoid
         (c) Nucleus—eccentric, round, large
            [1] Chromatin—clumped or finely dispersed
            [2] Nucleoli—commonly absent, but may contain one or more that are greyish blue in color
         (d) Cytoplasm
            [1] Not abundant
            [2] Medium to dark blue
            [3] Azurophilic granules—clusters or diffusely scattered, when present
            [4] Pale perinuclear area
      (4) Abnormal erythrocyte precursors (megaloblastoid cells) are seen in small numbers.
         (a) Large size (often up to 20 microns)
         (b) Presence of nucleus too immature for the age of the cytoplasm
         (c) Presence of hemoglobin-tinged cytoplasm in a cell that otherwise would not have been classified as an erythrocytic precursor
         (d) Cytoplasmic pseudopod projections sometimes seen
      (5) Lack of reticulocytes is a common finding.
   b. Erythremic myelosis
      (1) Large numbers of nucleated erythrocytes are seen in the peripheral blood.
         (a) All stages of the maturation series are represented.
      (2) There is an absence of reticulocytes or polychromatophilic erythrocytes.
      (3) Megaloblastoid rubricytes resulting from asynchronism between cytoplasm and nucleus may be present.
      (4) Marked anisocytosis or erythrocytes of normal size can be seen.
   c. Erythroleukemia
      (1) Proliferation of both granulocytic and erythrocytic cells in all stages, including the blast form
      (2) May represent the stage of progression from erythremic myelosis to granulocytic leukemia
   d. Granulocytic leukemia
      (1) Total leukocyte counts may range from a leukopenia, to normal, to a leukocytosis of 50,000/microliter or more.
         (a) Often there is a persistent leukocytosis with morphologically abnormal and immature cells.
            [1] Cells may be as primitive as the myeloblast, progranulocyte, and myelocyte.
            [2] Giant forms with odd-shaped nuclei or cells with lack of synchrony between maturation of the cytoplasm and nucleus may be present.
               [a] The young, giant forms can easily be confused with young monocytes.
      (2) Anemia is a common manifestation, with nucleated erythrocytes, but seldom showing reticulocytes.
      (3) Differentiation from leukemoid reaction resulting from infections
         (a) May result in a neutrophilic leukocytosis of over 100,000/microliter, but most of the neutrophils are mature forms, bands, or metamyelocytes
   e. Eosinophilic leukemia—rare variant of granulocytic leukemia
      (1) Total leukocyte count can exceed 100,000/microliter
      (2) Neutrophilic leukocytosis, with a left shift

(3) At intervals, more than 50% of leukocytes are eosinophils.
(a) Cell stage can vary from mature to myelocytes.
(b) A few will be abnormally large with odd-shaped nuclei.
(4) Anemia

B. Dog
1. Granulocytic leukemia
a. Occurrence—uncommon
(1) A tendency to involve young dogs
b. Clinical signs—vary, depending upon the extent and type of tissue involved
(1) Progressive weight loss
(2) Progressive weakness and depression
(3) Fever variable
(4) Vomiting
(5) Diarrhea
(6) Anemia
(7) Lymphadenopathy—slight to moderate
(8) Splenomegaly
(9) Hepatomegaly
c. Blood picture
(1) Cell line
(a) Neutrophilic type usually seen
(b) Basophilic type rare—only 5 cases reported
(c) Eosinophilic type could occur, but has not been reported
(d) All granulocytic types involved in some cases
(2) The total leukocyte count may vary from normal to several hundred thousand per microliter, and may be a problem in differentiating from a leukemoid reaction.
(3) All stages of granulocytes may appear in the blood and bone marrow.
(a) Myelocytes and metamyelocytes have a tendency to predominate.
(b) Unless accompanied by more mature cell types, it may be difficult to distinguish the primitive cells from lymphoblasts or monoblasts, unless the peroxidase reaction is used.
[1] Numerous granules are evident in all granulocytes, from the progranulocyte to the mature cell.
[2] The myeloblast does not have granules.
(c) Degenerative changes develop rapidly in blood specimens.
[1] Smudge easily
[2] Vacuolization of the cytoplasm
[3] Shrinkage of the cell and pyknotic nuclei
(4) Marked myelophthisic anemia is common from myeloid proliferation that interferes with erythrocyte production.
(5) Thrombocytopenia—terminal stages
d. Extramedullary hematopoiesis in lymph nodes, spleen, and liver
(1) Large numbers of granulocytes appear in various stages of maturation.
2. Erythremic myelosis
a. Occurrence—only 1 case reported in the dog
b. Blood picture—marked refractory anemia, no reticulocytosis
c. Bone marrow—maturation arrest of erythroid cells

15 THROMBOCYTOPENIA

I. Platelet numbers

A. The normal range is from 200,000 to 500,000/microliter of blood.
   1. In spite of the wide normal range, the number of platelets in circulation in individual animals is relatively constant.

B. Purpura, hemorrhage, prolonged bleeding time, and delayed clot retraction:
   1. Occur commonly when the number is below 10,000/microliter
   2. May occur when the count is between 40,000 and 70,000/microliter

II. Clinical signs

A. Petechiation and purpura will appear in areas where pressure is placed on blood vessels.
   1. Oral mucous membranes
   2. Ventral thoracic area and abdomen
   3. Inner thighs

B. Hemorrhaging may occur into the:
   1. Intestinal tract
   2. Urogenital tract
   3. Respiratory tract
   4. Brain

C. Scleral or retinal hemorrhages can occur.

III. Causes

A. Caused by decreased platelet production from megakaryocytes in the bone marrow
   1. Aplastic anemia—associated with leukopenia and anemia
      a. Bracken fern poisoning
      b. Ionizing radiation
   2. Bone marrow infiltration
      a. Leukemia
      b. Myelofibrosis
      c. Systemic fungal infection
   3. Ionizing radiation—decrease is preceded by lymphopenia and granulocytopenia
   4. Drugs that act on platelet production
      a. Estrogens—produce destruction of hemopoietic elements in the bone marrow. Initial response is thrombocytosis, followed by thrombocytopenia in 12 to 14 days from administration. A leukocytosis is followed by a leukopenia and a gradual anemia. Dogs are much more sensitive than man or primates.
         (1) Estradiol cyclopentylpropionate (ECP)—more rapid; is at least ten times more potent than diethylstilbestrol
         (2) Stilbestrol
      b. Thiazide diuretics
      c. Myelosuppressive drugs
         (1) Adriamycin
         (2) Alkylating agents
         (3) Antipurines

(4) Antimyrimadines
(5) Bleomycin
(6) L-asparaginase

5. Viral infections—the megakaryocytes provide an ideal site for viral replication; can affect vascular endothelium and platelets
   a. Equine infectious anemia
   b. Live measles vaccine in the dog
6. Rickettsial infections
   a. Ehrlichiosis (tropical canine pancytopenia)

B. Caused by enhanced platelet destruction
1. Nonimmune
   a. Infection
   b. Disseminated intravascular coagulation
      (1) Associated with low levels of fibrinogen, prothrombin, factor V, and factor VIII
      (2) Associated with increased fibrinogen degradation products (FDP's)
   c. Drug-induced idiosyncratic thrombocytopenia and pancytopenia
      (1) Antibacterial agents—isoniazide, sulfonamides
      (2) Antibiotics—chloramphenicol, streptomycin
      (3) Anticonvulsant drugs
      (4) Antirheumatic drugs
      (5) Tranquilizers—chlorpromazine, meprobamate, promazine
      (6) Miscellaneous—chlorothiazide, quinicrine, quinidine, acetaminophen
2. Immunologically mediated—the agent sensitizes the platelet and attaches itself as a hapten; the combination stimulates antibodies
   a. Primary
      (1) Idiopathic thrombocytopenic purpura (ITP)—cause unknown
   b. Secondary
      (1) Autoimmune hemolytic anemia
      (2) Systemic lupus erythematosus (SLE)
      (3) Virus—the virus adheres to the platelet and the antibodies are formed against the virus-platelet complex
         (a) Live virus vaccine—can be the cause
      (4) Drug-induced
         (a) Types of action (Fig. 15.1)

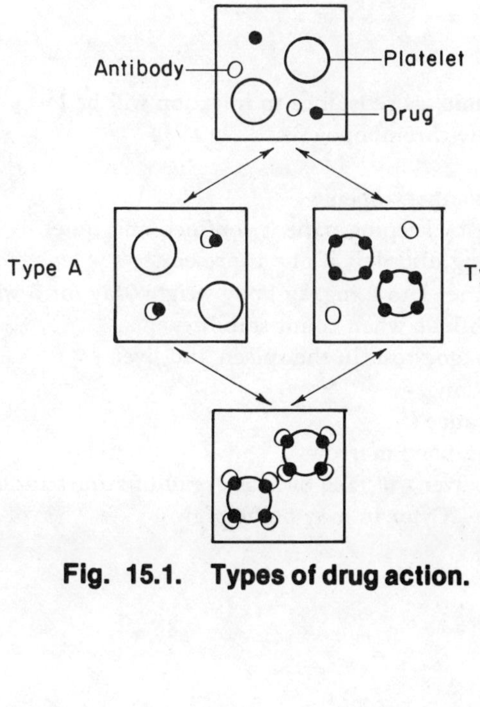

Fig. 15.1. Types of drug action.

[1] There is a chance affinity between the antigen (drug)-antibody complex and the membrane of the platelet in the immunological reaction, with the platelet acting as an "innocent bystander" (type A).

[2] The platelets are initially coated by the antigen (drug), which may act as a hapten when attached to a protein, and this combines with an antibody (type B).

(5) Lymphosarcoma—possible failure of neoplastic lymphocytes to recognize "self"

C. Caused by sequestration of platelets
   1. Endotoxin—leukopenia and thrombocytopenia develop rapidly due to aggregation and sequestration in the spleen, liver, and lungs.
      a. Salmonellosis and other gram-negative bacteria
   2. Hypersplenism—characterized by:
      a. Reduction in platelets, erythrocytes, or granulocytes
      b. Splenomegaly—increases the size of the platelet pool in the organ
      c. Cellular marrow indicating adequate marrow compensation in response to the reduction in cells
      d. Correction of the cytopenia by splenectomy
   3. Hypothermia

D. Caused by loss of platelets
   1. Massive hemorrhage

IV. Diagnostic tests

A. Platelet counts—reduced
   1. Direct—counting on a hemocytometer or in an automatic electronic counter
   2. Indirect—the number of platelets per oil immersion field can be estimated on a blood smear; 4 to 6 platelets or more per field is normal

B. Abnormal clot retraction—could be reduced number or abnormal platelet function
C. Prolonged bleeding time—could be due to platelet number, abnormal function, or vascular problem
D. Bone marrow aspiration—to determine if megakaryocytes are present
E. Platelet factor III test—to verify antiplatelet activity; has been characterized as an immunoglobulin in the gamma globulin fraction
F. Coombs' test and LE prep—the thrombocytopenia is frequently associated with these autoimmune conditions

V. Treatment

A. Estrogen toxicity
   1. Blood transfusions
   2. Antibiotics—if very leukopenic, as resistance to infection will be low
   3. Corticosteroids may stimulate thrombopoiesis.

B. Immunologically mediated thrombocytopenia
   1. Control or prevent bleeding by keeping patient confined and quiet.
   2. Detect and correct underlying disorder, if one is present.
   3. Glucocorticoids—prednisolone: 1 to 2 mg/kg body weight/day for 2 wk, then low maintenance dose of 2.5 to 5 mg/animal/day; discontinue when count stabilizes
      a. Suppressing effect on phagocytosis in the spleen and liver
      b. Inhibits antibody formation
      c. Enhances capillary resistance
      d. Thrombopoietic effect on bone marrow
   4. Splenectomy—if refractory; liver will take over as organ of sequestration
   5. Immunosuppressive therapy—Cytoxan may be helpful

6. Fresh whole blood transfusions—given within 12 hr of collection
7. Platelet transfusion
    a. Centrifuge whole blood in acid citrate dextrose at 1500 rpm for 3 to 5 min or 800 rpm for 10 to 15 min and administer platelet-rich plasma to the patient.
    b. Repeat in 3 to 4 days if platelets are not responding.

16 HEMOSTATIC DISORDERS

I. Hemostatic mechanism—hemostasis is a complex mechanism composed of a progression of physical and biochemical changes initiated by injury to the tissues and blood vessels and terminating in the transformation of fluid blood into a solid clot that seals the vascular endothelium. The three aspects of the hemostatic apparatus are (1) the blood vessel, (2) platelets, and (3) blood coagulation factors. (See Fig. 16.1.)

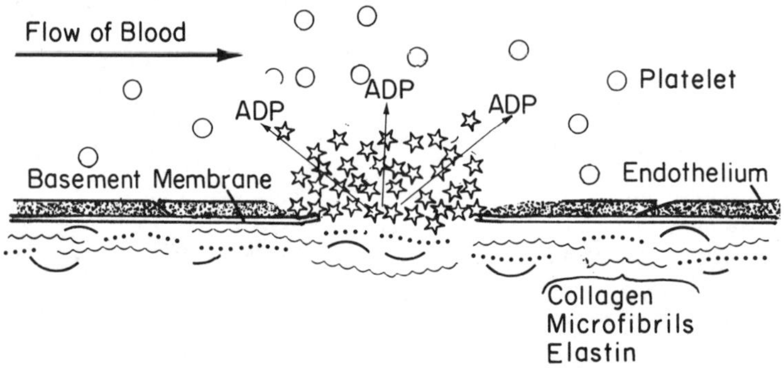

Fig. 16.1. Hemostatic mechanism.

A. Normal hemostatic sequence
   1. Vascular phase
      a. Vasoconstriction of the vessel wall
      b. Endothelial adherence
      c. Pressure of escaped blood in the surrounding tissue
   2. Platelets
      a. Platelets accumulate immediately at the site of blood vessel injury that is sufficient to expose the subendothelial structures to the flow of blood.
      b. Adhesion of platelets to the exposed basement membrane, collagen fibers, and microfibrils is the primary phase of hemostasis.
         (1) Platelets are transformed in shape from a disk to a sphere.
         (2) The interaction of platelets with subendothelial structures releases platelet internal constituents.
            (a) Adenosine diphosphate (ADP)
            (b) Serotonin
            (c) Histamine
            (d) Adenosine triphosphate (ATP)
         (3) Phospholipid (platelet factor 3) is released from platelets when activated by substances such as ADP, collagen, and thrombin. Although the exact nature of PF-3 is disputed, it is involved in blood coagulation, but not in the primary arrest of bleeding.
      c. Platelet aggregation is mediated by the release of ADP from the mass of platelets.
         (1) The process is self-perpetuating, for as more platelets aggregate, more ADP is released and the platelet mass becomes larger.
      d. Hemostatic plug formation is a mass of platelets sealing the blood vessel with a loose plug to stop the bleeding.
         (1) This primary hemostatic plug is measured by the bleeding time test in the skin or mucous membrane.

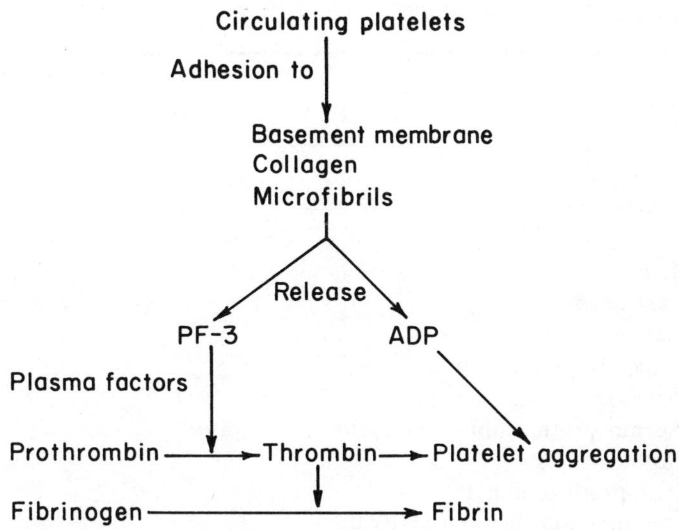

3. Plasma coagulation factors
   a. Two coagulation mechanism systems
      (1) Extrinsic system—tissue or extravascular
         (a) Active system, especially in animals, as it helps to promote speed of reaction
         (b) The extrinsic system consists of:
            [1] Tissue thromboplastin—factor III
            [2] Proconvertin—factor VII
            [3] Factors common to both systems
               [a] Factor X—Stuart factor
               [b] Factor V—proaccelerin
               [c] Prothrombin—factor II
               [d] Fibrinogen—factor I
               [e] Fibrin stabilizing factor—factor XIII
      (2) Intrinsic system—intravascular
         (a) The intrinsic system consists of:
            [1] Hageman factor—factor XII
            [2] Plasma thromboplastin antecedent—factor XI
            [3] Christmas factor—factor IX
            [4] Antihemophilic factor—factor VIII
            [5] Factors common to both systems
   b. Prothrombin is converted to thrombin through a sequential activation of clotting factors within the circulating blood.
      (1) The factors are activated through the extrinsic system or through the intrinsic system.
   c. Thrombin converts fibrinogen to fibrin.
      (1) Fibrin consolidates the platelet plug by a fibrin network around the plug and contracts over it to form a stable clot.
   d. To prevent the process from continuing and causing a complete occlusive thrombus, it is necessary to stimulate anticoagulant methods of the blood and also to activate the fibrinolytic mechanism, which will eventually dissolve the clot.
      (1) The forces for hemostasis and dissolution of the clot should be in dynamic equilibrium, otherwise there will be bleeding or excessive thrombus formation.
   e. The endothelium of the vessel wall grows over the fibrin plug; the fibrin is gradually converted to collagen, contracting until only a small scar marks the site of injury.

B. Blood coagulation factors and synonyms

International classification	Synonyms	Produced in the liver	Require vitamin K for synthesis
I	Fibrinogen	+	
II	Prothrombin	+	+
III	Tissue thromboplastin		
IV	Calcium		
V	Proaccelerin	+	
	Labile factor		
	Accelerator globulin		
VII	Proconvertin	+	+
	Serum prothrombin conversion accelerator		
	Stable factor		
	Autoprothrombin I		
VIII	Antihemophilic factor (AHF)		
	Antihemophilic globulin		
	Platelet cofactor I		
	Plasma thromboplastic factor A		
IX	Christmas factor	+	+
	Plasma thromboplastin component (PTC)		
	Platelet cofactor II		
	Autoprothrombin II		
	Plasma thromboplastic factor B		
X	Stuart factor	+	+
	Stuart-Prower factor		
XI	Plasma thromboplastin antecedent (PTA)	+	
XII	Hageman factor		
XIII	Fibrin stabilizing factor (FSF)	+	
	Laki-Lorand factor		
	Fibrinase		

C. Blood coagulation mechanism

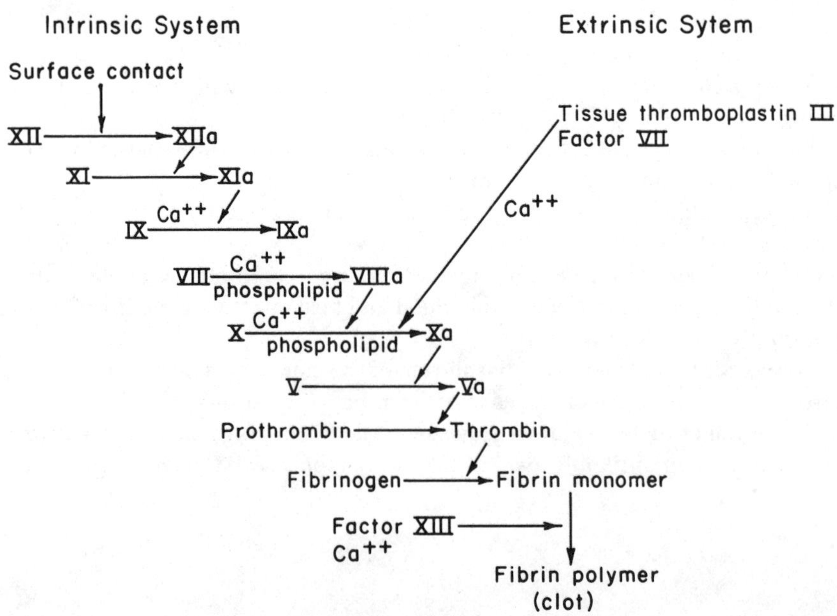

1. Simplified scheme of blood coagulation
   a. Stage I: thromboplastingenesis—3 to 5 min
   b. Stage II: thrombin formation—8 to 15 sec
   c. Stage III: fibrin formation—under 1 min
   d. Stage IV: fibrinolysis—variable

II. Clinical evaluation—since bleeding problems can be either inherited, acquired, or both, the initial approach to the successful differential diagnosis of a bleeding disorder must begin with a complete history and a thorough physical examination

A. History
1. Is the bleeding tendency pathological; i.e., is the amount and duration of bleeding not in proportion to the degree of injury from trauma or surgery?
   a. Prolonged bleeding following venipuncture, simple tooth extraction, tail docking, ear cropping, or other forms of surgery
2. Time of onset and duration of hemorrhagic phenomena and their possible relationship to:
   a. Age of patient
      (1) Young animals
         (a) More likely to have inherited than acquired problems
         (b) Newborn puppies have low prothrombin values and may have hemorrhagic lesions in the mouth, subcutaneous tissue, and intraperitoneal area.
         (c) Death can occur from umbilical vessel hemorrhage into the peritoneal cavity when the umbilical cord has been severed too short.
         (d) Number of littermates affected and sex and ratio of affected animals in litter—important in inherited and sex-linked coagulation defects
      (2) Mature animal
         (a) If the animal is an adult at the onset of the bleeding disorder, it is likely to be acquired.
3. Drug or chemical exposure to agents that cause a platelet, bone marrow, or liver alteration
   a. Warfarin—inhibits vitamin K, thereby inhibiting synthesis of prothrombin
   b. Aspirin—interferes with ADP release from platelets
   c. Estrogens
   d. Phenylbutazone
   e. Anticoagulants—heparin

B. Physical examination
1. Type of bleeding
   a. Purpura—hemorrhages in skin and mucous membranes
      (1) Petechial hemorrhages—platelet disorder (number or function), vascular disease, allergies
      (2) Ecchymotic hemorrhages—any abnormality in hemostasis
   b. Bleeding into tissues or body cavities—coagulation defect or trauma to vessels
      (1) Abdomen
      (2) Thorax
      (3) Joints—hemarthrosis with joint enlargement and lameness
      (4) Spinal canal
      (5) Muscle
      (6) Eye—hemorrhages in retina, sclera, iris
   c. Massive bleeding from a single site without a history of a previous bleeding episode or purpura—likely to be a surgical or anatomic defect rather than a coagulation disorder
   d. Sudden severe bleeding from multiple sites after prolonged surgery—suggests acquired fibrinogen deficiency
   e. Hemarthroses, hematomas, or large ecchymotic hemorrhages at trauma sites—suggest hemophilia
   f. Hematuria or melena—may indicate hemorrhage from mucous membranes
2. Signs of an underlying disease that may be associated with a secondary bleeding disorder
   a. Immunologic disease
   b. Leukemia

c. Liver disease
d. Splenic disorders—splenomegaly may be present in a number of blood dyscrasias
e. Uremia
f. Exposure to ionizing radiation
g. Neurological disorders
h. Disseminated intravascular coagulation (DIC)

III. Laboratory evaluation

A. General considerations
1. The selection of a test or battery of tests to characterize the hemostatic defect should be determined by the clinical evaluation.
2. Collection and handling of blood samples for coagulation studies
a. All blood samples should be obtained with plastic syringes by using careful venipuncture.
b. The anticoagulant of choice for coagulation and platelet studies is trisodium citrate or sodium oxalate.
(1) 1 part of 3.8% trisodium citrate to 9 parts of whole blood
(2) For total platelet counts, EDTA is preferred since it will lessen clumping, but it will inhibit platelet interactions.
(3) Heparin inhibits thrombin action.
c. Keep all samples in plastic or silicone-coated test tubes.
(1) Activation of factor XII and clumping of platelets are prevented by smooth surfaces.
d. Plasma samples should be obtained from fresh blood and tested immediately or should be frozen at −20°C for later testing.
(1) Platelet-poor plasma is provided by centrifuging at 2500 rpm for 15 min.
(2) Platelet-rich plasma for platelet function tests is obtained by slow centrifugation (800 rpm) for 5 to 10 min.
e. Samples for platelet tests should be kept at room temperature, as platelet shape is altered by heat or cold.
(1) Platelet tests must be done within 2 hr of blood collection.
(2) The ideal plastic surface for platelet preparations is polycarbonate.

B. Platelet count—the first aspect to be considered, as 75% of acquired bleeding problems affect platelets
1. Indirect method—the number of platelets per oil immersion field is estimated on the stained blood smear
a. 4 to 6 platelets/field is normal.
2. Direct methods
a. Several methods are described in Chapter 6, Counting of Blood Cells.
3. Interpretation
a. Normal values vary between 200,000 to 500,000/microliter
(1) In individual animals the number of platelets in circulation is relatively constant.
b. Thrombocytopenia—counts below 100,000/microliter; hemorrhages, purpura, prolonged bleeding, and clot retraction failure occur with platelet numbers below 10,000/microliter and may occur if the count is between 40,000 and 75,000/microliter
(1) Inherited
(2) Acquired
(a) Decreased or faulty production of platelets
[1] Bone marrow suppression by drugs
[a] Estradiol cyclopentylpropionate (ECP)
[2] Bone marrow suppression by viruses
[a] Viral septicemias can affect the vascular endothelium and the platelets.
[b] Live measles vaccine in the dog
[3] Bone marrow suppression by irradiation
(b) Increased destruction of platelets
[1] Hypersensitivity
[a] Platelet-hapten combinations—agent sensitizes the platelet and attaches itself as a hapten, the combination stimulating antibodies

1. Idiopathic thrombocytopenic purpura—cause is undetermined, but could be drugs, viruses, bacteria
2. Drugs

[b] Autoimmune
1. Autoimmune hemolytic anemia (AIHA)
2. Systemic lupus erythematosis (SLE)
3. Leukemia—abnormal clones of lymphocytes may produce antibodies

[c] Isoimmune
1. Incompatible blood transfusions

[d] Immunologically mediated thrombocytopenia—demonstrated by the PF-3 test in the globulin fraction of serum
1. Idiopathic thrombocytopenic purpura
2. AIHA with thrombocytopenia
3. SLE

[2] Agglutination of platelets by toxins
[a] Endotoxin—platelets agglutinate, producing platelet thrombi and thrombocytopenia

[3] Disseminated intravascular coagulation

(c) Massive hemorrhage—may use all available platelets, producing a severe reduction

c. Thrombocytosis—increase in the platelet count
(1) Regenerative anemia—total count usually will increase twofold
(2) Reactive thrombocytosis—mature megakaryocytes have a decreased size and fewer nuclei than normal due to increased maturation and release of platelets
(a) Malignancies
(b) Infection
(c) Iron deficiency
(d) Trauma
(3) Splenectomy—since the vast splenic reservoir is gone, there is a persistent elevation of circulating platelet numbers
(4) Thrombocythemia
(a) Megakaryocytic leukemia—one of the myeloproliferative disorders; commonly associated with increased erythrocyte and leukocyte production

C. Tests for platelet dysfunction (thrombocytopathies)—with platelet dysfunction, bleeding may occur despite normal platelet counts

1. Clot retraction methods—one of the functions of the platelet is to facilitate clot retraction or syneresis; if platelet numbers are in excess of 100,000 and have adequate function there will be good clot retraction

a. Method I
(1) Bleed the patient and a normal dog as a control.
(2) Place 1 to 2 ml of blood in a clean, dry *glass* test tube that measures 10 to 12 mm in diameter.
(3) Allow to stand at room temperature (25°C) for 4 to 8 hr or 2 to 4 hr at 37°C.
(4) Compare amounts of clot retraction by observing serum portion.

b. Method II—dilute whole blood clot retraction and lysis test
(1) Fill a plastic syringe with 4.5 ml of cold buffered saline.
(a) Keep in the refrigerator with the needle attached ready for use.
(2) Withdraw 0.5 ml of fresh whole blood from the patient directly into the saline-filled cold syringe.
(3) Mix quickly and thoroughly.
(4) Transfer 2 ml of this diluted whole blood into each of two 10 x 75 mm glass tubes containing 1 unit of bovine thrombin.
(a) Topical thrombin (Parke-Davis) 1000 units/vial
(5) Immediately cap with Parafilm or plastic wrap and invert gently to mix.
(6) Place in the refrigerator or an ice bath for 30 min, then transfer to a water bath at 37°C.
(7) Degree of clot retraction is recorded at 1 and 2 hr as 1+ to 4+.
(8) Check the length and diameter of the clot.
(9) Keep tubes in a water bath and check hourly for clot lysis.

(a) 6 to 8 hours will be an adequate time for observation, but since abnormal samples will not lyse properly, leave them in the water bath overnight and examine the following morning.

2. PF-3 test—verification of antiplatelet activity if clotting time is shortened by at least 10 sec; submit a serum sample to an expert in coagulation
3. Russell's viper venom or Stypven time
   a. Normal values—8 to 15 sec
      (1) Requires platelet lipid or a lipid substrate for activation of factor X
      (2) Similar to prothrombin time test but requires normal platelet function to have normal test—measures prothrombin, factors V and X, and platelets
4. Platelet adhesiveness
   a. Although a variety of tests measure the tendency of platelets to adhere to glass, the majority pass whole blood through a plastic tube containing glass beads.
      (1) Platelet counts are done on the blood before and after it has gone through the glass bead column, and the number of platelets adhering to the glass beads are usually expressed as a percentage of the initial platelet count.
   b. Interpretation
      (1) Abnormal in a number of platelet function disorders
         (a) Especially important, as it may be the only platelet function abnormal in von Willebrand's disease
5. Platelet aggregation

D. Bleeding time
1. Method
   a. Make a small, deep puncture in the skin with a lancet or no. 11 Bard-Parker blade and note the time when blood first appears.
   b. Remove the drops of blood with filter paper every 30 sec, being careful not to touch the skin.
      (1) The use of highly absorbent paper such as cleansing tissue tends to prolong bleeding time, due to the more effective removal of surface blood.
   c. When blood no longer appears from the puncture site, the end point is noted.
2. Interpretation
   a. Normal values—1 to 5 min in domestic animals
   b. Prolonged
      (1) Vascular lesions
      (2) Platelet defects
      (3) Capillary fragility
      (4) von Willebrand's disease
   c. Difficult test to standardize

E. Coagulation time—whole blood clotting time
1. Methods
   a. Lee-White method
      (1) Obtain at least 3 ml of blood in a plastic syringe by careful venipuncture.
         (a) As soon as the blood enters the syringe, start a stopwatch.
      (2) Place 1 ml of blood into each of three tubes (10 x 75 mm).
      (3) Place the test tubes in a water bath at 37°C.
      (4) After 2 min, one of the three tubes is tipped gently at 1-min intervals until the blood has clotted.
      (5) Test the third tube in the same manner.
      (6) The time elapsed between the first appearance of blood in the syringe and clot formation in the third tube is the clotting time.
   b. Capillary tube method
      (1) A skin puncture is made; after wiping away the first drop, fill a special capillary tube with blood, noting the time when blood first appeared.
      (2) Holding the tube between the thumb and index finger of both hands, gently break the tube every 30 sec until a strand of fibrin is seen extending across the gap between the ends of the tube.

(3) The interval between the appearance of the blood and the appearance of the fibrin strand is the coagulation time.

2. Interpretation
   a. Normal values
      (1) Lee-White method in glass tubes—3 to 12 min
      (2) Capillary tube method
         (a) Horse and cattle—3 to 15 min
         (b) Other animals—1 to 5 min
   b. Prolonged
      (1) Deficiency of coagulation factors—rough measure of intrinsic system
      (2) Generally normal in thrombocytopenia, but may be slightly prolonged

F. Prothrombin time

1. Principle—oxalated plasma is clotted by the addition of calcium in the presence of excess thromboplastin. The time required for clotting of the plasma is assumed to be directly related to the speed of conversion of prothrombin to thrombin, and depends upon the level of plasma prothrombin.
2. Interpretation
   a. Normal
      (1) Dog—9 to 14 sec
      (2) Cattle—18 to 28 sec
      (3) Horse—9 to 12 sec
      (4) Several of the commercial reagents (rabbit brain thromboplastin) produce extremely short clotting times with animal plasma.
         (a) Normal—6 to 10 sec
         (b) Prolonged—10 to 30 sec
   b. Prolonged—tests the extrinsic system
      (1) Deficiency of prothrombin and factors V, VII, and X
         (a) Liver disease
         (b) Vitamin K deficiency or malabsorption
         (c) After dicoumarol ingestion (vitamin K antagonist)

G. Partial thromboplastin time (PTT)—activated or nonactivated

1. Principle—the intrinsic system is tested with kaolin used to activate factor XII, and cephalin supplants the role of platelets
2. Interpretation
   a. Normal ranges
      (1) Dog—usually 17 to 30 sec, but may be shorter with some commercial reagents
   b. Prolonged
      (1) Most reliable method for a defect in the intrinsic system—tests all factors except VII and platelets
         (a) If prothrombin time is normal, detects factors VIII, IX, XI, and XII deficiency
      (2) von Willebrand's disease
      (3) Disseminated intravascular coagulation

H. Thrombin time

1. Principle—thrombin time is the time taken for plasma to form a fibrin clot on addition of thrombin. It is a rapid test for measuring plasma fibrinogen concentration and detecting the presence of fibrin or fibrin split products.
2. Method
   a. To a 10 x 75 mm test tube add 0.2 ml of patient's plasma.
   b. Place in 37°C water bath.
   c. 0.1 ml of commercial bovine thrombin (10 units/ml) is added rapidly; at the same time a stopwatch is started.
   d. The end point is a clot and is compared to a normal control plasma of the same species.
3. Interpretation

a. Normal values—15 to 20 sec
b. Prolonged
(1) Low plasma fibrinogen levels (less than 100 mg)
(2) Impaired fibrinogen function
(3) Inhibitors of thrombin-induced clot formation
(a) Fibrinolytic split products—disseminated intravascular coagulation
(b) Heparin

IV. Hemostatic disorders
A. Acquired
1. Vascular disorders
a. Trauma
(1) Accidental
(2) Surgical
b. Symptomatic purpura
(1) Bacterial septicemia—action of toxin on vessel wall
(2) Viremia—hemorrhages may be the result of viral replication in endothelial cells and platelets, resulting in widespread endothelial damage, thrombocytopenia, and exhaustion of coagulation factors in attempting to repair the vascular damage.
(a) Hog cholera
(b) Infectious canine hepatitis
(c) Live measles vaccine—in dogs
(d) African swine fever
(e) Rinderpest
c. Purpura hemorrhagica
(1) Can occur in any animal, but more commonly in the horse
(2) Usually a secondary disease to a respiratory infection associated with *Streptococcus* spp., such as strangles or pneumonia
(3) Edema more pronounced than the hemorrhages
(4) Thrombocytes and coagulation factors normal
d. Vitamin C deficiency
(1) Occurs in monkeys and guinea pigs, but not domestic animals, for they synthesize their own vitamin C.
(2) Hemorrhages are probably due to a defect in the "cement" between endothelial cells and the perivascular sheath.
e. Anaphylactoid purpura
(1) Results in increased vascular permeability, which is characterized by variable amounts of hemorrhage and subcutaneous edema
2. Platelet disorders
a. Thrombocytopenia—most common cause of bleeding problems
(1) Decreased platelet production
(a) Aplastic anemia
(b) Bone marrow infiltration
(c) Ionizing radiation
(d) Drugs that act on platelet production
(e) Viral infections—equine infectious anemia
(f) Rickettsial infections—*Ehrlichia*
(2) Enhanced platelet destruction
(a) Nonimmune
[1] Infection
[2] Disseminated intravascular coagulation
[3] Drug induced
(b) Immunologically mediated
[1] Primary
[a] Idiopathic thrombocytopenic purpura (ITP)

LABORATORY FINDINGS IN BLEEDING DISORDERS

Disorder	Platelet count	Clot retraction time	Bleeding time	Coagulation time	Prothrombin time	Partial thromboplastin time
Vascular	Normal	Normal	Prolonged	Normal	Normal	
Thrombocytopenia	Decreased	Increased	Prolonged	Normal	Normal	Normal
Thrombopathy	Normal	Increased	Prolonged	Normal	Normal	Normal
Deficiencies of vitamin K-dependent clotting factors (prothrombin, VII, IX, and X)	Normal	Normal	Normal	Normal or prolonged	Prolonged	Normal or prolonged
Hemophilia (VIII or IX)	Normal	Normal	Normal	Prolonged	Normal	Prolonged
von Willebrand's disease	Normal	Increased	Prolonged	Normal	Normal	Normal or prolonged
DIC	Decreased	Increased	Prolonged	Prolonged	Prolonged	Prolonged

[2] Secondary
[a] Autoimmune hemolytic anemia
[b] Systemic lupus erythematosus
[c] Virus
[d] Drug induced
[e] Lymphosarcoma

(3) Sequestration of platelets—in spleen, liver, and lungs
(a) Endotoxin
(b) Hypersplenism
(c) Hypothermia

(4) Loss of platelets
(a) Hemorrhage

b. Thrombasthenia—platelets defective in function
(1) Uremia—due to toxin
(2) Drugs
(a) Inhibit platelet aggregation by inhibiting ADH release from the platelet
[1] Aspirin (acetylsalicylic acid)
[2] Phenylbutazone
(b) Decrease platelet adhesion
[1] Dextran
[2] Clofibrate (Atromid-S)
[3] Local anesthetics
[4] Glyceryl guaiacolate

3. Coagulation factor disorders
a. Liver disease
(1) Major site of synthesis of coagulation factors—prothrombin; fibrinogen; factors V, VII, IX, X, XI, and XIII
(2) The extrinsic clotting mechanism is particularly compromised in liver disorders.
(3) Liver disease—infection, obstruction, neoplasia

b. Vitamin K deficiency
(1) Vitamin K acts in the hepatocyte to regulate the biosynthesis of prothrombin and factors VII, IX, and X.
(2) Inadequate bile salts interfere with the absorption of vitamin K from the intestine, since this vitamin is fat soluble.

c. Poisoning with coumarin derivatives—interferes with vitamin K metabolism and prevents synthesis of vitamin K-dependent coagulation factors (prothrombin, factors VII, IX, and X)
  (1) Warfarin (dicoumarol)—rodenticide
  (2) Moldy sweetclover—contains coumarin derivative
d. Disseminated intravascular coagulation
  (1) DIC is characterized by widespread intravascular fibrin deposition, principally within arterioles and capillaries, leading to:
    (a) Impaired organ function
    (b) Bleeding diathesis from:
      [1] Depletion of platelets
      [2] Depletion of coagulation factors—fibrinogen, prothrombin, factor V, and factor VIII
      [3] Anticoagulant effects of increased fibrinogen degradation products (FDP's) produced by the action of plasmin on fibrinogen in the fibrinolytic mechanism are shown below.

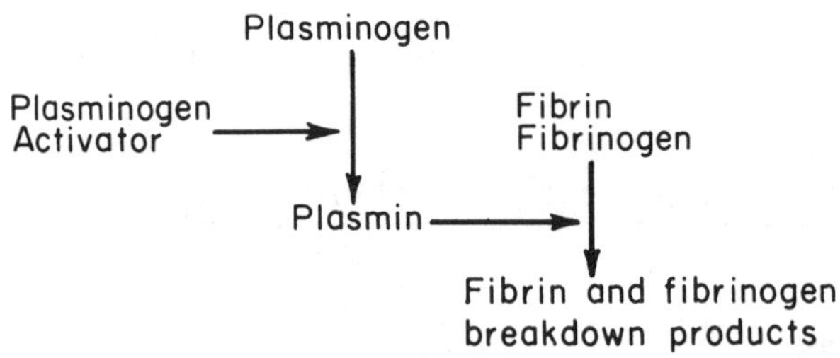

  (2) It is secondary to a variety of diseases:
    (a) Bacterial endotoxin
    (b) Anoxia—shock, massive trauma
    (c) Tissue extracts—neoplasia, tissue necrosis, heartworms
    (d) Physical and chemical agents—proteolytic enzymes, cancer chemotherapy
    (e) Endothelial damage—viruses, rickettsia, heat stroke
    (f) Intravascular hemolysis—hemolytic anemia, incompatible blood transfusion
    (g) Stagnant blood flow

B. Inherited defect or deficiency
1. Factor VII (proconvertin)
  a. Occurrence
    (1) Dog
      (a) Beagle—several strains
      (b) Alaskan Malamute—1 strain
  b. Clinical signs
    (1) Mild clinical condition in both sexes—no clinical bleeding
    (2) Susceptible to demodectic mange, as a coagulation defect in the extrinsic system promotes moist tissue environment in the skin
  c. Inheritance pattern—autosomal, incompletely dominant
2. Factor VIII (AHF)—hemophilia A or classical hemophilia
  a. Occurrence—responsible for 80% of hereditary bleeding disorders
    (1) Dog—all purebred and mixed breeds
    (2) Horse—Thoroughbred and Standardbred
    (3) Cat—2 cases
    (4) Swine—as von Willebrand's disease
  b. Clinical signs
    (1) Forms
      (a) Severe—less than 1% factor VIII activity
      (b) Mild to moderate—5 to 20% factor VIII activity
    (2) Mild
      (a) Traumatic injuries can cause bruising.

(b) Can survive to maturity, in spite of ear cropping or tail docking
(3) Severe
(a) Excessive bleeding—into soft tissues, joints, gastrointestinal tract, brain, spinal cord, and other organs and from the nose
c. Inheritance pattern—X-linked, recessive

3. Factor IX (Christmas factor)—hemophilia B, Christmas disease
a. Occurrence
(1) Dog—3 breeds
(a) Cairn Terrier
(b) Black and Tan Coonhound
(c) St. Bernard
b. Clinical signs
(1) Milder hemorrhagic problems than with hemophilia A
c. Inheritance pattern—X-linked, recessive

4. Factor X (Stuart factor)
a. Occurrence
(1) Only in Cocker Spaniel
b. Clinical sign
(1) Mild anemia syndrome in heterozygotes, lethal in homozygous animals
c. Inheritance pattern—autosomal, incompletely dominant

5. Factor XI (PTA)
a. Occurrence
(1) Cow
(2) Dog—Springer Spaniel
b. Clinical signs
(1) Mild—hematuria, small hematomas
c. Inheritance pattern—autosomal

6. von Willebrand's disease
a. Occurrence
(1) Swine
(2) Dog
(a) German Shepherd
(b) Golden Retriever
(c) Miniature Schnauzer
b. Clinical signs
(1) Severe in homozygous state and may be lethal
(2) Heterozygous state may have all forms of bleeding.
(a) Chronic intermittent bloody diarrhea
(b) Shifting leg lameness that disappears with age
(c) Chronic otitis externa
(d) Prolonged estrual bleeding
(e) Prolonged postpartum bleeding
(f) High morbidity and low mortality
c. Inheritance pattern—autosomal
d. Differentiation from hemophilia A
(1) Both have factor VIII deficiency, but not as severe in von Willebrand's disease.
(2) von Willebrand's disease has a platelet function defect that produces a prolonged bleeding time, while in hemophilia A the primary bleeding time is normal, as platelet function is normal.
(a) The defect is related to the initial stage of hemostasis because the platelets do not adhere to collagen fibers *in vivo* and are not retained by glass bead columns *in vitro*.

7. Hypofibrinogenemia
a. Occurrence
(1) Dog—St. Bernard (in Europe)
(2) Dairy goat—in the Netherlands

b. Inheritance pattern—autosomal, may be dominant or incompletely dominant depending upon the family

8. Thrombocytopathy—platelet function disorder
   a. Occurrence
      (1) Dog
         (a) Otter Hound
         (b) Basset Hound
         (c) Foxhound—isolated case
         (d) Scottish Terrier—isolated case
      (2) Laboratory rat
   b. Inheritance pattern—autosomal, incompletely dominant

Part two CLINICAL CHEMISTRY

17 KIDNEY FUNCTION TESTS

I. Kidney function tests in common use for clinical purposes

A. Blood urea nitrogen (BUN) or nonprotein nitrogen (NPN)
B. Creatinine
C. Concentration tests
D. Phenolsulfonphthalein (PSP)
E. Urinalysis
  1. Specific gravity
  2. pH
  3. Protein
  4. Microscopic examination of sediment

II. General considerations

A. Purpose of kidney function tests
  1. Determine the nature of an impairment of renal function
    a. Urinalysis is usually the only test that provides diagnostic assistance.
    b. Only in the case of severe renal disease is it possible to detect abnormal function, as the kidney has tremendous reserve capacity.
      (1) Only when more than 50% of the nephrons are not functioning is it possible to diagnose a renal impairment.
  2. Determine the extent of an impairment of renal function
    a. It is best to perform serial tests to determine the extent that an abnormal kidney function is reversible or to follow the course of chronic kidney impairment.
  3. Renal function tests provide part of the evidence upon which a prognosis should be based. Serial determinations, rather than single tests, are more reliable for purposes of prognosis.

B. Determination of the nonprotein group of nitrogenous substances, especially urea and creatinine, is important because significantly increased values are usually the result of accumulation of these substances in the blood because of defective kidney elimination.
  1. Nitrogen-containing constituents of blood
    a. Protein
      (1) Albumin
      (2) Globulin
  2. Nonprotein nitrogenous substances
    a. Metabolic waste products

(1) Urea
(2) Creatinine
(3) Uric acid
(4) Creatine
(5) Amino acids
(6) Ammonia

III. Blood urea nitrogen

A. Formation—urea is the principal end product of catabolism of protein formed by the liver
1. Ornithine combines with ammonia and carbon dioxide to form citrulline.
2. Citrulline combines with ammonia to produce the amino acid, arginine.
3. Arginase, a liver enzyme, hydrolyzes arginine to urea and ornithine, leaving the latter free to participate again in the cycle.

B. Excretion of urea—filtered through the glomerulus, then 25 to 40% is reabsorbed by the tubules
C. Methods
1. Urograph (BUN-o-graph, Haver-Lockhart Laboratories)—chromatography paper banded with reagents (Fig. 17.1)

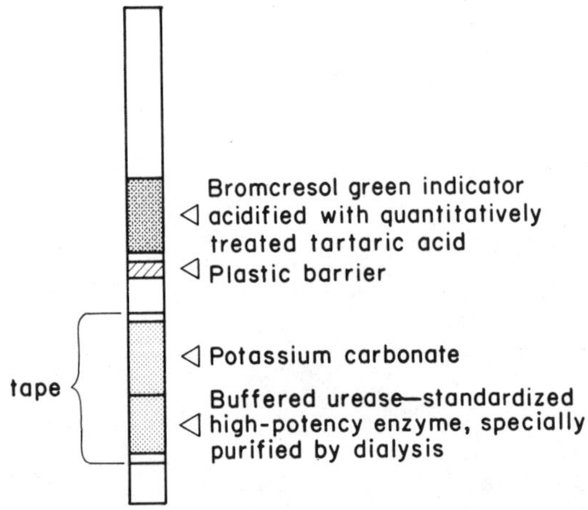

Fig. 17.1. Urograph strip.

a. With a long needle attached to a small syringe or with a long-tipped pipette, place 0.2 ml of fresh serum or plasma in a 10 x 75 mm test tube.
(1) Avoid wetting the sides of the tube.
b. Into the tube, place one Urograph strip with the taped end down.
(1) Do not touch the indicator band (upper yellow) with the fingers.
(2) Center the strip in the bottom of the tube; for if the strip is not properly positioned, serum may travel up between the edge of the strip and the wall of the tube by capillary action, bypassing the reagents and producing inaccurate results.
c. Allow to stand at room temperature for 30 min, away from drafts.
d. To estimate the urea nitrogen levels, compare the color height on the indicator band with the illustrations below at a point where the demarcation between black and white is sharpest (Fig. 17.2).
e. When the BUN concentration is too high to read directly (as the scale only reads to 75 mg/dl), mix the serum with equal volumes of Versatol (a standard serum with known urea nitrogen level).
(1) Example—the patient's serum is mixed 1:1 with Versatol (urea nitrogen level is 15 mg/dl), and the result for this mixture is 60 mg/dl:
(a) Patient's value = (2 x 60) − 15
(b) Patient's value = 120 − 15 = 105 mg/dl
2. Azostix (Ames Co.)—stick impregnated with urease that changes color when in contact with urea in the blood

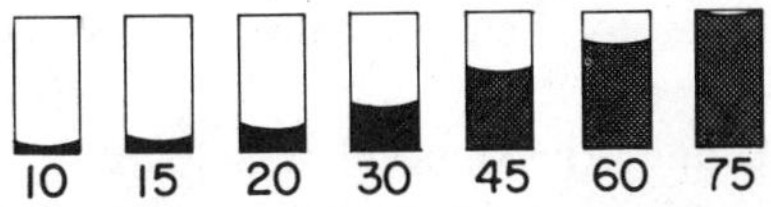

Fig. 17.2. Color heights for estimation of urea nitrogen levels.

a. Not a reliable test and therefore not recommended

3. Scribner kit (available from Rochester Products Co.)
   a. Method
      (1) Glycerol urease extract is added to serum to hydrolyze the urea to ammonia.
      (2) The mixture is diluted with physiological salt solution, and Nessler's reagent is added to produce a yellow color.
      (3) The depth of the color is compared to a set of color standards; this limits the usefulness of the test, as the standards are available only to 30 mg/dl.
4. Mercury-combining power (LaMotte Blood Urea Outfit employs this method)
5. Colorimetric methods—various methods are employed in the blood analyzer systems, or kits of reagents are available from a variety of sources

D. Interpretation
1. Normal values range from 10 to 30 mg/dl
2. Low values
   a. Protein malnutrition
   b. Hepatic insufficiency—ability of hepatic cells to form urea is one of the last functions to fail when extensive hepatocellular damage occurs
   c. Technical errors in conducting the test
3. Increased values
   a. Prerenal causes—elevations are seldom over 100 mg/dl
      (1) Reduced renal blood flow
         (a) Congestive heart failure
         (b) Shock—hypotension plus diversion of blood from the kidneys
      (2) Factors that reduce net filtration pressure in the glomerulus
         (a) Hypotension
         (b) Shock
         (c) Adrenocortical insufficiency
         (d) Heart failure—some types
         (e) Increased protein osmotic pressure
         (f) Dehydration (severe)—protein exerts a strong force to prevent fluid from leaving the glomerular capillaries
         (g) Increased protein in the diet—transient
   b. Renal disease—elevation of the BUN will occur when approximately 70% of the nephrons are nonfunctional
      (1) The correlation between the BUN level and the severity of renal disease is usually fairly good if one considers the duration of the condition.
   c. Postrenal uremia
      (1) Perforation of the urinary system allowing urine to escape
      (2) Obstruction of the urinary system
         (a) Obstruction of only one ureter will not result in uremia unless the opposite kidney is impaired.

IV. Creatinine

A. Formation—creatinine is formed in the metabolism of muscle creatine and phosphocreatine
1. Not affected by dietary protein, protein catabolism, age, sex, or exercise

B. Excretion—after being filtered by the glomerulus, it is excreted in the urine

1. Since it is not excreted or absorbed by the renal tubules to any degree, it can be used as a rough index of the glomerular filtration rate (GFR).
2. The quantity excreted depends upon the skeletal muscle mass and renal function.
3. Creatinine is eliminated more easily than urea nitrogen, so that an increase is not seen as early as the increase in urea nitrogen when there is renal impairment.

C. Methods

1. The alkaline picrate method of Jaffe is commonly used in commercial reagent kits and in automated methods.
   a. Although chromagens of noncreatinine nature are measured as well as creatinine, this does not present a serious problem.

D. Interpretation

1. Normal values range from 1 to 2 mg/dl.
2. Low values have no significance.
3. Increased values
   a. The glomerular filtration rate is reduced when creatinine is over 2 mg/dl.
   b. As with the BUN, there is only a rough correlation between the degree of elevation and the degree of renal impairment.
      (1) There is a tendency for the creatinine to be elevated later than the BUN in the progress of generalized renal disease.
   c. In addition to primary renal disease, creatinine will be elevated in prerenal and postrenal uremia.
      (1) Impaired blood flow
      (2) Obstruction of the urinary system
   d. For prognosis purposes, serial determinations are superior to a single test.
   e. In early renal disease or failure, neither creatinine nor BUN are sensitive.
   f. Fewer nonrenal factors influence creatinine than influence BUN, but the creatinine test is technically more difficult to perform.

KIDNEY FUNCTION TESTS

Anatomic unit	Physiologic function	Laboratory tests: Qualitative	Laboratory tests: Semiquantitative	Laboratory tests: Quantitative
Glomerulus	Protein-free filtration of plasma	Random urinalysis	Clearance tests: Urea, creatinine, mannitol	Glomerular filtration rate: Inulin; thiosulfate
Proximal convoluted tubule	Obligate conservation of essential materials; excretion of metabolic products	Urine glucose	PSP	*p*-aminohippuric acid (PAH) clearance Urate clearance
Henle's loop ascending limb	Sodium pump—regulated by aldosterone, which maintains the high, variable concentrations of Na within the tissue of the medulla required for the countercurrent phenomenon needed for concentrated urine	Urine specific gravity	Concentration test	Urine osmolality
Distal convoluted tubule	Acidification of urine—by K, Na, NH_3 excretion and reabsorption	Urine pH		24-hr urinary NH_3 and total acidity
Collecting tubule	Concentration of urine—under partial influence of antidiuretic hormone (ADH)	Urine specific gravity	Concentration test	Urine osmolality Effect of vasopressin on urine volume
Juxtaglomerular apparatus	Regulates the sodium pump of Henle's loop and the distal convoluted tubule through the action of aldosterone		Serum K Blood pH Serum CO_2	Urine aldosterone Plasma renin assay Angiotensin assay
Renal plasma flow	Regulates glomerular filtration rate, tubular excretion and reabsorption, acidification, and concentration of urine	Urinalysis		Inulin clearance Diodrast clearance PAH clearance

18 URINALYSIS

I. General considerations

A. The relatively simple procedures involved in urinalysis, conducted in a few minutes of time, can yield much valuable information in regard to the function of the urinary system as well as other organs or systems of the body.

B. A complete urinalysis should be a routine procedure for the following:

1. Surgical and geriatric patients
2. Disease problems as yet without a diagnosis, since abnormal urine findings could indicate the need for additional evaluation of a particular organ or body system
   a. Kidney disease—abnormal specific gravity, proteinuria, casts, leukocytes, erythrocytes
   b. End-stage renal disease—low specific gravity with failure to concentrate urine when water is withheld, pH decreased
   c. Bladder infection—proteinuria, leukocytes, bacteria
   d. Neoplasia—exfoliated neoplastic cells, hematuria
   e. Liver disease—bilirubinuria, altered urobilinogen, bilirubin crystals
   f. Hemolysis—hemoglobinuria, increased urobilinogen
   g. Diabetes mellitus—glycosuria and ketonuria
   h. Diabetes insipidus—low specific gravity with failure to concentrate urine when water is withheld
   i. Acidosis—low pH
   j. Alkalosis—increased pH

II. Collection

A. Containers

1. Collection container must be clean.
2. Glass vials or disposable plastic containers
   a. Opaque plastic or dark glass should be used if the specimen is not to be examined soon after collection, as sunlight will cause degradation of certain constituents such as bilirubin and urobilinogen in less than an hour.
3. Catheterization into a sterile container is mandatory for urine to be used for bacterial cultures and sensitivity testing.

B. Timing of collection

1. An early morning sample from house-trained pets is most likely to contain constituents of diagnostic significance.
   a. Fluid consumption during the day dilutes the urine (the resulting lowered specific gravity will cause disintegration of erythrocytes and leukocytes) and all the substances.
2. Avoid catching the first part of the urine stream of noncatheterized samples, as it will contain cellular debris, leukocytes, and exudate flushed from the urethra, prepuce, and genital tract.

C. Timing of analysis

1. A fresh sample is preferred.
   a. Bacteria are normally found in the urethra, so contamination with urea-splitting bacteria may result in loss of usefulness of urine for diagnostic purposes if it is allowed to stand several hours at room temperature.
      (1) Urea—split to ammonia; alkalinizes urine
      (2) Formed elements (cells and casts) dissolve as urine becomes more alkaline.
2. Urine preserved by refrigeration is suitable for examination for 2 to 3 hr.

a. Allow sample to warm to room temperature.
   (1) Low temperature will slightly increase specific gravity.
   (2) Low temperature can interfere with tests using enzymes for reactions.

3. Freezing—damages cells
4. Preservatives—may be used when immediate analysis or refrigeration is impossible, but may interfere with several chemical tests
   a. Toluene
      (1) Antimicrobial
      (2) Add sufficient quantity to just cover the surface of the urine.
      (3) The portion to be examined should be pipetted from beneath the surface film of toluene.
      (4) Does not interfere with chemical determination of protein or glucose, but changes the amount of ketones
      (5) Useful to preserve a 24-hr urine specimen obtained in a metabolism cage
   b. Thymol
      (1) Antimicrobial—often combined with sodium fluoride to preserve glucose
      (2) Use a small crytstal of thymol or 5 to 10 ml of a 10% solution in isopropyl alcohol for a 24-hr collection of urine.
      (3) A false-positive protein reaction will result with the sulfosalicylic acid method.
   c. Formalin
      (1) Prevents bacterial growth
      (2) One drop of 40% formalin in 30 ml of urine will preserve casts or cellular elements.
      (3) Interferes with glucose reaction
   d. Chloroform
      (1) Antimicrobial
      (2) 5 ml will be adequate to preserve a 24-hr urine collection.
   e. Boric acid
      (1) Antimicrobial
      (2) 1 g preserves a 24-hr urine sample.
      (3) Available in tablet form from many commercial laboratories and can be used when hormone analysis of the specimen is requested
   f. Metaphosphoric acid
      (1) 1 volume of aqueous 10% concentration is added to 5 volumes of urine to preserve vitamin C (ascorbic acid).

D. Analysis
1. Random sample
   a. Suitable for qualitative examination only, because concentration of any solute will vary with the quantity of water being excreted at that time
   b. Quantitative analysis requires a specific period of time for collection.
      (1) Phenolsulphonphthalein excretion—20-min test period
      (2) Hormones such as cortisol—24-hr urine collection

III. Physical examination of urine

A. Urine volume
1. The amount of urine produced per day by normal animals is dependent upon several variables.
   a. Diet
   b. Fluid intake
   c. Climate—temperature and humidity
   d. Exercise
   e. Size and weight
2. Normal ranges—accurate data not available

Species	Daily amount (L)	ml/kg/day
Horse	2-11 (4.7)	
Cattle (dairy)	8.8-22.6 kg (14.2)	14
Sheep and goat	0.5-2 (1.0)	
Pig	2-6 (4.0)	
Dog	0.5-2 (1.0)	31 (25-41)
Cat		26 (22-30)
Man	1-1.2	9-29

a. Dog in a controlled environment—12 to 20 ml of urine per pound of body weight per 24 hr is a rough approximation

b. Urine volume is usually inversely related to specific gravity.
   (1) High volume and low specific gravity
   (2) Low volume and high specific gravity
   (3) Exceptions
      (a) Diabetes mellitus—high volume and high specific gravity due to glycosuria
      (b) Severe or terminal nephritis—may be associated with low volume and low specific gravity

3. Increased volume—polyuria
   a. Nonpathologic—transient
      (1) Increased water consumption, including compulsive (psychogenic) water drinking
      (2) Diuretics—produce rapid formation of urine
      (3) Parenteral fluids
      (4) Sodium chloride or salty food—increase thirst
      (5) Corticosteroids and ACTH
   b. Pathologic—may be permanent
      (1) Chronic progressive renal failure—polyuria an early sign, as the kidney is unable to concentrate the urine
         (a) In a clinically dehydrated patient, polyuria and a low specific gravity indicates an inability of the kidney to conserve water.
      (2) Acute renal failure during the diuretic phase due to ischemia or tubular disease
      (3) Diabetes mellitus—strong osmotic activity of glucose in the distal tubules of the kidney does not allow water to be removed normally, and diuresis occurs.
      (4) Primary renal glycosuria
      (5) Diabetes insipidus—deficiency of antidiuretic hormone from the posterior pituitary results in failure to reabsorb water in normal quantities in the distal renal tubules
      (6) Renal diabetes insipidus
      (7) Renal cortical hypoplasia
      (8) Severe renal amyloidosis
      (9) Chronic pyelonephritis
      (10) Pyometra—sometimes produces polydipsia and reduced concentration of urine in the kidneys
      (11) Hyperadrenocorticism
      (12) Generalized liver disease—thought to be associated with unmetabolized aldosterone
      (13) Absorption of large amounts of serous effusions

4. Decreased volume—oliguria
   a. Physiologic—transient, with a small amount of urine and a high specific gravity (> 1.025)
      (1) Decreased water intake
      (2) High environmental temperature
      (3) Excessive hyperventilation (panting)
      (4) Exercise—sympathetic stimulation decreases flow of blood through the kidneys, and as a result the glomerular filtration rate is decreased
      (5) Dehydration due to any cause (vomiting, diarrhea, etc.)—the normal kidney conserves water to restore normal fluid balance

b. Pathologic
  (1) Fever from any cause—especially with low fluid intake
  (2) Acute renal failure—small volume of urine with low specific gravity due to ischemia or tubular disease
  (3) Chronic primary renal failure—small volume of low specific gravity
  (4) Edema secondary to circulatory dysfunction
    (a) Cardiac decompensation—interferes with renal circulation
  (5) Markedly reduced blood pressure
  (6) Obstruction of urinary passages—impairs flow of urine

B. Color
1. Method
  a. Record color of urine, while observing it in a test tube or urinometer cylinder, as:

Colorless	Yellow-brown	Reddish brown
Pale yellow	Greenish yellow	Brown
Yellow	Green	Blue
Dark yellow	Red	Milky

  b. Always consider color in association with specific gravity and volume.
  c. The normal color is yellow to light amber and depends primarily on the concentration of urochromes, whose output is relatively constant.
  d. The intensity of color varies inversely with the volume.
    (1) Large volume—decreased urochrome concentration per unit volume; pale yellow and often low specific gravity
2. Interpretation
  a. Yellow to amber—normal
  b. Colorless to pale yellow—usually dilute urine with low specific gravity and polyuria
    (1) End-stage renal disease
    (2) Excessive intake of water or solutions
    (3) Diabetes insipidus
    (4) Hyperadrenocorticism
    (5) Diabetes mellitus—in some cases
    (6) Pyometra
  c. Dark yellow to yellow-brown—concentrated urine with a high specific gravity and small quantity
    (1) Acute nephritis
    (2) Diminished intake of fluids
    (3) Dehydration—prolonged vomiting or diarrhea
    (4) Fever
  d. Yellow-brown or greenish yellow—yellow-green foam when urine is shaken
    (1) Urobilinoids—chromagen derived from heme
      (a) Green—biliverdin
      (b) Yellow brown—bilirubin and urobilin
  e. Red, wine, or brown
    (1) Cloudy—hematuria
      (a) Clearer after centrifugation
    (2) Translucent—hemoglobinuria
    (3) Burgundy, pinkish brown to reddish brown—porphyrins
  f. Brown to brownish black
    (1) Hemoglobin—upon standing
    (2) Bile—large amounts
    (3) Normal horse urine is a yellow color when voided, but it turns a deep brown color upon standing for a time due to oxidation of pyrocatechin.
    (4) Myoglobin—in azoturia
    (5) Methemoglobinuria

(6) Melanin—after urine stands
(7) Phenol derivatives—after urine stands
(a) Carbolic acid poisoning
(b) Decomposed protein
(8) Indican

g. Green
(1) Methylene blue—in urinary antiseptics; will decolorize with hydrochloric acid
(2) Bile—biliverdin
(3) Acriflavine
(4) Dizan

h. Red to pink
(1) Phenothiazine—usually excreted in colorless form but turns pink with oxidation on exposure to air
(2) Phenolsulfonphthalein dye—in alkaline urine
(3) Neoprontosil
(4) Phenolphthalein
(5) Cascara
(6) Pyridium

C. Transparency
1. Method
a. Record transparency, while observing in a test tube or urinometer cyclinder, as:
(1) Clear
(2) Cloudy
(3) Flocculent
2. Interpretation
a. Clear—freshly voided urine from the normal animal is usually clear, except in the horse where it is normally thick and cloudy due to calcium carbonate crystals and mucus
b. Cloudy—not necessarily pathological, as many samples may become cloudy upon standing; cause of loss of transparency best determined by microscopic examination of sediment
(1) Epithelial cells—if present in large numbers
(2) Blood—red to brown color and smoky
(3) Leukocytes—may produce milky, ropy appearance if present in large numbers
(4) Bacteria—produce a uniform turbidity if present in large numbers; the turbidity does not settle out and cannot be removed by filtration
(5) Mucus
(6) Crystals
(a) Calcium carbonate—in fresh horse urine or bovine urine after it stands
(b) Amorphous urates—white or pink cloud in acid urine upon standing or when chilled
(c) Amorphous phosphates—white cloud in alkaline urine

D. Specific gravity
1. Method
a. Fill the urinometer cylinder about three-fourths full with urine.
(1) The container used for flotation of the urinometer should be large enough in diameter to prevent adherence of the urinometer to its sides.
b. Place the urinometer in the urine and rotate it to prevent its touching the sides or the bottom of the cylinder.
c. Read the scale on the stem of the urinometer at the interface of the air and urine, and record it in decimals, e.g., 1.020.
(1) Before a new urinometer is used, its accuracy should be checked by testing in distilled water, and it should read 1.000 at its calibration temperature.
(2) Each urinometer is calibrated to give readings at a definite temperature, usually between 20°C and 25°C, so the urine specimen should be allowed to stand at room temperature for a few minutes before taking a reading.

(a) For greater accuracy, add 0.001 for each 3°C above the calibration temperature and subtract 0.001 for each 3°C below the calibration temperature.

d. If the quantity of urine is small, the specific gravity may be determined by

(1) Refractometer

(a) The use of an instrument such as the Goldberg Refractometer (American Optical Co.) provides a highly accurate means of determination of specific gravity of urine on a volume as small as a single drop.

2. Interpretation

a. Normal 1.015 to 1.050 (ave. = 1.025)

Species	Range	Average
Horse	1.020-1.050	1.035
Cattle	1.025-1.045	1.035
Sheep and goat	1.015-1.045	1.030
Pig	1.010-1.030	1.015
Dog	1.015-1.045	1.025
Cat	1.020-1.040	1.030
Man	1.010-1.030	1.020

(1) The normal kidney is able to dilute urine to a specific gravity of 1.001 and concentrate urine to a specific gravity of 1.060+. Factors causing variation in the normal dog are:

(a) Diet

(b) Fluid intake

(c) Climate

(d) Activity

(2) Interpretation of all other components of the routine urinalysis should be considered in association with the specific gravity of the specimen if conclusions are to be meaningful.

(a) Most tests are performed on a fixed volume (and thus rate of formation) of urine without regard to specific gravity of the specimen.

(b) Example—4+ proteinuria in the presence of low specific gravity implies a heavier loss of protein than 4+ proteinuria in a more concentrated (higher specific gravity) sample.

(c) Also true for formed elements of sediment, glucose, bilirubin, etc.

(3) The specific gravity reflects the concentrating or diluting ability of the kidney; work is required to dilute as well as to concentrate urine.

(a) Glomerular filtrate enters the proximal convoluted tubule at a specific gravity of 1.010 ± 0.002.

[1] Nephrons will dilute or concentrate this filtrate depending on the needs of the body.

[2] Renal tubules must be functional and remove solute to achieve a specific gravity below that of the glomerular filtrate.

[a] A specific gravity of 1.002 to 1.005 implies functional renal tubules.

(4) Specific gravity of a random sample

(a) Specific gravity varies with water consumption.

[1] A specific gravity in the fixed range (1.008 to 1.012) may be seen in any randomly obtained urine sample of a normal dog, since the ability of the normal kidney to change specific gravity overlaps this fixed range.

[2] The presence of a specific gravity of 1.008 to 1.012 in a random sample is justification for further reevaluation of the functional competence of the kidneys (not pathognomonic of chronic interstitial nephritis).

[a] Perform water concentration or Pitressin test.

[b] The presence of the following in association with a fixed specific gravity indicates that the animal cannot conserve needed body water and therefore concentration tests are not necessary.

1. Clinical dehydration
2. Uremia
3. Abnormally high packed cell volume

b. Causes of decreased specific gravity

(1) A low random sample specific gravity is usually unreliable for interpretation except to indicate the need for further evaluation of the animal's ability to concentrate urine. There are several exceptions.

(a) If the animal is already obviously dehydrated and yet the specific gravity of the urine is low, there is no justification for a concentration test. The answer is obvious—the animal cannot concentrate urine because of impaired kidney function.

(b) Marked elevation of packed cell volume may also imply dehydration and give more meaning to a low random sample specific gravity.

(c) If an animal is obviously uremic and yet has a low specific gravity urine, again the answer is clear—there is no remaining ability for concentration of urine by the kidneys that formed it.

(d) Acute renal failure can give exactly the same results as chronic renal failure; therefore, one should not be too hasty to regard a lesion as chronic and irreversible when in fact it may be acute and reversible.

(e) If random sample specific gravity exceeds 1.025, there is obvious evidence of concentrating ability on the part of the renal tubule and no need to do a concentration test.

(2) Nonpathologic—transient

(a) Excessive water consumption—most common cause

(b) Diuretics

(c) Parenteral fluids

(d) Corticosteroids and ACTH

(e) Following estrus and injection of female hormones

(3) Pathological

(a) End-stage renal disease—usually from 1.003 to 1.015, due to inability of the kidney to concentrate urine

[1] Fixed specific gravity may result and refers to the phase when the specific gravity is fixed between 1.010 and 1.012, which is the same molecular concentration as that of plasma dialysate; it is due to the inability of the kidney to dilute or concentrate urine beyond these points.

[2] A concentration test can be used to differentiate this condition from low specific gravity due to increased water intake and diabetes insipidus.

[a] The bladder should be emptied and the specific gravity of the urine determined.

[b] Withhold all fluids and food (unless dry) for at least 12 hr.

[c] Collect urine specimen and again determine specific gravity.

[d] Results

1. Normal kidney—specific gravity is above 1.020
2. Impaired kidney—the closer to 1.010, the less the amount of functioning kidney tissue
3. Diabetes insipidus—specific gravity will become higher, but not to normal limits

[e] Caution—animals verging on uremia should not have fluids restricted for this long a period, as the condition will be aggravated

(b) Acute nephritis—severe or terminal

(c) Severe renal amyloidosis

(d) Renal cortical hypoplasia

(e) Chronic generalized pyelonephritis

(f) Diabetes insipidus—usually from 1.002 to 1.006, due to loss of antidiuretic hormone from the posterior pituitary

[1] Administration of 0.5 to 1.0 ml of posterior pituitary solution will produce immediate but temporary cessation of thirst and polyuria.

[2] Restricting fluids for 12 hr will elevate the specific gravity, but not to normal limits, and less urine will be produced.

[3] With infusion of Ringer's solution, isotonicity will be preserved in both plasma and urine of healthy animals, while hypertonic plasma and hypotonic urine will occur if the animal has diabetes insipidus.(3)

(g) Renal diabetes insipidus

(h) Pyometra—from excessive water intake

(i) Hyperadrenocorticism
(j) Rapid absorption of edema fluid
(k) The ability of the kidneys to regulate specific gravity depends upon their competence at the time the urine was formed and not the length of time it took to achieve this level of function.
[1] Therefore cannot be used as sole means of prognosis
[a] Specific gravity of 1.010 can occur in:
1. Normal animal
2. Acute reversible renal disease
3. Chronic irreversible renal disease

c. Causes of increased specific gravity—usually associated with a small volume of urine except in diabetes mellitus
(1) Physiological—transient
(a) Decreased water intake
(b) High environmental temperature
(c) Excessive hyperventilation (panting)
(2) Pathological
(a) Dehydration due to any cause—vomiting, diarrhea, etc.
(b) Fever—any cause
(c) Edema due to circulatory dysfunction
(d) Exudation associated with burns—rare in veterinary medicine
(e) Initial stage of acute nephritis—any cause; may be associated with low specific gravity when severe or terminal
(f) Diabetes mellitus
(g) Primary renal glycosuria
(h) Shock
(i) Any disease state in which abnormal quantities of solids are added to urine
[1] Protein
[2] Glucose
[3] Inflammatory exudate—minor effect
[a] Specific gravity is inversely related to volume of urine per day in health and disease. Exceptions:
1. Diabetes mellitus—large volume and high specific gravity due to glycosuria
2. Severe or terminal nephritis—may be associated with small volume and low specific gravity
[b] Addition of considerable quantities of any type of solids will increase the specific gravity
1. Inflammatory exudate
2. Protein and glucose—each gram per deciliter increases the specific gravity by approximately 0.003

IV. Chemical examination of urine

A. Reaction (pH)
1. Methods
a. Nitrazine paper (E. R. Squibb & Sons)
(1) Dip the paper strip into urine several times.
(2) Match the color of the paper strip with the chart 1 min after wetting with urine.
b. Hydrion pH paper strips
(1) Wet the paper with urine and compare with the color chart within 30 sec.
c. pH section of multiple strips (e.g., Labstix)
2. Interpretation
a. Normal: Range varies in different species and individuals, depending upon the diet and metabolism. Urine tends to become less acid after meals (alkaline tide).
(1) Horse—alkaline (pH 8)
(2) Cattle—alkaline (pH 7.4 to 8.4)
(3) Sheep—alkaline

(4) Pig—acid or alkaline
(5) Dog—acid (pH 6 to 7)
(6) Cat—acid (pH 6 to 7
(7) Man—usually acid (pH 4.8 to 7.5)

b. Acid
(1) Normal in carnivorous animals
(2) Nursing calves and foals
(3) Diet with an excess of protein
(4) Starvation—catabolism of body proteins
(5) Fever
(6) Acidosis—both metabolic and respiratory
(a) Diabetes mellitus
(b) Uremia—any cause
(7) Prolonged muscular activity
(8) Administration of acid salts
(a) Sodium acid phosphate
(b) Ammonium chloride
(c) Sodium chloride
(d) Calcium chloride

c. Alkaline
(1) Normal in herbivorous animals
(2) Vegetable diet
(a) Cereals have a high protein content and tend to produce an acid urine.
(3) Cystitis—depending upon the type of bacteria
(4) Urine retention—decomposition of urea to ammonia
(5) Rapid absorption of transudates
(6) Alkalosis—both metabolic and respiratory
(7) Alkaline therapy
(a) Sodium bicarbonate
(b) Sodium and potassium citrate or acetate
(c) Sodium lactate
(d) Potassium nitrate
(8) Urine becomes alkaline when kept at room temperature because of ammonia formation as a result of decomposition of urea.

B. Protein
1. Methods
a. Robert's test
(1) Principle
(a) Precipitation of protein by a strong acid
(2) Procedure
(a) Place 2 ml of Robert's reagent in a test tube

Robert's reagent:

Concentrated nitric acid	1 part
Saturated magnesium sulfate	5 parts
(770 g to 1 L of water)	

(b) Layer 2 ml of clear urine on the reagent by inclining the tube and allowing the urine to run slowly down the side from a long dropper or pipette.
[1] Cloudy urine should be cleared by either centrifugation or filtration before being used.
(c) A positive test is indicated by a white ring at the zone of contact, which should be read against a dark background and reported as:

Negative	No ring at zone of contact
Trace	Barely perceptible ring
+	Distinct narrow ring
+ +	Wider, definite ring
+ + +	Very wide ring
+ + + +	Thick, dense ring occupies most or all of urine layer

(3) Comments
  (a) In many clinical laboratories, Robert's test is the routine method, as it is simple, quick, and easy to read, even when only a small amount of protein is present.
  (b) Limitation—cloudy urine specimens must be cleared by centrifugation or filtration

b. Sulfosalicylic acid test—Bumintest Reagent Tablets (Ames Co.)
(1) Principle
  (a) When Bumintest Reagent Tablets are dissolved in water, a sulfosalicylic acid solution is provided that precipitates urine proteins.
(2) Procedure
  (a) Make a 5% solution of sulfosalicylic acid by dissolving four Bumintest Reagent Tablets in 1 oz (30 ml) of water.
    [1] The reagent remains stable indefinitely under ordinary conditions.
  (b) Place equal parts of reagent solution and urine (not less than 10 drops each) in a small test tube.
    [1] Cloudy urine should be cleared by centrifugation or filtration.
  (c) Shake the tube gently and estimate the amount of protein by the degree of turbidity.
(3) Limitations
  (a) Small amounts of protein may be overlooked, as it is difficult to judge the degree of turbidity.
  (b) Cloudy urine cannot be used until centrifuged or filtered.

c. Albustix Reagent Strip (Ames Co.)—colorimetric strip test
(1) Principle
  (a) Formula—tetrabromphenol blue, citrate buffer, bibulous strip of cellulose
  (b) Action
    [1] At a fixed pH certain indicators will have one color in the presence of protein and another in the absence of protein. The citrate buffer provides a hydrogen ion concentration of approximately pH 3. At this pH, tetrabromphenol blue has a yellow color, while at this same pH in the presence of increasing amounts of protein the indicator will have a green to blue color.
(2) Procedure
  (a) Dip the yellow end of the strip in urine.
  (b) Compare the color of the dipped end with the color chart on the label of the bottle.
  (c) The intensity of the color is proportional to the amount of protein present in the urine and should be reported as:
    [1] Negative—yellow, as no color change occurs
    [2] Positive—the yellow end of the test strip changes immediately to a yellow-green to green to blue-green, depending upon the quantity of protein present
(3) Limitations
  (a) A slight color change on negative samples may be misleading.
  (b) Very highly buffered alkaline urine may give false-positive reactions, and for this reason the test is not recommended for use with urine of species having highly alkaline urine.

d. Albutest Reagent Tablet (Ames Co.)—colorimetric tablet test
(1) Principle
  (a) Formula—bromphenol blue, salicylate buffer, absorbent (cellulose)
  (b) Action
    [1] Same as that of Albustix, except that a different indicator and buffer are used in the tablet. When a drop of urine containing protein is placed on the tablet, the protein is absorbed on the tablet surface. Following addition of two drops of water, a considerable quantity of the

urine is washed away, but protein, indicator, and buffer remain at the surface of the tablet and the indicator produces a green to blue-green color. With a urine containing no protein, the tablet may show color change when the drop of urine is added because of the local effort of pH of the urine, but upon addition of two drops of water the yellow color of the indicator is restored.

(2) Procedure

(a) Place the tablet on a clean surface such as a paper towel, and place 1 drop of urine on the tablet.

(b) After the urine drop has been absorbed, add 2 drops of water and allow penetration before reading.

(c) Compare the color on top of the tablet with the color photograph on the insert of the package.

[1] Negative—the original color of the tablet will not be materially changed at the completion of the test

[2] Positive—a blue-green spot will remain on the tablet surface after the addition of water. The intensity of the color is proportional to the amount of protein present in the urine.

(3) Limitations

(a) A slight color change on negative samples may be misleading to a person first doing the test, but this can be overcome with a little practice.

(b) This test is not nearly as subject to highly alkaline buffered urine as Albustix and could be used with urines from species having alkaline urine.

2. Interpretation

a. Always interpret proteinuria in conjunction with the specific gravity.

b. Normally no protein can be demonstrated in urine by the usual methods.

(1) A small amount of protein normally passes through the glomerular capillaries, but most is reabsorbed by the proximal convoluted tubules.

(a) The small amount of protein that normally passes into the urine is composed primarily of globulins and is insufficient to give a positive reaction with the usual tests.

c. Physiological or functional proteinuria—transient and believed due to a temporary increased glomerular permeability as a result of capillary congestion

(1) Excessive muscular exertion

(2) Convulsions

(3) Emotional stress

(4) Ingestion of an excessive amount of protein

(5) First few days of life

d. Pathologic proteinuria

(1) Prerenal—the protein originates from nonrenal conditions and its loss in the urine is not due to primary renal disease

(a) Bence-Jones proteinuria

[1] Indicative of multiple myeloma

[2] Detected by heating urine, as it precipitates at 50° to 60°C

[3] Detection by urine electrophoresis is more reliable.

(b) Hemoglobinuria

(c) Myoglobinuria

(2) Renal

(a) Causes

[1] Increased permeability of glomerulus

[2] Impaired reabsorption of protein normally present in glomerular filtrate due to tubular disease

[a] If present, will be small in amount

[3] Blood or exudate of renal origin

(b) Although the degree of proteinuria is not always consistent with the cause or severity of the disease, the following conditions might be considered first in differential diagnosis.

[1] Marked—heavy proteinuria without hematuria usually originates in the kidneys and especi[illegible] through the glomerulus

[a] Marked hematuria from any cause—renal neoplasm will produce erythrocytes, leukocytes, and sometimes tumor cells
[b] Acute nephritis
[c] Glomerulonephritis
[d] Nephrosis—especially if due to chemical poisoning
[e] Amyloidosis
[2] Moderate
[a] Pyelonephritis—sometimes produces marked proteinuria, but if chronic may be slight
[b] Polycystic kidneys—slight to moderate proteinuria
[3] Slight
[a] End-stage renal disease—negative to moderate

(3) Postrenal (false, accidental)—protein gains entrance to urine after it leaves the renal tubules by contamination with exudates or blood
(a) A marked hematuria of any cause—produces moderate to marked proteinuria; often seen with improper catheterization
(b) Inflammatory exudate—results in slight to moderate amount of protein
[1] Pyelitis
[2] Ureteritis
[3] Cystitis
[4] Urethritis
[5] Urolithiasis

(4) Extra urinary causes of proteinuria
(a) Blood or exudate from the genital tract contaminates urine.
[1] Preputial or vaginal discharges
[2] Prostatitis
(b) Chronic passive congestion of kidneys can be produced by a number of conditions.
[1] Cardiac insufficiency
[2] Pressure increased within the abdomen from ascitic fluid or tumors
[3] Bacterial endocarditis
[4] Microfilaria of *Dirofilaria immitis*
[5] Liver disease
[6] Febrile reaction
(c) Neoplasms
(d) Emboli

C. Glucose

1. Methods

a. Clinitest Reagent Tablet (Ames Co.)—semiquantitative estimation of sugar in urine
(1) Principle
(a) Formula—copper sulfate, citric acid, sodium hydroxide, sodium carbonate
(b) Action
[1] Reducing sugars present in the urine react with the copper sulfate to reduce the cupric ions to cuprous oxide, giving a color change depending upon the amount of reducing substances present.
(2) Procedure
(a) Place 2 drops of urine and 10 drops of water in a test tube.
(b) Add one Clinitest Reagent Tablet.
(c) Wait 15 sec after boiling stops, then shake gently and compare color reaction with color chart.
[1] Negative—the fluid will be blue; the white sediment that may form has no bearing on the test
[2] Positive—change to green, tan, orange, or dark brown
(3) Limitations
(a) Other reducing substances besides glucose may give a positive reaction. The tablets are stable indefinitely when stored at room temperature in an unopened bottle. They are very

hydroscopic, and precautions should be observed in avoiding exposure to moisture. Keep bottle tightly stoppered. Tablets that show dark blue discoloration in spots or in overall appearance will not give accurate results.

b. Clinistix Reagent Strip (Ames Co.) and Tes-Tape (Eli Lilly & Co.)—colorimetric strip tests for glycosuria
  (1) Principle
    (a) Strips are impregnated with glucose oxidase, peroxidase, and an indicator base, *o*-tolidine.
    (b) Only glucose is oxidized by oxygen in the presence of glucose oxidase, giving rise to gluconic acid and hydrogen peroxide.
    (c) Hydrogen peroxide is decomposed by peroxidase producing nascent oxygen, which oxidizes the indicator base to a colored complex.
  (2) Procedure
    (a) Dip the test end of the strip in urine, or briefly pass it through the urine stream.
    (b) At 10 sec, compare the dipped end of the strip with the color guide.
      [1] Negative—no color change occurs
      [2] Positive—dipped end turns purple with Clinistix and blue with Tes-Tape
  (3) Comments
    (a) Both products provide an excellent screening test for urine glucose; when negative tests are obtained, it is not necessary to proceed with more time-consuming tests except in the dog.
      [1] False-negatives
        [a] High concentrations of ascorbic acid
          1. Diabetic dogs
          2. Normal dogs—in over 85% of all dog urine samples tested, the strip did not work efficiently in detecting low and high glucose concentrations. In over 50% of the cases, the test failed to demonstrate the presence of glucose concentration of 0.15 g/dl.
      [2] When a positive reaction is obtained, it should be followed by the use of Clinitest Tablets or Benedict's solution to determine the amount present, for neither Clinistix nor Tes-Tape is satisfactory for quantitative determinations. Normally, a urine specimen that gives a positive test for glucose with Clinistix will also give a positive test with one of the standard methods. Occasionally, because of the greater sensitivity of Clinistix or Tes-Tape, a urine specimen is positive with these products and negative with metalloreduction tests. This indicates the presence of such small amounts of glucose that it is considered of no clinical significance. A positive reaction with reduction tests and a negative reaction with the glucose oxidase tests may result from the presence of nonglucose reducing substances, such as lactose, or less often from large concentrations of substances that inhibit enzyme reactions, such as ascorbic acid.

c. Diastix (Ames Co.)
  (1) Principle
    (a) A plastic strip with a pale blue area of reagent-impregnated paper on one end, containing the enzymes glucose oxidase and peroxidase. The indicator is potassium iodide, and in conjunction with a blue dye it effects a color change when glucose is present in the urine specimen.
  (2) Procedure
    (a) Dip the reagent end of the strip in the urine specimen for 2 sec and remove, or wet the reagent area of the strip for 2 sec by passing it through the stream of urine.
      [1] Refrigerated urine specimens must be allowed to reach room temperature before testing, since Diastix is dependent upon a temperature-sensitive enzymatic reaction.
      [2] Preservatives containing formaldehyde are known to have an adverse effect upon the test; but chloroform, merthiolate, toluene, or sodium fluoride-thymol do not affect the test.
    (b) Tap the edge of the strip against the side of the container to remove the excess urine.
    (c) Exactly 30 sec after removing the strip from the urine, compare the reagent side of the strip to the closest matching color block. Disregard color changes that occur after 30 sec.
    (d) Results
      [1] Original color of reagent area is blue.
      [2] Six color blocks range from pale blue to dark brown and correspond to urinary concentrations of:

0	
Trace	1/10%
+	1/4%
++	1/2%
+++	(1%)
++++	(2%)

(3) Specificity
- (a) Diastix is specific for glucose.
- (b) Large quantities of ascorbic acid have no effect on the reaction, but large quantities of ketone bodies may depress color development and result in a false-negative reaction, or may depress the color response up to one color block across the entire spectrum of the color chart.
- (c) Hypochlorite, chlorine, or peroxide may cause a false-positive reaction.

FALSE-POSITIVE AND FALSE-NEGATIVE REACTIONS WITH VARIOUS TESTS FOR GLYCOSURIA

Urine constituents causing false-positive or false-negative reactions with tests for glycosuria	Enzyme strip tests: Glucose test area of Clinistix	Enzyme strip tests: Glucose test area of Diastix	Copper reduction tests: Benedict's solution	Copper reduction tests: Clinitest
Sugars other than glucose				
Galactose	No effect	No effect	Reacts positively	Reacts positively
Lactose	No effect	No effect	Reacts positively	Reacts positively
Levulose (fructose)	No effect	No effect	Reacts positively	Reacts positively
Maltose	No effect	No effect	Reacts positively	Reacts positively
Pentose	No effect	No effect	Reacts positively	Reacts positively
Urine constituents				
Creatinine	No effect	No effect	May cause false +	No effect
Uric acid	No effect	No effect	May cause false +	No effect
Ketone bodies	No effect	Large quantities may depress color development	No effect	No effect
Drug metabolites or contaminants in urine				
Salicylates (aspirin)	No effect	No effect	May cause false +	No effect
Penicillin (massive doses)	No effect	No effect	May cause false +	No effect
Chloral hydrate	No effect	No effect	May cause false +	No effect
Menthol	No effect	No effect	May cause false +	No effect
Phenol	No effect	No effect	May cause false +	No effect
Turpentine	No effect	No effect	May cause false +	No effect
Glucosamine	No effect	No effect	May cause false +	No effect
Streptomycin	No effect	No effect	May cause false +	No effect
Isoniazid	No effect	No effect	May cause false +	No effect
Para-aminosalicylic acid*	No effect	No effect	May cause false +	No effect
Ascorbic acid	Large quantities may inhibit reaction	No effect	May cause false + with large quantities	May cause false + with large quantities
Nalidixic acid (RegGram)	No effect	No effect	May cause false +	May cause false +
Cephalosporins (Keflin, Keflex, Loridine)	No effect	No effect	May cause false +	May cause false +
Probenecid (Benemid)	No effect	No effect	May cause false +	May cause false +
Hypochlorite or chlorine	May cause false +	May cause false +	No effect	No effect
Peroxide	May cause false +	May cause false +	No effect	No effect

*Now designated aminosalicylic acid USP.

Notes:

1. If the enzyme test for glucose is positive and Clinitest is negative on the same specimen, it may be due to a concentration of glucose below the sensitivity range for which Clinitest is designed.

2. A positive Clinitest and negative enzyme test on the same specimen are usually due to the presence of nonglucose-reducing substances, i.e., lactose, galactose, etc.

3. False-positive can occur with Benedict's solution more frequently than with Clinitest because of differences in sensitivities of the two tests.

4. By design, Clinitest will detect approximately 0.25% levels of reducing substances. In contrast, Benedict's solution has a senstivity range from 0.07% to 0.15% and may react with the interfering substances listed.

2. Interpretation
   a. Normal urine does not contain glucose, for although glucose passes through the glomerulus, it should be reabsorbed by the proximal convoluted tubules.
   b. Glycosuria with hyperglycemia
      (1) Glycosuria occurs in dogs when the blood glucose levels exceed 180 mg/dl of blood.
      (2) Diabetes mellitus—association of hyperglycemia and ketosis as a result of a deficiency of insulin leading to faulty utilization and storage of carbohydrates
      (3) Acute pancreatic necrosis—when associated with deficiency of insulin
      (4) Hyperadrenocorticism
      (5) Increased secretion or injection of epinephrine
      (6) Solutions administered that contain glucose or fructose
      (7) Excessive intake of carbohydrates in the diet
      (8) Hyperpituitarism or hypothalamic lesions
      (9) Intracranial pressure increased
         (a) Tumor
         (b) Hemorrhage
         (c) Encephalitis
         (d) Fracture
      (10) Enterotoxemia in sheep due to *Clostridium perfringens*, type D
      (11) Hyperthyroidism—due to rapid absorption of carbohydrate from the gastrointestinal tract
   c. Glycosuria without hyperglycemia
      (1) Renal glycosuria—not often seen because of progressive destruction of nephrons
         (a) Due to impaired tubular reabsorption or lowering of renal threshold for glucose
         (b) Only small quantities of glucose seen
      (2) False-positive reaction for glucose when using reducing methods with a number of drugs that have been administered to the patient
         (a) Antibiotics—streptomycin, aureomycin, terramycin, chloramphenicol, penicillin
         (b) Lactose, pentose, or other reducing sugars
         (c) Ascorbic acid
         (d) Morphine
         (e) Salicylates
         (f) Chloral hydrate
         (g) Phlorizin

D. Acetone (ketone)
   1. Methods
      a. Acetest Reagent Tablets (Ames Co.)
         (1) Principle
            (a) Formula—sodium nitroprusside, aminoacetic acid (glycine), disodium phosphate, lactose
            (b) Action
               [1] Based on the nitroprusside reaction, with sodium phosphate to provide the optimum pH for the reaction and lactose to enhance the color quality
         (2) Procedure
            (a) Place the tablet on a clean surface such as a paper towel, and place 1 drop of urine on the tablet.
            (b) Take reading of color on the tablet at 30 sec and compare to color chart.
               [1] Negative—tablet color is unchanged or turns a cream color
               [2] Positive—tablet color varies from lavender to deep purple, representing trace, moderate, or strongly positive reactions
      b. Ketostix Reagent Strip (Ames Co.)—colorimetric strip test specific for diacetic acid
         (1) Principle
            (a) Formula—sodium nitroprusside, aminoacetic acid (glycine), sodium phosphate
            (b) Action—based on the nitroprusside reaction and is specific for diacetic (acetoacetic) acid
         (2) Procedure
            (a) Dip the test end of the strip in urine, or briefly pass it through the urine stream.

(b) Compare color of the dipped end with the color chart on the label of the bottle at 1 min.
[1] Negative—color of test strip remains unchanged or appears cream colored from wetting with urine
[2] Positive—test end of strip develops color varying from pink to purple, representing small, moderate, or large amounts of diacetic acid

c. Ross test
(1) Principle
(a) Sodium nitroprusside is decomposed to sodium ferrocyanide, sodium nitrite, and ferric hydroxide in an alkaline solution. These products are oxidizing agents that form a complex having a purple color in the presence of diacetic acid and acetone. The test is much more sensitive for diacetic acid than for acetone.
(2) Procedure
(a) The reagent consists of a powdered mixture of:

Sodium nitroprusside	1 part
Ammonium sulfate	100 parts

(b) Place ½ in. of the powdered reagent in a dry test tube (13 x 100 mm).
(c) Add 5 ml of urine to the test tube and agitate.
(d) Add 1 to 2 ml of concentrated ammonium hydroxide to form a layer above the mixture.
[1] In the field, a flake of sodium hydroxide can substitute for the ammonium hydroxide solution and should be added before the tube is agitated.
(e) The reaction is reported as:

Trace	Very slight purple color
+	Slight purple color
+ +	Moderate purple color
+ + +	Dark purple color
+ + + +	Dark purple color or black

(f) This test is also effective when applied to milk.

2. Interpretation
a. The ketone bodies include acetone, acetoacetic acid (diacetic acid), and beta-hydroxybutyric acid. A state in which these substances are present in increased amounts in the blood and urine is called ketosis. Acetoacetic acid and beta-hydroxybutyric acid, from which acetone is derived, are normal intermediate products of fat metabolism. When greater amounts of fatty acids are utilized with the production of more acetoacetic acid and beta-hydroxybutyric acid than can be oxidized by the tissues, these bodies accumulate in the blood and are excreted in the urine. Ketosis develops in any of the clinical states of deficient carbohydrate metabolism because optimum carbohydrate metabolism inhibits ketosis.
(1) Ketosis (acetonemia)—in pregnant or lactating cows and pregnant ewes (pregnancy disease)
(a) Associated with a hypoglycemia
(b) A marked positive acetone test in bovine urine is abnormal, as the urine of cattle usually contains a negligible quantity of ketone bodies.
(c) It is important to differentiate severe ketosis from mild ketosis caused by an animal going off feed from other pathological conditions.
(2) Diabetes mellitus—associated with a hyperglycemia, as normal carbohydrate utilization is lacking
(a) Clinical ketosis is rarely seen in the dog; when it is observed, it is usually associated with diabetes, so this should be the first condition to investigate as a possible cause in this species.
(3) Acidosis
(4) High fat diet
(5) Starvation or fasting—carbohydrate stores are depleted and metabolism of fat predominates
(a) The adult dog is comparatively resistant to the development of ketosis during fasting, but puppies develop a marked ketosis.
(6) Impaired liver function
(7) After ether or chloroform anesthesia

(8) Prolonged vomiting and diarrhea—a type of starvation ketosis
(9) Infectious diseases—associated with caloric imbalance
(10) Milk fever—if prolonged
(11) Endocrine disorders
(a) Hyperfunction of the anterior pituitary or adrenal cortex
(b) Excess of female sex hormones

E. Blood
1. Methods
a. Occultest Reagent Tablet (Ames Co.)
(1) Principle
(a) Formula—orthotolidine, strontium peroxide, calcium acetate, tartaric acid, sodium bicarbonate, red dye
(b) Action
[1] Oxygen is liberated from strontium peroxide when reduced by peroxidase of hemoglobin and is detected by the orthotolidine.
(2) Procedure
(a) Place 1 drop of well-mixed urine in the center of a filter paper square.
[1] Have a paper towel under the filter paper to avoid contamination from the working area.
(b) Place the tablet in the center of the moist area.
(c) Drop 2 drops of water on the tablet so that they run down onto the paper.
(d) A positive reaction for blood is characterized by a distinct blue area that forms within 2 min on the paper surrounding the tablet; if the reaction is negative, the paper will not change color even though the tablet may turn slightly blue.
(3) Comment
(a) More sensitive and less expensive than Hematest Reagent Tablets. The sensitivity is 1 part of blood in 100,000.
b. Hematest Reagent Tablet (Ames Co.)
(1) Principle
(a) Formula—orthotolidine, strontium peroxide, calcium acetate, tartaric acid
(b) Action
[1] Same as for Occultest Reagent Tablet
(2) Procedure and results
(a) Same as for Occultest Reagent Tablet
(3) Limitations
(a) Less sensitive and more expensive than Occultest Tablet, the test is specifically designed to detect occult blood in feces, as the sensitivity is 1 part of blood in 20,000 to 30,000.
c. Hemastix (Ames Co.)
(1) Principle
(a) The reagent portion of the strip is impregnated with a buffered mixture of organic peroxide and orthotolidine.
(2) Procedure
(a) Dip the test end of the strip into well-mixed urine, or briefly pass it through the urine stream. Observe at 30 sec.
(b) Results
[1] Negative—no blue color is present on the test end of the strip at 30 sec.
[2] Positive—test end of the strip turns blue within 30 sec; the color blocks on the bottle label indicate reactions obtained with small, moderate, and large amounts of excreted occult blood
(3) Specificity
(a) Hemoglobin, myoglobin, and erythrocytes give a positive reaction. The test is more sensitive to free hemoglobin and myoglobin than to intact erythrocytes.
(b) False-positive reaction—oxidizing agents such as hypochlorites
(c) False-negative reaction—ascorbic acid, large quantities

2. Interpretation—distinction between hematuria and hemoglobinuria is of tremendous diagnostic significance
   a. Hematuria—intact erythrocytes incorporated in the urine
      (1) Acute nephritis
      (2) Nephrosis—marked degeneration
      (3) Renal infarction
      (4) Passive congestion of kidney
      (5) Neoplasm of kidney, bladder, or prostate
      (6) Urolithiasis—urethral, cystic, or renal
      (7) Abscess of kidney
      (8) Pyelitis
      (9) Pyelonephritis
      (10) Ureteritis
      (11) Cystitis
      (12) Urethritis
      (13) Trauma to urethra—usually from improper catheterization
      (14) During estrus or postpartum in female—from contamination by uterine or vaginal discharges
      (15) Prostatitis
      (16) Severe infections—anthrax, leptospirosis, infectious canine hepatitis
      (17) Chemical agents
         (a) Copper poisoning
         (b) Mercury poisoning
         (c) Sulfonamides
         (d) Phenol
         (e) Methenamine
      (18) Thrombocytopenia
      (19) Sweetclover poisoning
      (20) Parasites
         (a) *Dioctophyma renale*—in the canine
         (b) *Dirofilaria immitis*—in the canine
      (21) Acute vegetative endocarditis and congestive heart failure—in the canine
   b. Hemoglobinuria—hemoglobin in the urine is due to excessive hemolysis of erythrocytes
      (1) Parturient hemoglobinuria
      (2) Bacillary hemoglobinuria—*Clostridium hemolyticum*
      (3) *Clostridium perfringens*, type A
      (4) Leptospirosis
      (5) Piroplasmosis or babesiasis
         (a) **Hemoglobinuria is an important sign in the differentiation of this disease from anaplasmosis because hemoglobinuria is absent in anaplasmosis.**
      (6) Feeding large amounts of beet pulp—aphosphorosis
      (7) Hemolytic disease of the newborn
      (8) Incompatible blood transfusion
      (9) Photosensitization
      (10) Severe burns
      (11) Chemical hemolytic agents
         (a) Sulfonamides
         (b) Copper
         (c) Mercury
      (12) Plants
         (a) Broom
         (b) Savin
         (c) Mercury
         (d) Hellebore
         (e) Ranunculus

(f) Convolvulus
(g) Colchicum
(h) Oak shoots
(i) Ash
(j) Hazel
(k) Frosted turnips and other roots
(l) Privet

c. Myoglobinuria—myoglobin from muscle cells will produce a positive reaction with blood tests, imparts a brown to black color to the urine, and is differentiated from hematuria by the absence of intact erythrocytes in the urine sediment
(1) Azoturia—paralytic equine myohemoglobinuria

F. Bilirubin (bile)
1. Methods
a. Foam test
(1) Shake a few milliliters of urine vigorously in a test tube.
(2) Results
(a) Normal urine will foam slightly and the foam is white.
(b) Bile pigment produces a yellow, greenish yellow, or brown color to urine, and this color is imparted to the foam.
(3) Limitations
(a) There is a marked increase in the foaming quality of urine with proteinuria. The foam test is not sensitive or specific.

b. Icotest Reagent Tablet (Ames Co.)—to detect bilirubinuria
(1) Principle
(a) Formula—*p*-nitrobenzene diazonium *p*-toluene sulfonate, sulfosalicylic acid, sodium bicarbonate, absorbent asbestos-cellulose mat
(b) Action
[1] The reaction of bilirubin in the urine with the diazo compound in the tablet produces a blu or purple color.
(2) Procedure
(a) Place 5 drops of urine on 1 square of the special mat.
(b) Place the Ictotest Reagent Tablet in the center of the moistened area.
(c) Allow 2 drops of water to flow over the tablet onto the mat.
(d) Results
[1] Negative—mat shows no color within 30 sec; a slight pink or red color that sometimes appears should be called negative
[2] Positive—the mat around the tablet turns blue or purple; the amount of bilirubin is propor tional to the speed and intensity of the color reaction

c. Ictostix (Ames Co.)
(1) Principle
(a) A plastic strip has affixed to one end a small square of filter paper impregnated with stabiliz diazotized 2, 4-dichloroaniline as the reagent. When bilirubin is present, it reacts with the reagent to form azobilirubin, and the reagent area changes in color from buff to light tan or light brown, depending upon the amount of bilirubin present.
(2) Procedure
(a) Dip the reagent area of the strip in fresh, well-mixed, uncentrifuged urine and remove immediately.
(b) Tap the edge of the strip against the side of the container to remove any excess urine.
(c) 20 sec after moistening compare the color of the reagent area to the color chart on the bottle label. Hold the strip close to the color blocks and match quickly.
(d) Results

Result	Color	Approximate mg bilirubin/dl urine
Dry	Buff	
Negative	Pale lemon	
+ (small)	Light tan	0.2
+ + (moderate)	Dark tan	0.5
+ + + (large)	Light brown	1.0

(3) Specificity
(a) The Ictostix is specific for bilirubin in biological material, but with animal urine it does not appear to be as sensitive as the Ictotest Tablet.
(b) False-positive reaction—chlorpromazine (e.g., Thorazine) metabolites
(c) False-negative reaction
[1] Using a urine specimen that has not been freshly voided
[2] Pyridium and other brightly colored compounds may give a reddish color to the urine and could mask the reaction.

d. Gmelin test
(1) Principle
(a) Bile pigments are oxidized by acids to colored derivatives.
(2) Procedure
(a) In a test tube place 2 ml of nitric acid that has become yellow from age and partial oxidation. A piece of applicator stick placed in nitric acid will give the yellow nitric acid required for the test.
(b) Overlay the acid with 2 ml of urine.
(c) When bile is present, a ring will form at the junction of the two fluids, and the colors green and violet can best be seen by holding the tube against a white background.
(3) Limitations
(a) This is not a satisfactory test to apply to bovine urine, which contains a pigment other than bile that turns pinkish red on contact with an acid; this color is not significant.

2. Interpretation
a. Always interpret in association with specific gravity.
b. The threshold for bilirubin in the normal dog kidney is low.
(1) Urine from the normal dog often contains some bilirubin, especially if the sample is concentrated.
(a) Tests for bilirubin will frequently be slightly positive in the absence of liver disease.
c. Pathologic bilirubinuria
(1) Bilirubin must be conjugated by liver to pass through normal glomeruli.
(2) Conjugated bilirubin may spill into urine following excessive accumulation in blood.
(a) Causes
[1] Hepatocellular disease
[a] Infectious canine hepatitis
[b] Leptospirosis
[c] Cirrhosis
[d] Neoplasia
[e] Toxicities
[2] Obstruction of bile ducts—any cause
(3) In jaundice due to hemolysis, bilirubinuria is usually not present until liver damage results.

G. Urobilinogen
1. Methods
a. Wallace-Diamond test

(1) Principle
  (a) Depends upon the reaction of urobilinogen and other chromagens with Ehrlich's benzaldehyde reagent to form a red color
(2) Procedure
  (a) To 5 ml of urine in a test tube add 0.5 ml of Ehrlich's benzaldehyde reagent.

Ehrlich's benzaldehyde reagent:	
para-dimethylaminobenzaldehyde	2 g
20% aqueous solution of concentrated hydrochloric acid	100 ml

    [1] It is essential that the urine be fresh, since urobilinogen on exposure to light and air is changed into urobilin, which does not react.
    [2] If large amounts of bile are present, equal parts of urine and 10% aqueous solution of barium chloride should be mixed and filtered to remove all precipitate, as bilirubin interferes with reading the results of the urobilinogen reaction.
  (b) Allow the tube to stand for 5 min and observe for pink to red color development by viewing lengthwise through the tube against a white background.
    [1] Normal—pink to light red color
    [2] No urobilinogen—absence of pink or red color
    [3] Increased urobilinogen—cherry red color
  (c) When the undiluted urine shows an apparent increase in urobilinogen, as noted by a cherry red color, it may be of value to conduct a semiquantitative determination by making dilutions of the urine and repeating the test.
    [1] Place 6 to 8 test tubes of the same diameter in a rack.
    [2] Add 5 ml of water to each test tube.
    [3] Add 5 ml of fresh urine to the first tube, mix, and pipette 5 ml of the mixture into the second tube. Repeat this procedure serially until the final test tube, from which 5 ml of the mixture should be removed and kept if further dilution is required.
    [4] Add 0.5 ml of Ehrlich's reagent to each tube and mix thoroughly.
    [5] Allow the tubes to stand for 5 min.
    [6] The last tube dilution in which a faint pink color appears should be recorded as the end point.
    [7] When barium chloride is used to remove the bilirubin, allowance should be made for this dilution, for then the first tube in the semiquantitative determination should be diluted 1:4 (rather than 1:2), the second tube 1:8, etc.

b. Urobilistix (Ames Co.)
(1) Principle
  (a) The plastic strip has affixed to one end a small square of paper impregnated with 2.9% para-dimethylaminobenzaldehyde and 97.1% buffer as a dry reagent. The method is based on the Ehrlich reaction of the reagent with urobilinogen in a strongly acid medium to form a reddish color.
(2) Procedure
  (a) Dip the reagent area of the strip in fresh urine that has been well mixed.
    [1] The test should be made on urine within 1 hr after collection, as urobilinogen is quite unstable when exposed to room temperature or light.
    [2] No preservative or additive should be used, as preservatives do not prevent deterioration of urobilinogen.
  (b) Remove the strip from the urine. Tap the edge of the strip against the side of the container to remove excess urine.
  (c) Allow the reaction to continue for exactly 60 sec from dipping; immediately compare the reagent area to the color chart, holding it close to the chart. Interpolate the result if the color produced falls between two color blocks.
  (d) Results
    [1] The dry test area is yellow.
    [2] Color blocks representing 0.1, 1, 4, 8, and 12 Ehrlich units/dl vary from a yellow-green to a reddish brown.

(3) Specificity
  (a) The main indication for the test is in the diagnosis of biliary obstruction where there is an absence of urine urobilinogen. The absence of urobilinogen cannot be determined with this strip.
  (b) False-positive reaction
    [1] Strongly alkaline urine will have higher urine urobilinogen values than would be normal.
      [a] Herbivorous animals
      [b] Patients with a urinary tract infection such as cystitis
      [c] Patients on medication
    [2] *p*-aminosalicylic acid metabolites, Gantrisin, and Azo-Gantrisin all give an orange color that matches the 4 Ehrlich units/dl block, but the reaction is immediate rather than gradual.
    [3] Pyridium metabolites
    [4] Porphobilinogen
  (c) False-negative reaction
    [1] Urine not fresh
    [2] Urine specimen greatly diluted by polyuria
    [3] Amount of urobilinogen in the urine varies with the time of day.
      [a] It is preferable to test urine for urobilinogen on a 2-hr specimen collected between 2 to 4 in the afternoon, when the urobilinogen may be maximal.
    [4] A strongly acid urine will have lower urobilinogen values than normally seen.
    [5] Patients on antibiotic therapy producing suppressed intestinal flora

2. Interpretation
  a. Normal urobilinogen
    (1) Urobilinogen is a chromagen that is formed in the intestines by the reducing action of bacteria on bilirubin. A portion is excreted in the feces, but some is absorbed into the portal circulation and returned to and removed by the liver through the bile. Some of the urobilinogen enters the kidney during the period it is in the general circulation, and a small amount is excreted in the urine.
    (2) Canine and feline urine will have a color production in dilutions up to 1:32 and occasionally up to 1:64.
  b. Decreased amount or absence of urine urobilinogen
    (1) Obstruction of biliary passages
      (a) Urine urobilinogen is of greatest value in differentiating obstructive jaundice from jaundice caused by hepatic disease or hemolysis. In animals with complete obstruction, bilirubin does not reach the intestinal tract and urobilinogen is not formed. Urobilinogen is absent in the urine and in the feces, producing a clay-colored stool, for the oxidation product of urobilinogen (urobilin) contributes to the normal brown color.
    (2) Decreased destruction of erythrocytes
    (3) Impaired intestinal absorption—as in diarrhea
    (4) Certain antibiotics—especially aureomycin; inhibition of intestinal bacteria interferes with the formation of urobilinogen
    (5) Nephritis—sometimes; due to dilution of urobilinogen by the polyuria associated with end-stage renal disease
  c. Increased amount of urine urobilinogen
    (1) Hepatitis—damaged liver cells cannot effectively remove urobilinogen from the portal circulation
    (2) Cirrhosis of the liver
    (3) Hemolytic jaundice
      (a) Excessive hemolysis of erythrocytes results in an increased amount of bilirubin, with an increase in the production of urobilinogen in the intestines and an abnormally large amount of urobilinogen excreted in the urine.
    (4) It is helpful to use the presence of urine urobilinogen in combination with urine bilirubin in testing, although it should be noted that these disorders often occur concomitantly and any test or combination of tests for them may not give classical results and may be confusing to interpret.

Substance	Normal patient	Hemolytic disease	Hepatic disease	Biliary obstruction
Urine urobilinogen	Normal	High	High	Low
Urine bilirubin	Negative	Negative	Positive	Positive

d. Substances that interfere with testing
   (1) Indole—also gives a red color with Ehrlich's reagent
   (2) Bile and nitrites—produce a green color with Ehrlich's reagent
      (a) Nitrites may be produced by bacteria in urinary tract infections.
   (3) Sulfonamides and procaine—produce a greenish yellow color with Ehrlich's reagent
   (4) Formalin

H. Indican
1. Method
a. Obermayer's test
   (1) Principle
      (a) Indican is derived from indole, a product of intestinal putrefaction of protein. Indole is absorbed by the blood and oxidized by the liver to indoxyl, which combines with potassium sulfate to form indican (indoxyl potassium sulfate), which is eliminated in the urine. Obermayer's reagent oxidizes indican to indigo-blue, which is absorbed in the chloroform layer to produce a blue color.
   (2) Procedure
      (a) To 5 ml of urine in a test tube add 5 ml of Obermayer's reagent.

Obermayer's reagent:	
Concentrated hydrochloric acid	1000 ml
Ferric chloride	2 g

      (b) Mix thoroughly by inverting the tube several times.
      (c) Add 2 ml of chloroform and mix by inverting the tube several times, but avoid violent shaking.
      (d) Allow the chloroform to settle in the bottom of the tube.
      (e) A blue color in the chloroform layer indicates the presence of indican.

Negative	No color
+	Pale blue color
+ +	Moderate blue color
+ + +	Dark blue color
+ + + +	Black

2. Interpretation
a. Normal
   (1) Indican is absent or present as a trace in the urine of the dog and cat.
   (2) Indican is always present in heavy concentration in the urine of herbivorous animals and has no clinical significance.
b. Increased amount
   (1) Is of questionable diagnostic significance, as it does not differentiae between intestinal conditions and many preferable methods are available for identifying the conditions characterized by an indicanuria
   (2) Constipation
   (3) Indigestion
   (4) Intestinal obstruction
   (5) Gastritis
   (6) Enteritis
   (7) Diminished bile flow

(8) Diet rich in protein
(9) Decomposition of protein in other parts of body
(a) Large abscess
(b) Empyema
(c) Peritonitis

I. Calcium
1. Method
a. Sulkowitch test
(1) Principle
(a) Urine calcium is precipitated as insoluble calcium oxalate.
(2) Procedure
(a) Add 5 ml of distilled water to an equal quantity of urine and mix well.
(b) In a second tube of the same diameter, mix equal parts of urine and Sulkowitch reagent.

Sulkowitch reagent:	
Oxalic acid	2.5 g
Ammonium oxalate	2.5 g
Glacial acetic acid	5.0 ml
Water, to make	150 ml

(c) Compare the two test tubes in transmitted light in 2 min and again in 10 min.
(d) Results
[1] Low—no visible precipitate
[2] Normal—precipitate just detectable or seen as fine white cloud
[3] High—heavy white precipitate
2. Interpretation
a. Normal urine calcium (7)

Species	Excretion mEq/day	Concentration mEq/L
Dog	1.3(0.1-7)	2.1(0.2-76)
Cat	0.11	3.0
Cattle	18(4.5-74.3)	
Man	8(2-18)	7.5(1.4-13)

b. Decreased urine calcium—serum calcium level is below the renal threshold of 7.5 mg/dl
(1) Bovine hypocalcemia—the Sulkowitch test does not give an indication of the serum calcium level and is not a reliable aid in the field diagnosis of this condition. (6)
(2) Canine puerperal tetany
(3) Hypoparathyroidism
(4) Osteomalacia
c. Increased urine calcium—serum calcium level is above 10.5 mg/dl
(1) After administration of calcium solutions—the Sulkowitch test is reliable in indicating an excess of calcium in the blood
(2) Renal osteodystrophy—parathyroid hyperplasia with renal failure
(3) Hyperthyroidism
(4) Hypervitaminosis

J. Sulfonamides
1. Methods
a. Lignin test
(1) Principle

(a) The arylamine group in the sulfonamide reacts with crude cellulose in the presence of acid to produce a yellow to orange color.

(2) Procedure

(a) Place 1 or 2 drops of urine or dissolved crystals on a strip of newspaper or paper towel.

[1] Filter paper or bond paper should not be used.

(b) Apply a drop of 25% hydrochloric acid to the center of the moistened area.

(c) The presence of sulfonamide is indicated by the appearance of an orange color.

K. Multiple Reagent Strips (Ames Co.)—available in the following combinations:

Substance	Time read	Uristix	Combistix	Hema-Combistix	Labstix	Bili-Labstix	Multistix	N-Multistix
Protein	Not critical	X	X	X	X	X	X	X
Glucose								
Clinistix	10 sec	X	X	X	X	X		
Diastix	10-30 sec						X	X
pH	Not critical		X	X	X	X	X	X
Blood	30 sec			X	X	X	X	X
Ketones	15 sec				X	X	X	X
Bilirubin	20 sec					X	X	X
Urobilinogen	60 sec						X	X
Nitrite	30 sec							X

L. Comments

1. The most useful combination in veterinary medicine appears to be Labstix Reagent Strip and Ictotest Tablets.

   a. Ictotest Reagent Tablets are 4 to 8 times more sensitive to bilirubin than the bilirubin test area on the multiple strips.

   b. The urobilinogen test area does not indicate the absence of urobilinogen, and since it has limited application (biliary obstruction), it is not a routine test in urinalysis.

   c. The nitrite test in the N-Multistix has not been especially reliable for detection of urinary tract infections in domestic animals.

2. It should be kept in mind that these are screening tests and can be verified by other methods when more sensitivity is desired:

Substance	Recommended confirming tests
Protein	Robert's test Sulfosalicylic acid (Bumintest)
Glucose	Clinitest (in diabetic animals with large quantities of ascorbic acid in the urine)
Blood	Occultest Microscopic examination of urine sediment
Ketones	Acetest tablets
Urobilinogen	Wallace-Diamond or Watson method

V. Microscopic examination of urine

A. General considerations

1. The microscopic examination of urine is of great clinical importance and should never be omitted.
2. Recognition of significant objects in urine sediment can only be accomplished by experience.
   a. Important structures to identify include casts, erythrocytes, leukocytes, and bacteria.
   b. Disregard objects that have no significance, as urine may be contaminated by every conceivable type of debris.
3. If the urine sample is small, it should be centrifuged first to insure an adequate amount of sediment; the supernatant can be used for the chemical tests.
4. Casts and erythrocytes disappear upon standing, so examination should be made on fresh specimens.
5. Normal urine usually contains little sediment. There may be an occasional leukocyte, epithelial cells, mucus, crystals, and bacteria if the urine was not collected aseptically.

B. Method

1. Agitate the urine to suspend any sediment that may have settled to the bottom.
2. Fill a centrifuge tube with urine to within ¾ in. of the top and centrifuge for 3 min at a low rate of speed.
3. Pour all the urine out of the tube. When the tube is placed in an upright position, there is sufficient urine on the sides to drain to the bottom and suspend the sediment.
4. Mix the sediment with the urine by striking the bottom of the tube with a finger, pour a drop on a glass slide, and cover with a coverglass that has been wiped clean of oil and lint.
5. Examine under the microscope with the low power objective and subdued light; then examine with the high power objective to identify smaller objects.
6. Findings should be reported as the average number seen per low power or high power field, or few, many, or abundant.
7. If necessary, stain with new methylene blue or Sternheimer-Malbin stain.

C. Organized sediment (See Fig. 18.1.)

1. Epithelial cells
   a. Types
      (1) Squamous epithelial cells
         (a) Largest of the cells appearing in urine sediment
         (b) Have an irregular outline and occur singly or in sheets
         (c) Contain a small, round nucleus
         (d) Derived from the superficial layer of the urethra and vagina
      (2) Transitional epithelial cells
         (a) Various forms, including round, oval, spindle-shape, and caudate
         (b) Intermediate in size between the squamous epithelial cell and the renal cell
         (c) Often granular in texture and contain a small nucleus
         (d) Derived from part of the urethra, bladder, ureters, and pelves of the kidneys
      (3) Renal epithelial cells
         (a) Small, round cells with a single nucleus
         (b) Slightly larger than leukocytes
         (c) Even when the urine is freshly collected, cellular structure is insufficiently defined due to degeneration.
         (d) Usually can be identified with certainty only when the renal cells are incorporated in epithelial casts
   b. Significance
      (1) A certain number of epithelial cells in urine is normal.
         (a) Squamous epithelial cells may appear in large numbers, especially in voided samples from female animals.
         (b) Occasional transitional cells are normally present.

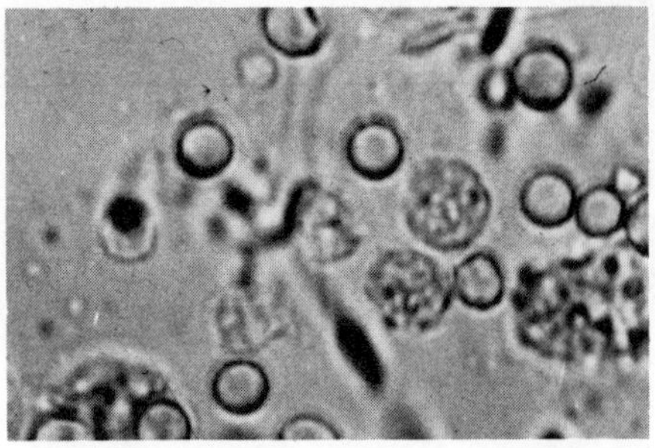

Erythrocytes, leukocytes, and spermatozoa.

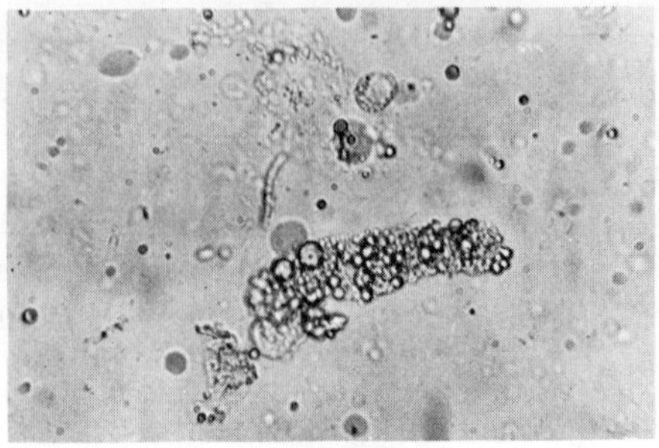

Fatty cast.

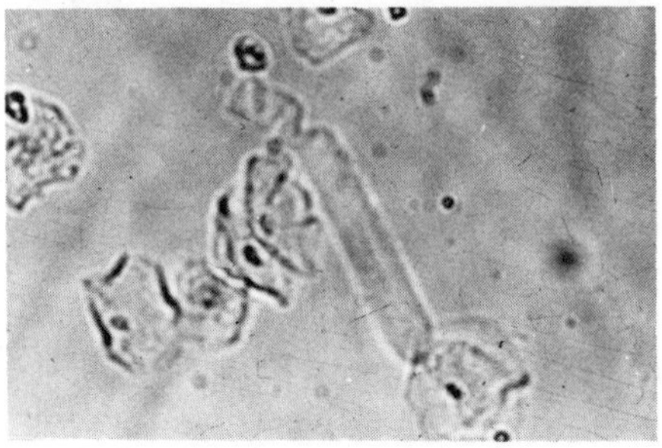

Squamous epithelial cells and hyaline cast.

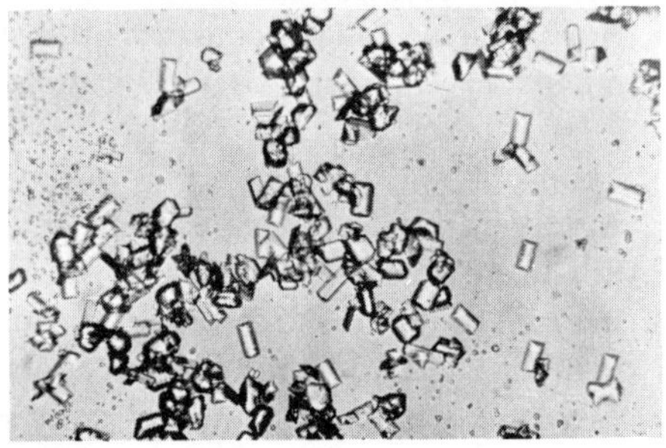

Triple phosphate crystals.

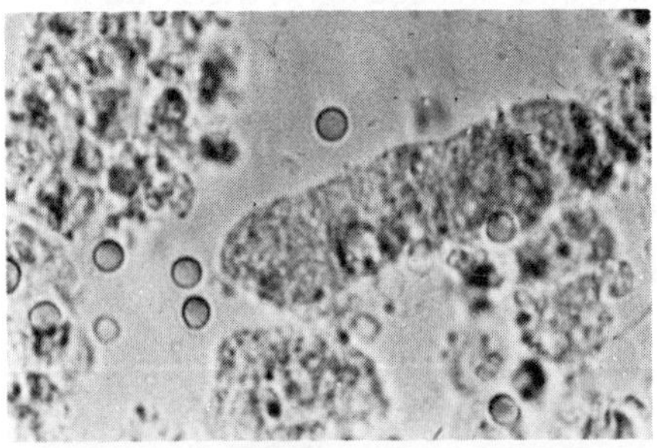

Granular cast and erythrocytes.

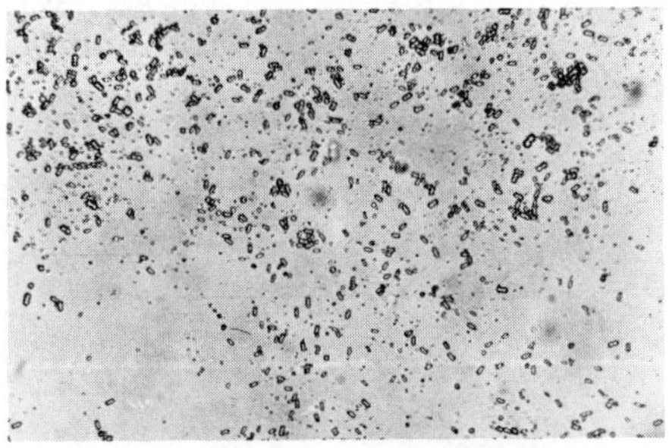

Calcium carbonate crystals (low power).

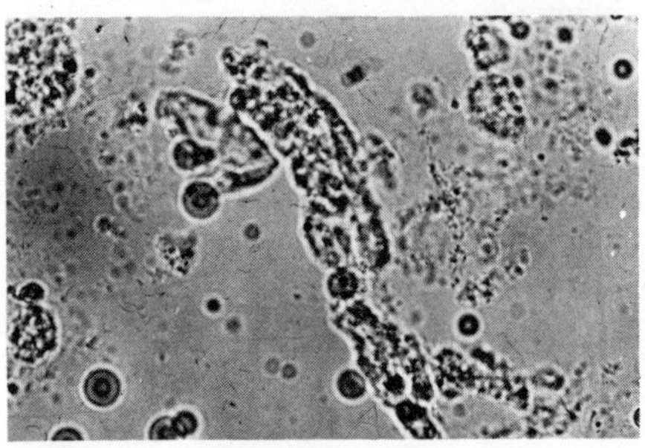

Epithelial cast.

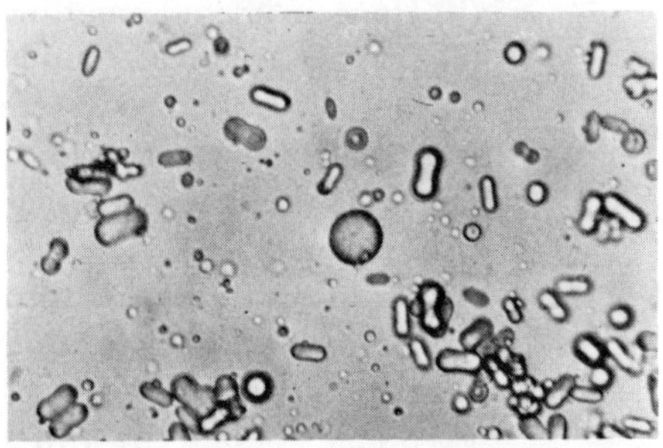

Calcium carbonate crystals (high power).

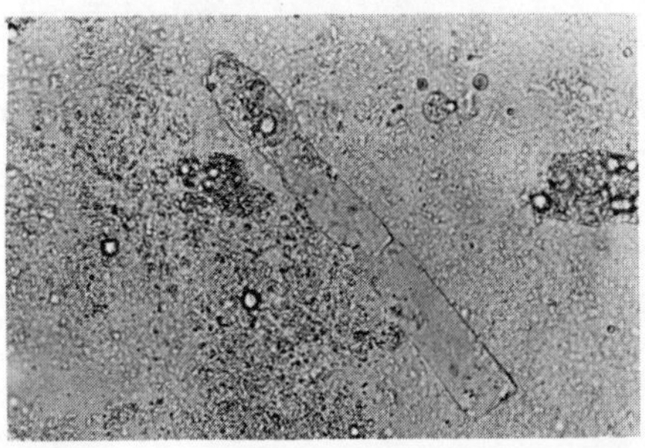

Waxy cast.

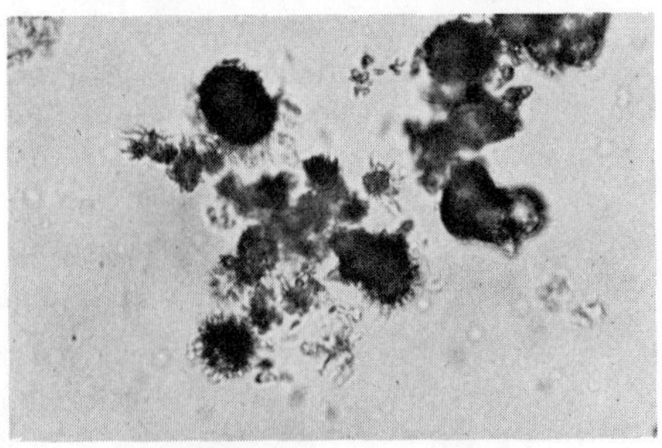

Ammonium urate crystals.

Fig. 18.1. Urine sediment.

(2) In certain pathological conditions, cells are greatly increased in number.

(a) Renal cells are present in acute interstitial nephritis, but usually cannot be recognized.

(b) Transitional cells are increased in cystitis and pyelonephritis.

2. Erythrocytes

a. Yellow to orange, but may be colorless if they have been in the urine long enough for hemoglobin to dissolve out

b. Smaller than leukocytes and contain no internal structure, so are often confused with oil droplets or amorphous urates

c. Usually round, but may vary greatly in appearance according to the physical and chemical properties of the urine

(1) In concentrated urine the erythrocytes are likely to be crenated.

(2) In dilute urine they are swollen and appear as faint colorless rings.

d. If in doubt about the identification, add a drop of dilute acetic acid or saponin solution, which dissolves the erythrocytes, or use one of the chemical tests for blood on the sediment left in the tube.

e. Significance—denotes hemorrhage somewhere in the genitourinary tract

(1) If catheterization was employed to obtain the urine, this may account for the presence of fresh blood.

3. Leukocytes or pus cells

a. Appear as granular cells that are larger than erythrocytes but smaller than epithelial cells

b. It may be possible to distinguish the nucleus, usually segmented, but often it has degenerated.

c. Significance

(1) A few leukocytes may be present in normal urine.

(2) Pyuria indicates a purulent process at some point in the genitourinary tract.

(a) Contamination from the genital tract—vulvitis, vaginitis, balanitis, metritis

(b) Urethritis

(c) Cystitis

(d) Pyelitis or pyelonephritis

(e) Nephritis

4. Casts

a. Formation

(1) Casts are cylindrical bodies appearing in the urinary sediment; they are so named because their shape represents an actual cast of the tubular lumen.

(2) They are formed principally in the lumen of the distal tubules and in the collecting tubules of the kidneys.

(a) It is here that the urine is likely to reach its maximum concentration and acidity, which favors the precipitation of protein.

(3) When cells and cellular debris are present in the tubules, they are included in the hyaline matrix at the time of its formation as casts, giving rise to a variety of types.

b. Types of casts

(1) Hyaline cast

(a) Made of protein alone

(b) Colorless, homogeneous, semitransparent, cylindrical structures with parallel sides and usually rounded ends

(c) Readily soluble in alkaline urine, which probably accounts for their uncommon occurrence in the sediment of large animals

(d) Can only be seen in a well-darkened field, since the refractive index of hyaline is nearly identical with the surrounding medium

(2) Granular cast

(a) Hyaline casts containing fine or coarse granules that are chiefly derived from the disintegration of tubular epithelial cells

(b) The most common type of cast seen in domestic animals

(3) Epithelial cast

(a) Formed from desquamated cells from the epithelial lining of the renal tubule

(b) Often appears as two rows of epithelial cells

(4) Waxy cast
(a) Yellow or gray in color, broader than hyaline casts, highly refractive, and usually found broken off with square ends
(5) Fatty cast
(a) Contains numerous fat globules that are very refractive
(b) Colorless, or will stain orange to red with Sudan III stain
(6) Blood casts (4)
(a) Blood cast—homogeneous cylindrical mass that is deep yellow or orange in color
(b) Hyaline red blood cell cast—deep yellow-orange color; cellular margins of erythrocytes incorporated in the cast can be seen
(7) Leukocytic cast
(a) Leukocytes adhere to the hyaline matrix.

c. Significance of casts—generally indicate varying degrees of renal changes: renal irritation, renal inflammation, renal degeneration (1)
(1) Hyaline cast
(a) Indicates the mildest form of renal irritation
(b) A few may be present in normal urine.
(c) May be seen with more severe types of renal damage, but usually other types of casts will also be present
(d) Any febrile condition
(e) After anesthesia
(f) After strenuous exercise
(g) Circulatory disturbances
(2) Granular cast
(a) Indicates a more severe type of renal disease than the hyaline cast, for it represents the disintegration of renal tubular epithelium
(b) Large numbers are usually associated with more severe renal disease involving necrosis of tubular cells.
[1] Nephritis—any cause
[2] Infarcts—bacterial endocarditis
(c) Occasional granular casts are usually seen in chronic interstitial nephritis, for the large volume of urine limits cast formation.
(3) Epithelial cast
(a) Formed as a result of desquamation of tubular cells that have not disintegrated
(b) Acute nephritis
(c) Degeneration of tubular epithelium
(4) Waxy cast
(a) Advanced severe nephritis and renal degeneration
(b) Amyloidosis—not frequently
(5) Fatty cast
(a) Degenerative tubular disease associated with deposition of lipoidal material in the renal tubules
(b) Occasionally seen in cats with renal disease, as lipuria is common in cats
(c) Occasionally seen in dogs with diabetes mellitus
(6) Blood cast
(a) Blood cast—glomerulitis
(b) Hyaline red blood cell cast—hemorrhage has occurred within the nephron of the kidney
(7) Leukocytic cast
(a) Occurs in association with inflammation that involves renal tubules
(b) Indicates a suppurative process in the kidney
(c) Pyelonephritis
(d) Kidney abscess
(8) Bile-stained cast
(a) Any cast may be pigmented with bile when large quantities of bilirubin are present.

5. Cylindroid
   a. Resembles a hyaline cast, except that one end tapers off to a fine filament
   b. Significance—same as that of the hyaline cast
6. Mucus and mucous threads
   a. Mucous threads have a long, narrow, wavy, twisted, ribbonlike appearance.
   b. Mucus in horse urine has a homogeneous appearance.
   c. Requires reduced illumination, as the refractive index is much the same as the surrounding medium
   d. Would often be overlooked except for objects that adhere to the mucous threads and help to outline them
   e. Significance
      (1) In the horse a large amount of homogeneous mucus is normal, for it is the only animal with mucus-secreting glands in the renal pelvis and in the ureter close to the kidney.
      (2) In other animals mucous threads may indicate an irritation of the urethra, but their presence is usually due to contamination of the urine specimen by genital secretions.
7. Microorganisms
   a. Bacteria
      (1) With use of the high power objective, bacteria are seen as small objects displaying true motility or Brownian movement.
      (2) It is often possible to ascertain the morphology of the bacteria present, but staining will increase the accuracy of the identification.
      (3) Significance
         (a) Little, unless the urine was collected aseptically by catheterization or aspiration from the bladder through the abdominal wall by means of a needle and syringe
         (b) Normally, no bacteria are seen in urine.
         (c) Large numbers of bacteria that are observed in catheterized or midstream urine or in samples obtained by paracentesis suggest bacterial infection anywhere along the urinary tract (cystitis, pyelonephritis), especially when associated with abnormal quantities of WBC and RBC.
            [1] Urinary bladder most common site
            [2] Bacteria observed with the microscope in a noncentrifuged sample of urine suggest a concentration of 1,000,000 + bacteria per millimeter or urine and infection.
            [3] Gram's stain may facilitate detection.
         (d) Infections of the genital tract may result in bacteria being seen in urine sediment; included here would be metritis, vaginitis, and prostatitis.
   b. Yeast
      (1) Colorless, round to ovoid, budding, and variable in size
      (2) Larger than bacteria, but smaller than leukocytes
      (3) Significance—exist in urine as a contaminant, since yeast infections of the urinary tract of domestic animals are rare
   c. Fungi
      (1) Usually characterized by distinct hyphae, are segmented, and may be colored
      (2) Significance—none, as fungi are common contaminants from the exterior
8. Parasites
   a. Parasite ova that may be seen in urine sediment include:
      (1) *Stephanurus dentatus*—swine kidney worm
      (2) *Dioctophyma renale*—giant kidney worm of the dog and mink
      (3) *Capillaria plica*—bladder worm of the dog, cat, and fox
      (4) *Dirofilaria immitis* microfilaria may appear in urine—rare
      (5) Urine samples contaminated by feces may contain a variety of parasite ova.
   b. Protozoa
      (1) Trichomonads and *Giardia* are usually the result of fecal contamination or contamination by genital secretions.
9. Spermatozoa
   a. Easily recognized by their characteristic structure
   b. Significance—none, except that the urine has been mixed with varying amounts of semen
   c. Commonly encountered in urine collected from the male dog; less common in other species

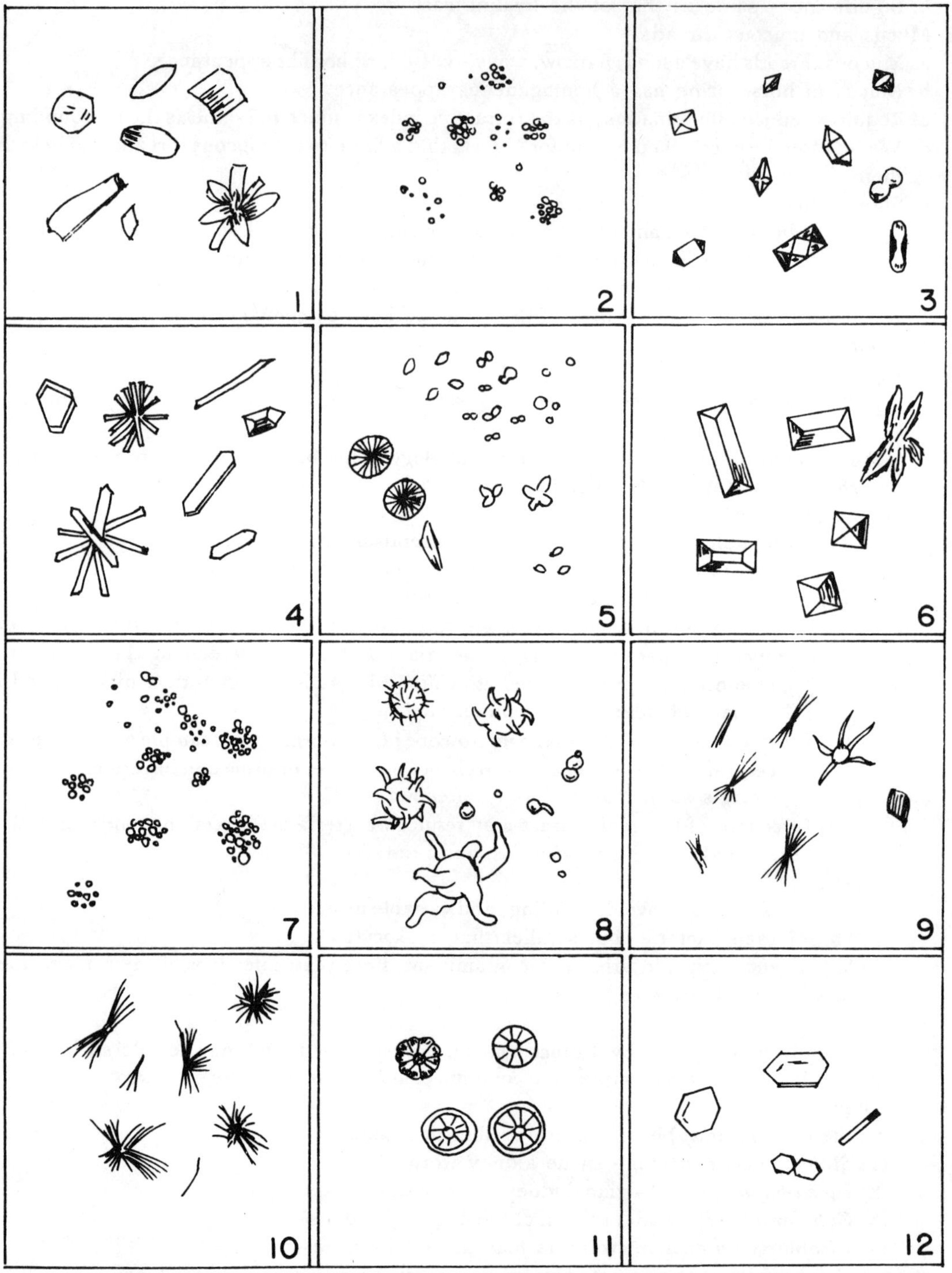

1. Uric acid
2. Amorphous urates
3. Calcium oxalate
4. Hippuric acid
5. Calcium carbonate
6. Triple phosphates
7. Amorphous phosphates
8. Ammonium urate
9. Bilirubin
10. Tyrosine
11. Leucine
12. Cystine

Fig. 18.2. Crystals in urine.

D. Unorganized sediment
1. Crystals (See Figs. 18.1, 18.2.)
a. See chart for morphology of crystals.
b. Significance
(1) The presence of crystals in urine depends upon the pH, the solubility and concentration of the crystalloid, and colloids and seldom has clinical significance.(2)
(2) Normal
(a) Acid urine may contain amorphous urates and uric acid and, less commonly, calcium oxalate and hippuric acid.
(b) Alkaline urine contains triple and amorphous phosphates, calcium carbonate (especially in the horse), and rarely ammonium urate crystals.

CRYSTALS IN URINE SEDIMENT

Crystal	Urine reaction	Color	Forms	Dissolved by	Not dissolved by
Normal					
Uric acid	Acid	Yellow	Rhombic or irregular plates, prisms, rosettes; or oval with pointed end	Sodium hydroxide	Acetic acid Hydrochloric acid Heat
Amorphous urates	Acid	Pink (grossly) Yellow (microscopically)	Granules	Heat	
Calcium oxalate	Acid, neutral, or alkaline	Colorless	Octahedral or envelope (small squares crossed by 2 intersecting diagonal lines), dumbbell	Hydrochloric acid	Acetic acid
Hippuric acid	Acid, neutral, or slightly alkaline	Colorless	Prisms, plates, or needles	Acetic acid	
Calcium carbonate	Alkaline	Colorless	Spheres, ovals, and dumbbells	Acetic acid	
Triple phosphate (ammonium magnesium phosphate)	Alkaline, neutral, or slightly acid	Colorless	Prisms with oblique ends ("coffin-lids"), feathery	Acetic acid	
Amorphous phosphates	Alkaline	Colorless	Granules in masses	Acetic acid	Heat
Ammonium urate	Alkaline	Yellow	Spheres, often covered with spicules, dumbbells, or sheaves of needles	Acetic acid	
Abnormal					
Bilirubin (hematoidin)	Acid	Yellow or dark red	Needles, plates, or granules		
Leucine	Acid	Yellow	Spheres with radial and concentric striations	Sodium hydroxide	Hydrochloric acid Ether
Tyrosine	Acid	Colorless	Fine needles usually arranged in sheaves with a constriction at middle	Ammonium hydroxide Hydrochloric acid	Acetic acid
Cystine	Acid	Colorless	Hexagonal plates	Hydrochloric acid Ammonia	Acetic acid

(3) Abnormal

(a) Crystals in urine are of minor significance, except in cases of urolithiasis and a few metabolic disturbances.

(b) Leucine and tyrosine crystals are encountered in acute liver disease.

(c) Cystine crystals indicate a disturbance in protein metabolism and may result in cystine calculi. (5)

2. Fat

a. Fat droplets appearing in urine are round, highly refractile, and of varying sizes, which helps to differentiate them from erythrocytes.

b. Fat droplets stain orange to red with Sudan III stain.

c. Significance

(1) Fat droplets usually enter the urine from extraneous sources such as a lubricated catheter or a greasy container.

(2) Lipuria of some degree is present in most cats, and may be due to fatty metamorphosis of the renal tubules. (8)

(3) Obesity

(4) High-fat diet

(5) Hypothyroidism (2)

(6) Diabetes mellitus

19 FLUID AND ELECTROLYTES

I. Water

A. Fluid compartments of the body (Fig. 19.1)
1. Intracellular water—consists of approximately 50% of the body weight
2. Extracellular water—20% of body weight and is further divided into:
a. Interstitial water—15%; water in the tissues between the vascular spaces and the cells
b. Intravascular water—5%

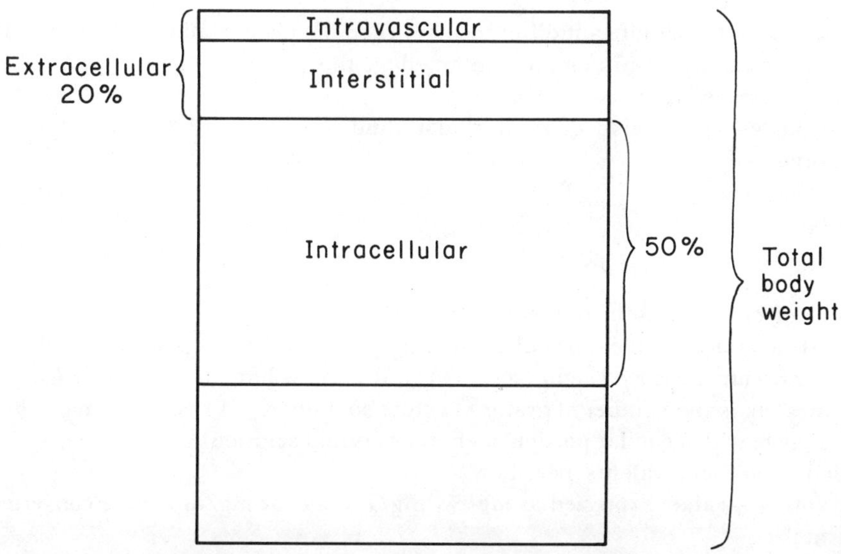

Fig. 19.1. Fluid compartments of the body.

B. Sources of water
1. Preformed water—water taken into body as liquids and contained in solid foods
2. Water of oxidation—water derived from oxidation of foods to carbon dioxide and water
a. Continues to be formed from endogenous sources even though no exogenous water might be available
b. Produces about 12 ml of water from the metabolism of each 100 calories

C. Water lost from body—boundary organs
1. Kidneys—urine accounts for slightly more than half the total fluid output of the body
2. Lungs
3. Skin—perspiration
4. Gastrointestinal tract—minimal loss in feces and saliva

II. Electrolytes—substances that become ionized when placed in water

A. Cations and anions—when electrolytes are placed in a wet electric cell, the ions will move in opposite directions, depending upon their charge
1. Cations—positive ions that migrate to the negative electrode or cathode
a. Cations of plasma and interstitial fluid include:
(1) Sodium—chief cation of the plasma and interstitial fluid
(2) Potassium—small amount

(3) Calcium
(4) Magnesium

b. Cations of the intracellular fluid
(1) Potassium—chief cation of the intracellular fluid
(2) Sodium—small amount
(3) Calcium
(4) Magnesium—relatively large concentration

2. Anions—negative ions that migrate to the positive electrode or anode
a. Anions of plasma and interstitial fluid include:
(1) Chloride—chief anion of plasma and interstitial fluid
(2) Bicarbonate
(3) Phosphate
(4) Sulfate
(5) Organic acids
(6) Proteinate—the significant difference between the plasma and the interstitial fluid is the much greater quantity of proteinate contained in the plasma

b. Anions of intracellular fluid
(1) Phosphate—chief anion of intracellular fluid
(2) Chloride
(3) Bicarbonate
(4) Sulfate
(5) Proteinate

B. Measurement of electrolytes in milliequivalents (5)

1. Milliequivalent values are measures of combining power and are replacing the old method of measuring electrolyte concentrations by weight (such as mg/dl) and volume (such as vol %).
2. A milliequivalent is the number of grams of solute contained in 1 cc of a normal solution, and thus can combine equally with a similar portion of another normal solution.
3. Conversion of milliequivalents per liter
a. Milligrams %—values expressed as mg %, mg/100 ml, or mg/dl can be converted to mEq/L by using the formula:

$$\frac{\text{mg/100 ml x 100}}{\text{atomic weight}} \text{ x valence} = \text{mEq/L}$$

b. Volume %—in the case of gases, a quantity of gas equal in weight to its molecular weight in grams occupies 22.4 L under standard conditions. The formula for conversion to mEq/L is:

$$\frac{\text{vol \% x 10}}{22.4} = \text{mEq/L}$$

4. The total concentration of cations always equals that of the anions in all fluids. (4)
a. Example given in Fig. 19.2.

III. Acid-base balance

A. Buffer systems (1,13) (See Fig. 19.3.)

1. The state of acid-base balance or imbalance of the extracellular fluid depends primarily upon the relative quantities of carbonic acid and base bicarbonate present in the extracellular fluid.
a. Normally these are present in a *ratio* of 1 part of carbonic acid to 20 parts of bicarbonate.
(1) When this ratio is disturbed, the acid-base balance is also upset, and there is a deviation from the normal pH (7.35 to 7.45) of the body fluid.
2. Other buffer systems—play only a minor role in the regulation of acid-base balance
a. Monosodium phosphate:disodium phosphate system
b. Plasma protein system

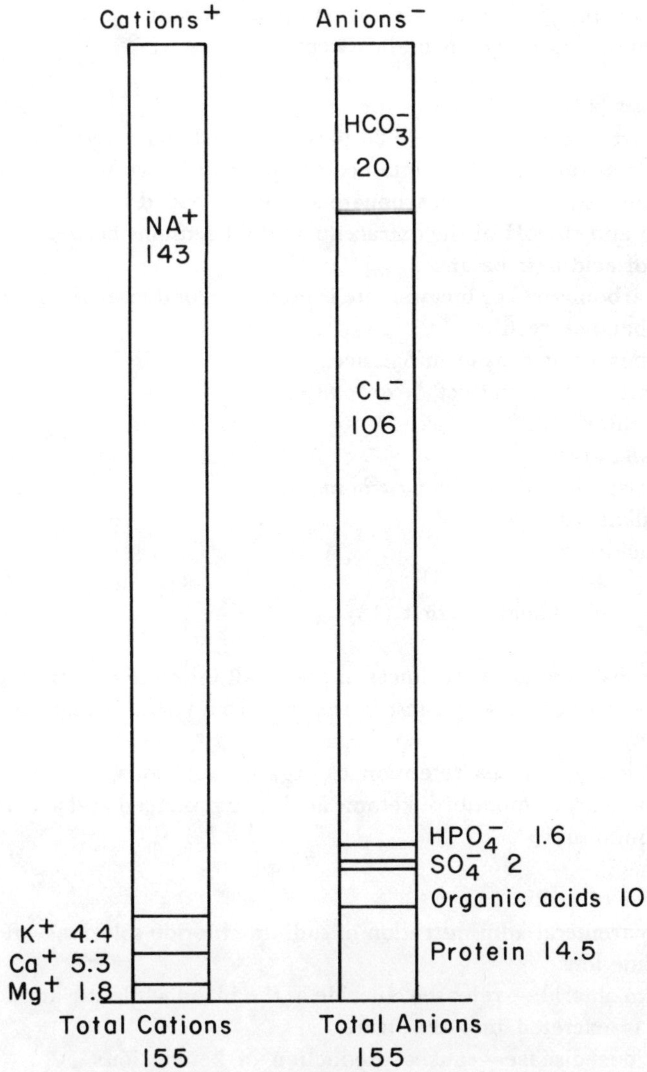

Fig. 19.2. Concentration of cations and anions.

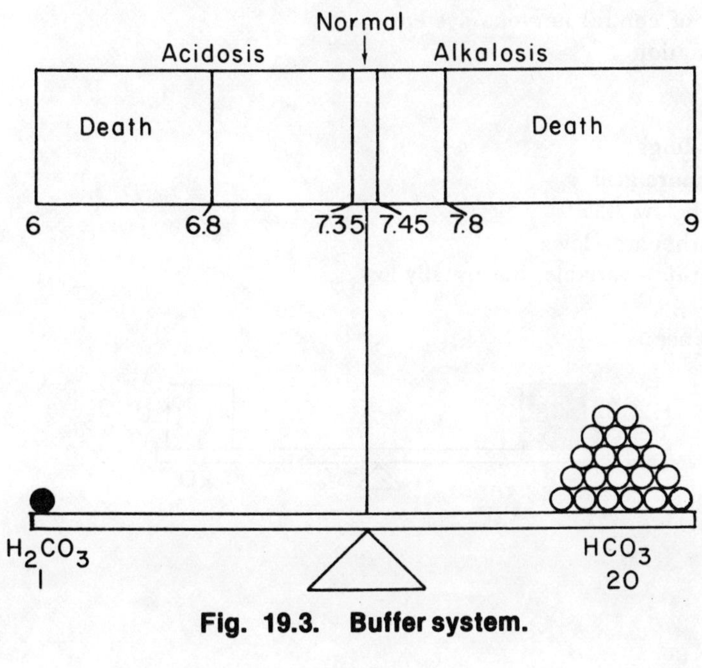

Fig. 19.3. Buffer system.

c. Monopotassium phosphate:dipotassium phosphate system
d. Oxyhemoglobin:reduced hemoglobin system

B. Acidosis and alkalosis (13)
1. The ratio of 1 part of carbonic acid to 20 parts of bicarbonate determines the pH of the extracellular fluid, and as long as this ratio is maintained the pH will lie within the normal range of 7.35 to 7.45.
a. If the carbonic acid and the bicarbonate are both divided by 2 or both multiplied by 2, the ratio remains 1:20 and the pH of the extracellular fluid remains between 7.35 and 7.45, so that the animal is in a state of acid-base balance.
b. If either the carbonic acid or bicarbonate is increased or decreased so that the ratio no longer holds, an acid-base imbalance results.
2. Two general types of acid-base imbalances occur.
a. Metabolic disturbances—affect *bicarbonate*
(1) Deficit—acidosis
(2) Excess—alkalosis
b. Respiratory disturbances—affect *carbonic acid*
(1) Deficit—alkalosis
(2) Excess—acidosis

C. Metabolic acidosis—bicarbonate deficit (13)
1. Causes
a. Extreme diarrhea—the digestive juices in the small intestine contain large amounts of sodium bicarbonate, and when these are lost in the feces as a result of diarrhea, the body is depleted of sodium ions (8)
b. Renal insufficiency—causes retention of organic acid ions
c. Ketosis in which large amounts of ketonic acids are produced and accumulate in the tissues
(1) Diabetes mellitus
(2) Starvation
d. Administration of acidic drugs
(1) Excessive parenteral administration of sodium chloride solutions—floods the extracellular fluid with chloride ions
(2) Ammonium chloride—releases chloride in the blood while the ammonium ion is synthesized into urea and is excreted into the urine
e. Severe infectious disease—causes production of ketone ions
2. Clinical signs
a. Hyperpnea—rapid rate and increased depth of respiration
b. Depression of central nervous system
(1) Disorientation
(2) Stupor
(3) Coma
3. Laboratory findings
a. Urine pH—more acid
b. Blood pH—below 7.35
c. Plasma bicarbonate—low
d. Plasma chloride—variable, but usually low
4. Pathogenesis
a. Normal balance

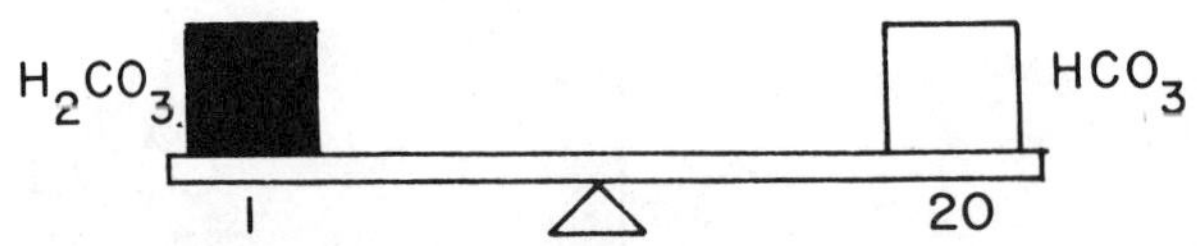

b. Acidosis—ketone and/or excess chloride ions replace bicarbonate ions

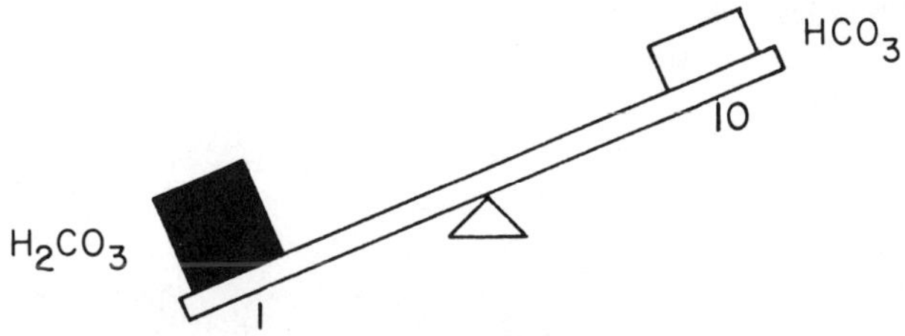

c. Body compensatory action
  (1) Breathing hyperactive—to remove carbonic acid
  (2) Kidneys conserve bicarbonate ions and excrete hydrogen ions and nonbicarbonate anions—urine becomes more acid

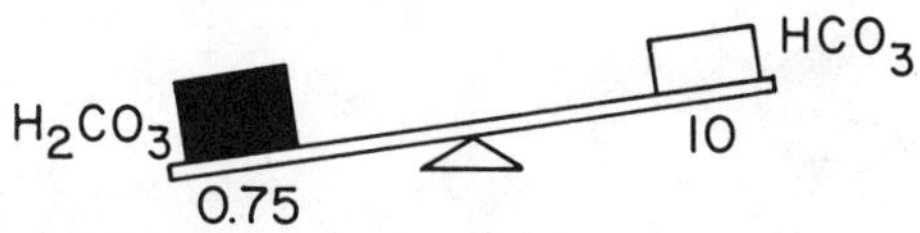

d. Therapy—administer bicarbonate ions
  (1) Sodium bicarbonate solution—the bicarbonate portion will be blown off through the lungs in the form of carbon dioxide, leaving behind sodium hydroxide, which causes the reaction of the body fluids to change toward the alkaline side
    (a) Can be given orally, which will be slower, or intravenously, which may be rather toxic, especially in small animals due to less dilution by the blood
  (2) Sodium lactate—converted to bicarbonate ions in the liver
    (a) Not as alkaline as sodium bicarbonate, so it is not as important to be as cautious in administration
    (b) Orally or intravenously
  (3) Sodium gluconate

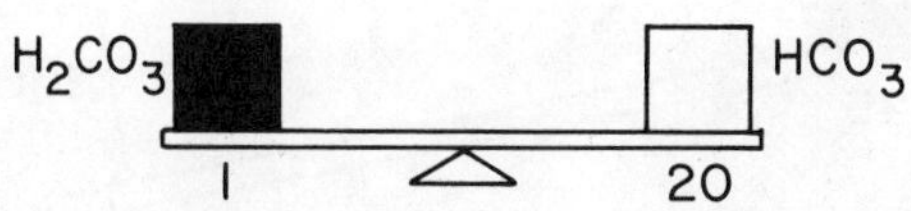

D. Metabolic alkalosis—bicarbonate excess (13)
1. Causes
  a. Excessive loss of acid
    (1) Excessive vomiting, such as occurs in pyloric obstruction and high intestinal obstruction
      (a) Loss of chloride causes a compensatory increase in bicarbonate, for the total of the anion column of electrolytes must always equal the total height of the cation column.
  b. Potassium loss—causes bicarbonate excess but manner is not known
    (1) X-ray therapy
    (2) Prolonged administration of K-deficit solutions
    (3) Hyperadrenocorticism
      (a) Overactivity of anterior pituitary
      (b) Adrenal tumor
      (c) Overdosage of ACTH or adrenal corticoids
  c. Alkaline therapy
2. Clinical signs
  a. Depressed breathing—slow and shallow
  b. Overexcitability of the nervous system
    (1) Tetany
    (2) Convulsions

3. Laboratory findings
   a. Urine more alkaline
   b. Blood pH—above 7.45
   c. Plasma bicarbonate—high
   d. Plasma potassium—may be low
   e. Plasma chloride—low
4. Pathogenesis
   a. Normal balance

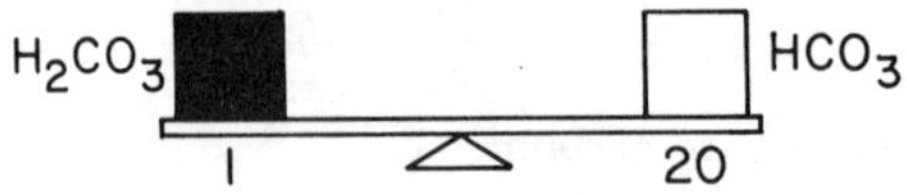

   b. Alkalosis—bicarbonate ion increased due to loss of chloride ion or to excess ingestion of bicarbonate

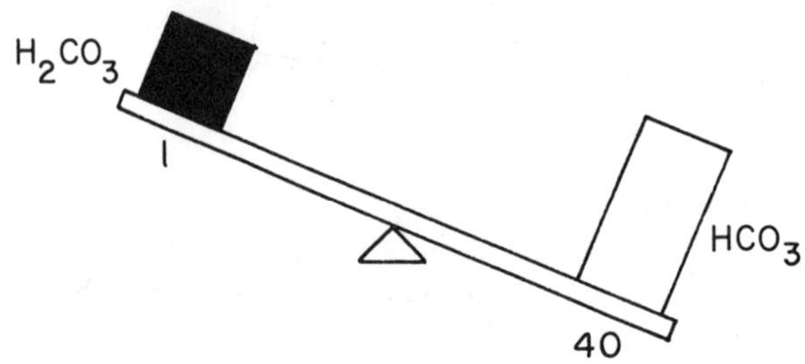

   c. Body compensatory action
      (1) Breathing suppressed—lungs hold carbon dioxide
      (2) Kidneys excrete bicarbonate ions and retain hydrogen ions and nonbicarbonate anions to produce more alkaline urine.

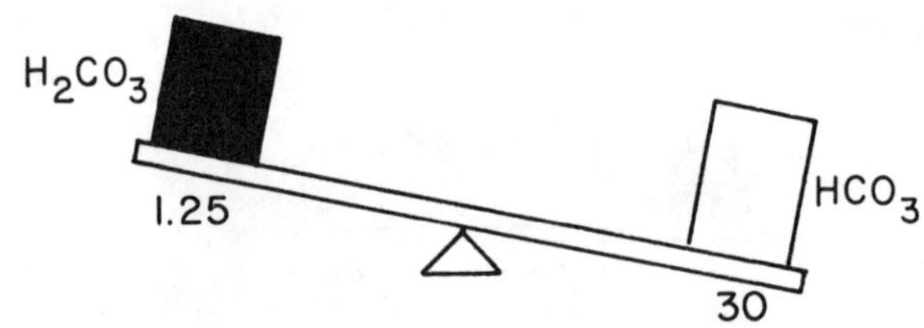

   d. Therapy—use chloride ions to replace bicarbonate ions
      (1) Sodium chloride
      (2) Ammonium chloride

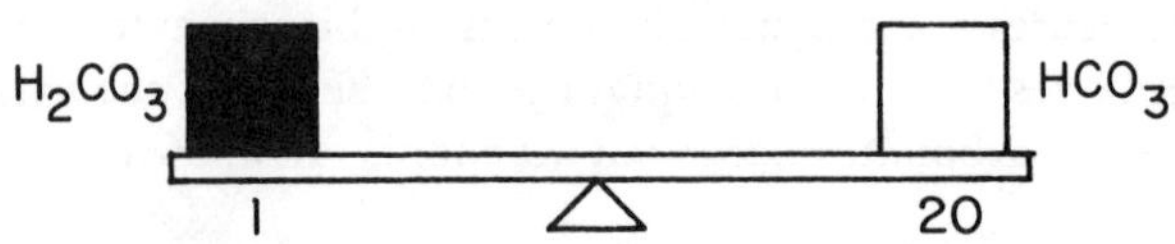

E. Respiratory acidosis—carbonic acid excess (hypoventilation) (13)
1. Causes
   a. Impaired respiration causing retention of carbon dioxide
      (1) Pneumonia
      (2) Emphysema
      (3) Pulmonary edema
      (4) Pneumothorax
      (5) Paralysis of respiratory muscles
      (6) Morphine poisoning
      (7) Barbiturate poisoning
      (8) Occlusion of breathing passages

2. Clinical signs
   a. Respiratory embarrassment
   b. Depression of central nervous system
      (1) Disorientation
      (2) Coma
3. Laboratory findings
   a. Urine pH—more acid
   b. Blood pH—below 7.35
   c. Plasma bicarbonate—high
   d. Plasma chloride—low; increased excretion of chloride by kidney to make more sodium available for bicarbonate
4. Pathogenesis
   a. Normal balance

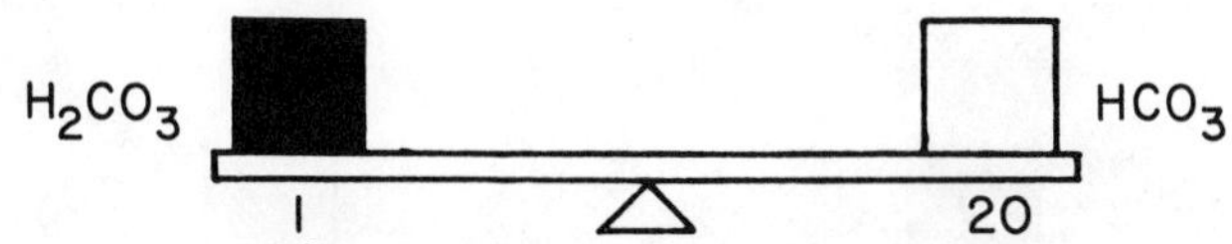

   b. Acidosis—carbonic acid excess due to hypoventilation

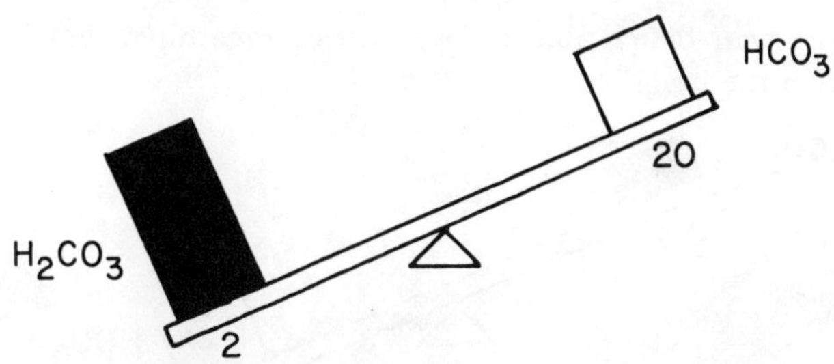

   c. Body compensatory action
      (1) Kidneys—conserve bicarbonate ions and excrete hydrogen ions and nonbicarbonate anions to produce more acid urine

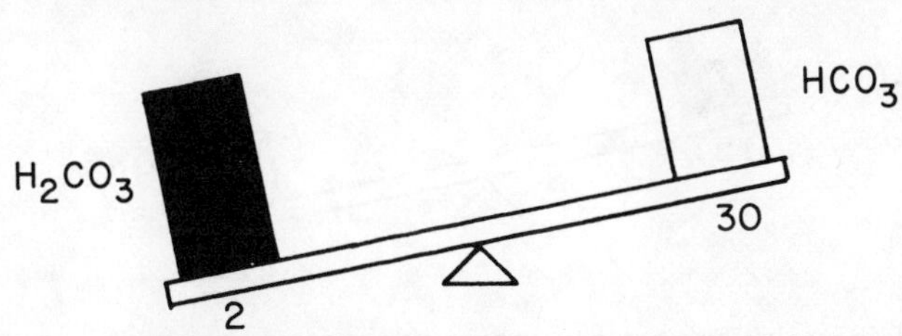

   d. Therapy—do not use alkalinizing solutions, as they decrease cerebral blood flow and decrease ability of hemoglobin to release oxygen to the tissues; instead, change the respiratory rate by treating the primary condition

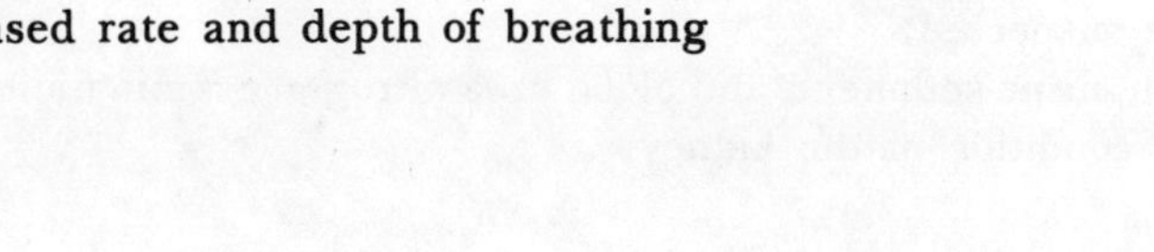

F. Respiratory alkalosis—carbonic acid deficit (hyperventilation) (13)
   1. Causes—increased rate and depth of breathing
      a. Fever

   b. Oxygen lack
   c. Respiratory center stimulation
      (1) Encephalitis
      (2) Drugs—salicylates
   d. Hysteria and anxiety
2. Clinical signs
   a. Deep, rapid breathing
   b. Tetany, progressing to convulsions
3. Laboratory findings
   a. Urine pH—more alkaline
   b. Blood pH—over 7.45
   c. Plasma bicarbonate—low
   d. Plasma chloride—normal to high
4. Pathogenesis
   a. Normal

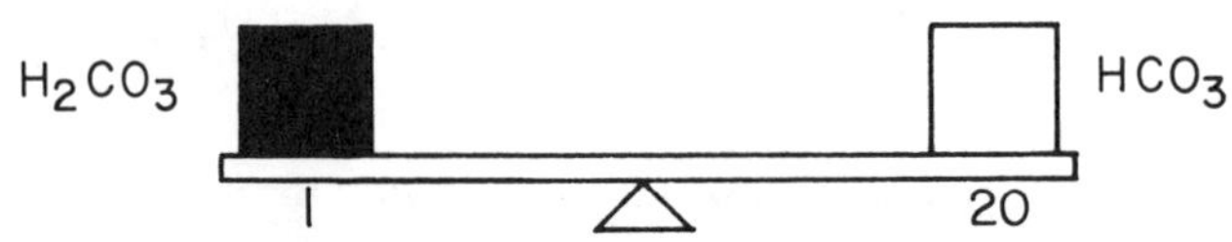

   b. Alkalosis—carbonic acid deficit due to hyperactive breathing, which results in an increased loss of carbon dioxide from the lungs

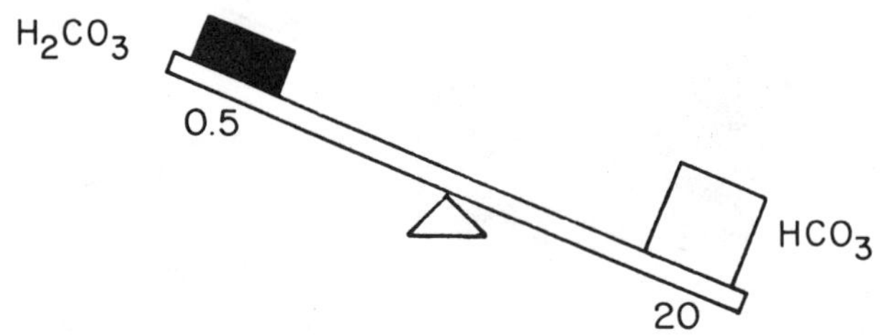

   c. Body compensatory action
      (1) Kidneys—excrete bicarbonate ions and retain hydrogen ions and nonbicarbonate anions

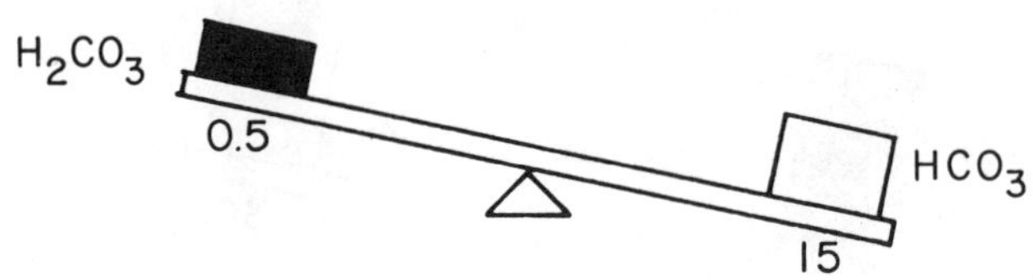

   d. Therapy—acidifying solutions are not indicated; increase the pCO_2 in the atmosphere

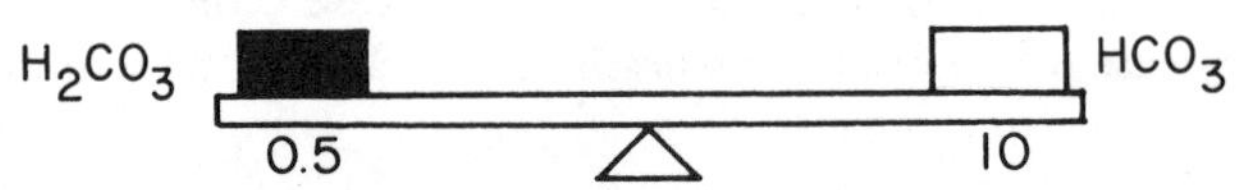

IV. Laboratory tests of value in evaluating fluid and electrolyte balance (15)

A. Urinalysis
1. Specific gravity
   a. Specific gravity is high and urine volume is low—indicates dehydration when kidney function is adequate
   b. Specific gravity is low, but clinically the animal appears to be dehydrated—chronic interstitial nephritis must be suspected
      (1) Urine protein, urine sediment, and blood urea nitrogen examinations must be conducted to determine the condition of the kidney.

(2) Replacement solutions must be selected with caution when renal disease is present.
(a) Avoid solutions containing potassium when anuria is present.

c. As treatment is administered, subsequent specific gravity determinations are important.
(1) A decreasing specific gravity usually indicates that hydration is being accomplished.

2. pH
a. If the animal has relatively normal kidney function and no cystitis is present, which might be responsible for alkaline urine, the reaction of the urine usually indicates the general acid-base balance of the plasma.
(1) When an animal normally has acid urine and it is now alkaline, it can be assumed that an alkalosis exists in the plasma.
(a) This should be correlated with the plasma bicarbonate to further evaluate the condition.

Alkaline urine + high plasma bicarbonate = metabolic alkalosis
Alkaline urine + low plasma bicarbonate = respiratory alkalosis

(2) When an animal has acid urine that becomes more acid or when an animal has normally alkaline urine that becomes acid, it can be assumed that an acidosis is present in the plasma.
(a) When correlated with the plasma bicarbonate

Acid urine + low plasma bicarbonate = metabolic acidosis
Acid urine + high plasma bicarbonate = respiratory acidosis

3. Protein and microscopic sediment
a. May indicate the presence of renal disease and thus suggest the necessity for caution in fluid and salt administration

4. Glucose
a. If glycosuria is present and the animal has not received glucose therapy, the possibility of a diabetic acidosis must be considered and confirmed or eliminated by blood glucose determination.
b. Repeated determinations of urinary glucose while solutions containing glucose are being administered will be of value in avoiding glucose diuresis.
(1) The amount of dextrose or glucose administered should not exceed 0.22g/lb/hr for total utilization. (6)
(2) When the concentration of glucose in the urine is found to be persistently high, the rate of administration or the concentration of glucose of the fluids being administered should be reduced.

5. Acetone
a. Acetone in the urine is a frequent finding in acidosis.

6. Chloride
a. Methods
(1) Similar to method for plasma chloride (see V,B)
(a) Place 1 ml of urine in flask.
(b) Acidify with 1 ml of 0.1 N nitric acid.
(c) Add a few drops of diphenylcarbazone.
(d) Titrate with mercuric nitrate solution.
(e) Every hundredth of a milliliter of solution used to reach the end point equals 1 mEq of chloride per liter of urine.

b. Significance
(1) A decreased quantity or absence of chloride in the urine may be the first sign of a salt depletion, as urine chloride output generally drops before the decrease in plasma chloride.
(a) A 24-hr composite urine specimen is required for a reliable evaluation, as a single urine collection does not necessarily reflect the true picture of chloride excretion.
(b) Using the decline in urine chloride as a guide for parenteral saline therapy may be dangerous because the urine chloride in many conditions is not a reliable indicator of internal conditions.
(2) Potassium deficiency is characterized by a low plasma chloride, a high plasma bicarbonate, and a high concentration of chloride ions in the urine.

(a) It is possible to tentatively diagnose a potassium deficiency by this combination of findings.
(b) In these cases, the decreased plasma chloride level will not respond to treatment with sodium chloride or ammonium chloride solutions until potassium chloride is also given.

B. Blood examination
1. Packed cell volume (PCV)
a. Provides information about the degree of hydration or dehydration.
b. A low PCV would suggest the need for blood transfusions rather than parenteral solutions.
c. Subsequent PCV determinations made during the course of hydration are of value.
(1) As hydration occurs, the PCV will fall, indicating that the therapy is adequate or that further solutions should be administered.
(2) As hydration progresses and the PCV readings fall below normal, the need for blood transfusions may be apparent.
2. Serum or plasma bicarbonate and chloride (10, 11, 12, 15)—screening method when more precise methods are not readily available
a. Equipment and reagents
(1) Four 60-ml dropper bottles—one each for sodium hydroxide, nitric acid, distilled water, and mercuric nitrate
(a) Remove the glass droppers.
(b) Cut the tops off the rubber dropper bulbs so that 1-ml tuberculin syringes can be inserted into the caps and hang down into the bottles.
(2) Four 1-ml tuberculin syringes
(a) Used for measuring serum or plasma and reagents, rather than using pipettes
(3) Two 30-ml dropper bottles with caps
(a) Used for the phenolphthalein and diphenylcarbazone indicators
(4) One 10- or 25-ml Erlenmeyer flask
(5) Two short 24- or 25-gauge needles
(6) Reagents must be accurately prepared and standardized.
(a) 0.1 N sodium hydroxide
(b) 0.1 N nitric acid
(c) Mercuric nitrate solution

Powdered mercuric nitrate	17.13 g
Nitric acid (concentrated)	2 ml
Distilled water, to make	1000 ml

(d) Diphenylcarbazone—120 mg in 130 ml of 95% ethyl alcohol (available in tablet form from Cambridge Chemical Products, Inc.)
(e) Phenolphthalein—150 mg in 30 ml of 95% ethyl alcohol
(f) 0.1 N. hydrochloric acid or potassium acid phthalate—to standardize sodium hydroxide and mercuric nitrate solutions
b. Standardization
(1) Standardization of all the reagents and the tuberculin syringes must be done initially and periodically, using 0.1N hydrochloric acid or potassium acid phthalate as the standard solution.
(2) The sample syringe is filled to the 1-ml mark with the 0.1 hydrochloric acid, and the contents are placed in the Erlenmeyer flask. Three drops of diphenylcarbazone are put in the flask. Next the mercuric nitrate syringe is filled to the 1-ml mark and the solution titrated into the flask until a purple end point is reached. If this has required exactly 1 ml of the mercuric nitrate, the concentration of this solution is correct. If it has required less than 1 ml of mercuric nitrate, the solution must be adjusted by the addition of water; that is, if 0.92 ml were used, then 920 ml of the mercuric nitrate solution should be taken and distilled water added to make 1000 ml. If more than 1 ml of the mercuric nitrate solution is required to reach the end point, then a small quantity of the powdered mercuric nitrate should be added to the stock solution until less than 1 ml is required to reach the end point; then the adjustments as described above are made.

(3) For standardization of the sodium hydroxide solution, 1 ml of hydrochloric acid is again added to the Erlenmeyer flask and 3 drops of phenolphthalein solution are added. Then the sodium hydroxide syringe is filled to the 1-ml mark and titrated into the flask. This should require 1 ml to reach the *faint* permanent pink end point. If the required quantity to reach the end point is not exactly 1 ml, a procedure similar to that described for the mercuric nitrate solution standardization should be used.

(4) It must be determined how much of the 0.1 N nitric acid is necessary to react with 1 ml of the standardized sodium hydroxide. One ml of the nitric acid is placed in the Erlenmeyer flask and 3 drops of phenolphthalein solution are added. The sodium hydroxide syringe is filled to the 1-ml mark and titrated into the flask. This should require 1 ml to reach the pink end point. If such is not the case, the following formula may be used to ascertain the volume of 0.1 N nitric acid needed to neutralize exactly 1 ml of the standardized sodium hydroxide:

$$\text{Vol 0.1 N nitric acid needed} = \frac{1.0}{\text{vol 0.1 N sodium hydroxide used}}$$

This volume of nitric acid will then be used in all subsequent determinations.

(5) Standardization should be made every month or when any of the solutions or syringes are replaced.

c. Method

(1) A 4- or 5-ml sample of venous blood is drawn from the patient and placed in a heparinized Vacutainer tube and centrifuged.

(2) Plasma is immediately drawn into the sample syringe to the 1-ml mark and discharged into the Erlenmeyer flask.

(3) One ml of 0.1 N nitric acid is drawn into its tuberculin syringe and added to the contents of the flask.

(4) The flask is swirled for 2 min and allowed to stand for 1 min.

(5) Three drops of phenolphthalein indicator are then added.

(6) The 0.1 N sodium hydroxide is then drawn into its syringe to the 1-ml mark and titrated into the flask to the permanent pink end point.

(a) With the 25-gauge needle on the syringe, each drop will equal 0.01 ml or 1 mEq.

(b) The quantity of sodium hydroxide remaining in the syringe is read in hundredths of a milliliter. This figure represents the *bicarbonate* in the sample in milliequivalents per liter.

(7) Next, the contents of the flask are acidified by the addition of 1 ml of the 0.1 N nitric acid, and 3 drops of the diphenylcarbazone indicator are introduced.

(8) The mercuric nitrate solution is drawn to the 1-ml mark in its syringe and titrated into the flask until the purple end point is reached, and the quantity *used* is determined in hundredths of a milliliter. This figure represents *concentration of chloride* in the sample in milliequivalents per liter.

3. Estimation of serum or plasma sodium (5, 15)

a. Accurate determination of sodium requires the use of a flame photometer, so it is often necessary to arrive at a fairly accurate estimation by an indirect method.

(1) The total anions must equal the total cations in the extracellular fluid. The sum of values for bicarbonate and chloride ions normally is about 126 mEq in the dog. The difference between this value and the concentration of sodium is 17 mEq/L. Therefore, in the absence of abnormal accumulations of other anions, the sum of the bicarbonate and chloride ions plus 17 is an approximation of the sodium concentration.

Bicarbonate + chloride = 20 + 106 = 126
Sodium = 143, therefore 143 − 126 = 17
Bicarbonate + chloride + 17 = sodium concentration

b. The other ions must be in relatively normal concentrations for this estimation of sodium to be of value.

(1) When calcium is disturbed more than 3 or 4 mEq/L, obvious signs of tetany will result.

(2) Alteration of potassium by more than 2 or 3 mEq/L will produce definite clinical signs, sometimes fatal.

(3) Magnesium levels are seldom disturbed.
(4) Renal insufficiency may introduce a significant error, due to the retention of organic acids, sulfates, and phosphates.

V. Replacement therapy (15)

A. Water
1. Replace deficit
a. Signs of clinical dehydration are not evident until the animal has lost water equal to about 5% of its body weight, so three classifications of clinical cases can be made.
(1) No clinical evidence or slight symptoms of dehydration, but with history of vomiting and/or diarrhea—replace water in amount of 4% of body weight
(2) Moderate clinical evidence of dehydration—replace water in amount of 6% of body weight
(3) Severe dehydration—replace water in amount of 8% or more of body weight and use diagnostic aids to evaluate further need
2. Maintenance needs
a. Water for urinary excretion—approximately 20 cc/kg body weight
(1) Daily amounts of urine (3)
(a) Horse—4.7 L (2 to 11)
(b) Large dog—1.0 L (0.5 to 2)
(c) Sheep and goats—1.0 L (0.5 to 2)
(d) Pig—4.0 L (2 to 6)
(e) Bovine—14.2 kg (8.8 to 22.6 kg)
b. Insensible loss (lungs and skin)—approximately 16 to 30 cc/kg of body weight
c. Water in vomitus and liquid stools—equal quantities

B. Electrolytes (See Table.)
1. Chlorides
a. Volume of extracellular fluid (20% of body wt) x (normal value of plasma chloride in mEq/L—patient's chloride in mEq/L) = amount of chloride needed (in mEq)
(1) Example—a dog weighing 44 lb (20 kg) is found to have a concentration of 86 mEq/L of plasma chloride. To estimate the amount of chloride needed to replenish the deficit:

$$(20/5) \times (106-86) = 4 \times 20 = 80 \text{ mEq of chloride needed}$$

b. If a large quantity of fluid is to be administered to the patient to replace the deficit of water, this fluid should also enter into the calculations. It is reasonably accurate to assume that the extracellular fluid comprises approximately one-third of the total water of the body. Therefore, one-third of the water given to replace the deficit will enter and increase the extracellular fluid. The water given to repair the deficit is the amount that has been estimated to be sufficient to return the patient to normal hydration. This amount is considered *water retained* for this formula. The number of liters of fluid given to repair the deficit is divided by 3 and the result multiplied by milliequivalents of electrolyte in 1 L of extracellular fluid. Adding this quantity to the previously determined deficit produces the formula:

$$\frac{\text{Body wt in kg}}{5} \times 106 \text{ (patient's chloride/L)} + \frac{\text{liters water retained}}{3} \times 106$$
$$= \text{chloride needed for repair to normal hydration (mEq)}$$

(1) Example—the dog in the previous example displayed moderate clinical evidence of dehydration, so water is to be replaced at the rate of 6% of body weight: 6% x 20 kg (20,000 g) = 1200 ml

$$(20/5) \times (106-86) + (1.2/3) \times 106 = (4 \times 20) + (0.4 \times 106) = 80 + 42.4$$
$$= 122.4 \text{ mEq chloride necessary to replace deficit}$$

NORMAL BLOOD ELECTROLYTES

Electrolyte	Dog	Cat	Horse	Cattle	Sheep	Pig	Ref.
pH	7.36(7.31-7.42)	7.35(7.24-7.4)	7.20-7.55	7.35-7.50	7.44(7.32-7.54)		(14)
	7.32-7.68		7.20-7.55	7.35-7.50			(3)
				7.42			(7)
Sodium—serum	143(137-149)	151(147-156)					(2)
(mEq/L)			149(146-152)	142(132-152)		155(140-160)	(14)
				142			(7)
Plasma	150(135-160)						(2)
	147(140-154)	153(150-156)	135		153(146-161)		(14)
Blood	127(116-136)						(2)
Potassium—		4.3(4.0-4.5)					(2)
serum (mEq/L)			3.3(2.7-3.5)	4.8(3.9-5.8)		5.9(4.9-7.1)	(14)
				4.85			(7)
Plasma	4.4(3.7-5.8)						(2)
	4.4(3.7-5.8)				4.8		(14)
Blood	6.0(4.9-9.6)						(2)
Calcium—serum	4.9(4.2-5.6)						(2)
(mEq/L)			6.1(5.6-6.7)	5.4(4.7-6.1)	5.7	5.5-5.7	(14)
				5.42			(7)
Plasma	5.3(4.7-6.1)						(2,14)
Magnesium—	1.9(1.4-2.4)	2.2	2.2(1.6-2.5)	2.3(1.0-2.9)		2.2(1.9-3.2)	(2)
serum (mEq/L)			1.5-2.1	2.3(1.0-2.9)		2.2(1.9-3.2)	(14
Plasma	1.8(1.3-2.0)		2.0		1.9(1.7-2.1)		(2)
	1.8(1.3-2.0)				1.9(1.7-2.1)		(14)
Blood	2.7	3.1	3.6	1.7(1.6-1.8)	2.3(2.2-2.4)	4.4(4.2-4.7)	(2)
Chloride—serum				104(97-111)		103(100-105)	(14)
(mEq/L)				103.7			(7)
Plasma	106(99-110)				116		(2)
	114(108-119)	120(117-123)	102(98-106)		103(98-109)		(14)
	106(99-110)		96				(14)
Blood	87(82-91)						(2)
Bicarbonate or carbon dioxide combining power (mEq/L)							
Serum				29.47			(7)
Plasma	20.5(18-24)						(2)
			28.6	27.7	25		(3)
	18.6	18	23.0	21.5	20.5		(14)
Phosphate (mg/dl)— serum (mEq/L)	5.6		3.1-5.6	5.6-6.5	6.9	5.3-9.6	(14)
Plasma	1.6(1.3-2.0)						(2)
Sulfate—plasma (mEq/L)	2.0						(2)

2. Sodium
   a. The sum of the bicarbonate and chloride ions plus 17 is an approximation of the sodium concentration for the dog:

      Bicarbonate + chloride + 17 = sodium concentration

   b. A formula similar to the one for chloride replacement can be used to determine the quantity of sodium necessary to replace the deficit:

$$\frac{\text{Body wt in kg}}{5} \text{ x } (143 - \text{patient's sodium/L}) + \frac{\text{liters water retained}}{3} \text{ x } 143$$

= sodium needed for repair to normal hydration (mEq)

      (1) Example—a dog weighing 20 kg was found to have a plasma bicarbonate of 32 mEq/L and plasma chloride of 85 mEq/L
      Using the formula for estimation of sodium:

      Bicarbonate + chloride + 17 = sodium = 32 + 85 + 17 = 134

      Knowing that the kidney function is normal and that the other ions are in relatively normal concentration, the same formula can be used:

$$\frac{\text{Body wt in kg}}{5} \text{ x } (143 - \text{patient's sodium/L}) + \frac{\text{liters water retained}}{3} \text{ x } 143$$

= mEq sodium necessary to repair deficit

$$(20/5) \text{ x } (143 - 134) + [(1.2/3) \text{ x } 143] = 93.2 \text{ mEq sodium needed}$$

3. Potassium
   a. Since potassium is essentially an intracellular ion, no attempt should be made to calculate potassium needs from the serum level.
4. Bicarbonate
   a. If the plasma or serum bicarbonate of the animal is known, the dose of one-sixth molar sodium lactate may be estimated by the following formula:

      Dose in ml = (normal bicarbonate in vol % — animal's bicarbonate in vol %) x (0.8 body wt in lb)

      (vol % = mEq/L x 2.24)

   b. another formula that may be used is:

      (Normal bicarbonate in mEq — animal's bicarbonate in mEq) x 0.5 body wt in kg
      = mM of sodium bicarbonate or sodium lactate necessary to correct the deficit

      (1 mM = 1 ml of a molar solution)

C. Composition of parenteral solutions (1, 5)

Solution	g/L	mEq/L cations	mEq/L anions	Calories	Tonicity
Sodium chloride (0.9% NaCl)	9.0	154 Na	154 Cl	...	Isotonic
Half-strength saline (0.45% NaCl)	4.5	77 Na	77 Cl	...	Hypotonic
Sodium chloride (5% NaCl)	50.0	850 Na	850 Cl	...	Hypertonic
Dextrose 2.5% in half-strength saline	25 Dextrose 4.5 NaCl	77 Na	77 Cl	85	Isotonic
Dextrose 5% in half-strength saline	50 Dextrose 4.5 NaCl	77 Na	77 Cl	170	Hypertonic
Dextrose 5% in saline	50 Dextrose 9.0 NaCl	154 Na	154 Cl	170	Hypertonic
Dextrose 5% in water	50 Dextrose	...	...	170	Isotonic
Ringer's	8.6 NaCl 0.3 KCl 0.33 $CaCl_2$	147 Na 4 K 6 Ca	157 Cl	...	Isotonic
Ringer's lactate	6.0 NaCl 0.3 KCl 0.2 CaCl 3.1 Na lactate	130 Na 4 K 4 Ca	111 Cl 27 mM lactate	...	Isotonic
Dextrose 2.5% in half-strength Ringer's lactate	25 Dextrose 3.0 NaCl 0.15 KCl 0.1 $CaCl_2$ 1.5 Na lactate	65 Na 2 K 2 Ca	55 Cl 13 mM lactate	85	Isotonic
Sodium lactate (one-sixth molar)	18.66 Na lactate	166 Na	166 mM lactate	...	Isotonic
Sodium bicarbonate 1.5%	15.0 $NaHCO_3$	178 Na	178 mM bicarbonate	...	Isotonic
Inpersol (peritoneal lavage solution)	15 or 70 Dextrose	140.5 Na 3.5 Ca 1.5 Mg	101 Cl 44.5 lactate		

D. Effects of administering too little or too much water and certain solutes (16)

Substance	Amount administered	
	Too little	Too much
Water	Serum solute and sodium concentration increased Highly concentrated urine Thirst Oliguria Fever Circulatory failure	Serum solute and sodium concentration decreased Very dilute urine Polyuria Intracranial hypertension Headache, confusion, nausea, and vomiting Weakness Muscle twitchings and cramps Convulsions Coma
Sodium	Extracellular fluid volume decreased Hemoconcentration Lost tissue elasticity Microcardia Hypotension Circulatory failure Uremia	Extracellular fluid volume increased Edema formation and congestive heart failure Tendency to potassium deficiency
Potassium	Apathy Lethargy Muscle weakness Electrocardiographic changes Ileus or diarrhea Hypopotassemia Metabolic alkalosis	Hyperpotassemia Electrocardiographic changes Muscle weakness Cardiac arrest
Phosphorus	Hypophosphatemia ? Other effects	Hyperphosphatemia Hypocalcemia Tetany
Carbohydrate	Ketosis Protoplasmic catabolism augmented Tendency to greater water and electrolyte losses	Hyperglycemia Glycosuria Hepatic failure

20 CLINICAL ENZYMOLOGY

I. Fundamental concepts in enzymology

A. Nature of enzymes

1. Enzymes are proteins that catalyze chemical reactions essential to life.
   a. The enzyme combines temporarily with the substance upon which it acts (the substrate) to form an enzyme-substrate complex.
   b. The complex breaks down to form the reaction products and liberates the enzyme to continue its catalytic function.
   c. Each enzyme can only catalyze a certain type of reaction and is more or less specific in its substrate requirements.
   d. Enzymes are named and classified according to the type of reaction and their substrate specificities.
      (1) Transferases—enzymes catalyzing the transfer of groups (e.g., amino, phosphate) from one compound to another
         (a) Glutamic oxaloacetic transaminase (GOT)
         (b) Glutamic pyruvic transaminase (GPT)
         (c) Creatine phosphokinase (CPK)
      (2) Dehydrogenases—enzymes catalyzing electron transfer
         (a) Lactic dehydrogenase (LDH)
         (b) Isocitric dehydrogenase (ICD)
      (3) Hydrolases—enzymes catalyzing substrate breakdown with water fixation
         (a) Amylase
         (b) Lipase
         (c) Alkaline phosphatase
         (d) Acid phosphatase
         (e) Cholinesterase
      (4) Lyases—enzymes that split carbon to carbon bonds without group transfer
         (a) Aldolase
2. Enzymes are produced intracellularly in all living cells and are released into the plasma and body fluids, where their activities are measured by their abilities to accelerate the particular chemical reactions they catalyze.
3. In general, it is preferable to make determinations on serum rather than plasma, as some anticoagulants used in the collection of plasma interfere with enzyme activity or in color development.

B. Mechanisms of serum enzyme alteration due to release of enzymes into the circulation

1. Alteration in cell membrane permeability
   a. Inflammatory reaction
   b. Degeneration of the cell
   c. Cellular activity increased
   d. Fatty metamorphosis
2. Cell necrosis results in release of intracellular enzymes into the bloodstream.
3. Impaired clearance of enzymes from the serum
4. Impaired synthesis by the tissue with resulting decrease in enzyme concentration in the serum
5. Enzyme production is increased from an extracellular site of activity.

C. Methods of enzyme assay

1. Enzymes are measured by their activity rather than their concentration because they are present in such minute concentrations in serum and other biological fluids and are so similar chemically.

2. The three main methods of assay are:
   a. Measurement of the disappearance of the substrate or change in substrate concentration
      (1) Amylase
   b. Measurement of an end product that is produced
      (1) Alkaline phosphatase
   c. Measurement of the change in amount of a coenzyme or cofactor at a specified time, with the rate of change being the measure of enzyme activity
      (1) Isocitric dehydrogenase

D. Method of reporting results as units of enzyme activity
   1. International unit, as defined by the Commission on Enzymes of the International Union of Biochemistry, is "one unit (U) of enzyme is that amount which will catalyze the transformation of one micromole of substrate per minute under defined conditions."
      a. The recommended reaction temperature is 30°C.
      b. By custom, the enzyme activity in body fluids, mainly serum, is related to a volume of 1 ml. Therefore, results are usually expressed as milliunits (mU)/ml. However, when 1 L is the reference volume, the activity is expressed in U/L, which is identical to mU/ml.
      c. International units are comparable only when the methods used to measure them are identical.
   2. A variety of units have been used for certain enzymes, and even though conversion factors are available for many of them, their use is not recommended.
      a. Normal ranges should be established for the method and unit being used.
      b. Whenever possible, it is better to use the international unit.

II. Factors governing the use of enzyme tests in diagnosis

A. Enzyme distribution in the tissues
B. Intracellular localization
C. Release of enzymes from damaged tissues
D. Alterations in membrane permeabilities
E. Clearance of enzymes from serum
F. Duration of elevation of serum enzyme activities
G. Serial serum enzyme patterns
H. Correlation of results with tests other than enzymes

III. Classification of enzymes

A. *Specific plasma enzymes* are almost exclusively synthesized in the liver and then excreted into the blood. Coagulation factors and cholinesterase are examples of this group. The activity of these enzymes in the plasma is decreased in liver cell damage, since their continuous synthesis and excretion is no longer maintained.
B. *Plasma nonspecific enzymes* have no known biological function in the blood. The normal level of these enzymes in the blood is maintained by a steady state of release from the cells and elimination from the serum.
   1. *Excretion enzymes* are excreted from parenchymatous cells into the extracellular and extravascular space. Some of these enzymes are regarded under certain conditions as cellular enzymes as well. Examples of this group are pancreatic and parotic alpha-amylase, lipase, and alkaline and acid phosphatase. The increase in serum activity if there is an obstruction is more important than the somewhat increased activity in acute cellular damage.
   2. *Cellular enzymes*
      a. *Organ specific enzymes* are localized either in one organ or are present in much higher concentrations in only one tissue compared with others. These indicator enzymes allow a fairly accurate diagnosis of specific organ damage. Examples of this group are glutamic pyruvic transaminase, arginase, sorbitol dehydrogenase, and glutamic dehydrogenase for the liver, and lipase for the pancreas.

b. *Organ nonspecific enzymes* include all the enzymes of the main metabolic cycles and chains, as they are present in almost all cells in the body. An increased serum activity of one of these enzymes may require isoenzyme studies to identify the tissue of origin. Examples in this group include lactic dehydrogenase and alkaline phosphatase.

IV. Enzyme distribution in tissues

Enzyme	Principal sources
Enzymes of high specificity	
Glutamic pyruvic transaminase	Liver (small animals)
Arginase	Liver
Sorbitol dehydrogenase	Liver (horse), kidney
Aldolase	Muscle
Ornithine carbamyl transferase	Liver
Lipase	Pancreas, intestinal mucosa
Enzymes of moderate specificity	
Glutamic oxaloacetic transaminase	Liver, heart, skeletal muscle
Creatine phosphokinase	Skeletal muscle, heart, brain
Isocitric dehydrogenase	Liver, heart
Enzymes of low specificity	
Lactic dehydrogenase	All tissues
Alkaline phosphatase	Liver, bone, intestinal mucosa, placenta, kidney

V. Intracellular localization

A. Significance

1. Soluble enzymes of the cytoplasm (cell-sap or supernatant) are more likely to be released into the circulation by increased membrane permeability than the mitochondrial enzymes are, which may suggest reversible inflammatory processes.
2. In necrotic conditions destruction of large numbers of cells will result in the appearance of mitochondrial, microsomal, and nuclear enzymes.

B. Localization of enzymes in intracellular structures

1. Enzymes present mainly in the supernatant or cytoplasm are:
   a. Glutamic pyruvic transaminase
   b. Lactic dehydrogenase
   c. Aldolase
2. Enzymes present mainly in the mitchondria are:
   a. Glutamic oxaloacetic transaminase—occurs in cytoplasm and mitochondria in different forms
   b. Glutamic dehydrogenase
   c. Ornithine carbamyl transferase
   d. Arginase
   e. Acid phosphatase
3. Enzymes present mainly in the microsomes are:
   a. Cholinesterase
   b. Alkaline phosphatase

VI. Removal of enzymes from the circulation

A. The variation in the rates of clearance has an important bearing on the use of enzyme tests in diagnosis, as the time factor must be considered in the evaluation of the disease process.

1. Following liver damage, arginase is removed more rapidly than transaminase from the serum. If the arginase and transaminase levels remain elevated, liver necrosis is still occurring. When the liver cells are undergoing repair, rapid decline in arginase levels should occur, followed by a more gradual decrease in transaminase activity.

B. Not much is known about the fate of the enzymes.
   1. A possible mechanism is intravascular inactivation through inhibition by small molecules, for which there is evidence.
      a. The protein is taken out of the bloodstream, not simply inactivated, as tissues have built-in mechanisms for degrading protein.
   2. It is possible that the reticuloendothelial system may participate in enzyme removal.
   3. Only minor amounts of serum enzymes are excreted through the urine, except in renal disease.
      a. The main exception is amylase, which is readily filtered by the kidney due to its relatively low molecular weight.
   4. Excretion in bile is a minor factor for most enzymes.
   5. It is possible that serum enzymes may find their way into the small intestine, where they could be digested and their constituent amino acids returned to the amino acid pool.

VII. Isoenzymes

A. Many enzymes exist in a variety of molecular forms, known as isoenzymes, that show similar substrate specificity yet differ in their physical and chemical properties.
B. Separation by electrophoresis is the method generally employed for clinical purposes.
C. Isoenzyme determination permits more precise recognition of the tissue of origin than is possible by determination of total serum enzyme activity alone. For clinical purposes, the isoenzyme separation and recognition most commonly requested include:
   1. Lactic dehydrogenase
   2. Alkaline phosphatase
   3. Creatine phosphokinase

D. Sources of isoenzyme fractions
   1. Lactic dehydrogenase—most species of animals
      a. LDH-1, LDH-2—heart, erythrocytes, kidney, brain
      b. LDH-3—lung, pancreas, adrenals, spleen, thymus, thyroid, lymph nodes, leukocytes
      c. LDH-4, LDH-5—skeletal muscle, liver
   2. Alkaline phosphatase—liver, bone, intestine, steroids
   3. Creatine phosphokinase—myocardium, skeletal muscle, brain

21 LIVER FUNCTION TESTS

I. General considerations

A. There are over a hundred laboratory tests for liver function.
  1. Most of these are obsolete, insensitive, or cumbersome.
  2. Only a few are useful in clinical practice, while others are better suited for research purposes.

B. The selection of one particular liver function test as a reliable index of liver function under all conditions is subject to severe limitations.
  1. The functions of the liver are varied and are not equally affected in disease.
  2. Hepatic functional reserve is so great that 80% of the organ may be destroyed before some abnormalities can be detected.
  3. Liver cell regeneration is so highly active that the function of new tissue will quickly compensate for the loss unless damage is generalized.
  4. Functional impairment of the liver may occur before a lesion is detected by histopathological examination, but the reverse may also be true.

C. It is usually necessary to use a battery, or profile, of several liver function tests to define the problem; since liver function varies with the type and extent of disease, repeated observations may be necessary.

II. Tests based upon the metabolism and excretion of biliary pigments (See Fig. 21.1.)

A. About 85% of bilirubin is formed from hemoglobin liberated from senescent erythrocytes destroyed by reticuloendothelial cells in the spleen. The remaining 15% is derived from other hemoproteins, which are mainly hepatic cytochromes.
  1. Protoporphyrin ring $\xrightarrow{\text{heme oxygenase}}$ biliverdin + iron + globin (Iron and globin are stored for reuse in Hb synthesis.)
  2. Biliverdin $\xrightarrow{\text{biliverdin reductase}}$ bilirubin
  3. Bilirubin is carried in the plasma loosely bound to albumin and an alpha-1 globulin and in this form is known by a number of different terms.
    a. Free bilirubin
    b. Indirect-reacting bilirubin—will not react with van den Bergh diazo reagents until the protein is removed
    c. Unconjugated bilirubin
    d. Water-insoluble bilirubin—cannot be excreted by the liver or kidney because of its low solubility in aqueous solutions
  4. Free bilirubin is acted upon by the hepatocyte to increase its solubility by removing the protein and conjugating the bilirubin with glucuronic acid, with glucuronyl transferase as the enzyme required for the conjugation. Conjugated bilirubin is also known as:
    a. Bilirubin glucuronide
    b. Direct-reacting bilirubin—will react directly with the van den Bergh diazo reagents
    c. Water-soluble bilirubin
  5. Conjugated bilirubin is carried to the small intestine by the biliary system after being secreted into the biliary canaliculi by the hepatocytes. In the intestine the bacterial flora reduce bilirubin to compounds of similar structure, which are collectively called urobilinogen.
  6. Fecal urobilinogen
    a. Oxidized to urobilin, which is an orange substance and is excreted in the feces
      (1) Stools containing no urobilin are clay colored.

b. Reabsorbed by the portal blood system and will either:
   (1) Be removed by the hepatocytes and excreted into the bile, thus completing the enterohepatic circulation of bile pigments
   (2) Reach the kidney through the general circulation and be excreted as urinary urobilinogen

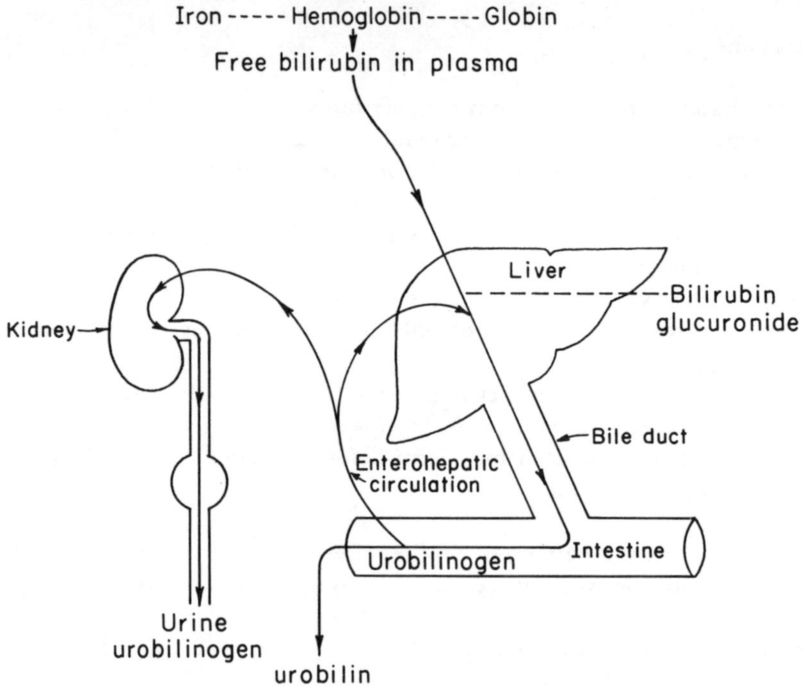

Fig. 21.1. Metabolism and excretion of biliary pigments.

B. Serum bilirubin
1. Icterus index
   a. Principle
      (1) The yellow color of serum or plasma is due chiefly to the presence of bilirubin. The intensity of the yellow color is compared with a standard potassium dichromate solution. The standards are expressed as units and numbered according to the quantity of potassium dichromate in 10,000 parts of water.
   b. Method
      (1) Obtain 5 ml of blood and allow to clot.
      (2) Separate the serum from the clot, centrifuge the serum, and place in a test tube of the same diameter as the standard; compare with the standard.
         (a) The plasma in the Wintrobe hematocrit tube can be used, or the plasma in the microhematocrit capillary tube can be judged if one is familiar with normal colors.
      (3) If the color is too intense to be compared, dilute the serum with equal parts of distilled water, and multiply the reading by 2 to express the icterus index.
      (4) Icterus index values can be read more accurately in a photoelectric colorimeter.
   c. Interpretation
      (1) Normal values
         (a) Dog—under 5 units
         (b) Cat—under 5 units
         (c) Pig—under 5 units
         (d) Sheep—under 5 units
         (e) Man—2 to 6 units
         (f) Horse
            [1] Varies directly with the packed cell volume and type of ration

PCV	Icterus index	
(%)	Low plant pigment ration	Alfalfa hay or pasture
25-30	5-7.5	15-20
30-40	7.5-15	20-25
40-55	12-20	25-30

[2] Varies with age

10 min to 24 hr	25-100 units (ave. 40)
2-5 days	10-50 (20)
7-21 days	10-25 (18)
1-3 mo	10-20 (15)

(g) Cattle—5 to 25 units
[1] Dry feed—pale plasma
[2] Green feed—up to 25 units

(2) Increased
(a) Increased blood destruction due to hemolysis
(b) Hepatocellular damage
(c) Biliary obstruction
(d) Fasting or reduced fluid intake in large animals
[1] Fasting a horse for 48 hr produces an increase up to 50 to 100 units and is especially pronounced when the gastrointestinal tract is involved.
[2] Hemoconcentration in cattle can raise the icterus index level to 25.

(3) Decreased
(a) Bone marrow depression

(4) Disadvantages
(a) The icterus index is a relatively crude test, as it measures a color that may result from other substances than bilirubin, such as carotene, carotenoids, and xanthophyll from ingested plants. These pigments do not affect the color of pig or goat plasma, but caution is necessary in the interpretation of readings in large animals.
(b) It does not differentiate between the sources of increased bilirubin.

2. van den Bergh's test
a. Principle
(1) Bilirubin in the serum from obstructive jaundice reacts immediately with Ehrlich's diazo reagent, while serum with hemolytic jaundice requires the addition of alcohol and a longer time interval for the reaction. Measurement of direct (1-min) bilirubin demonstrates the glucuronide compounds, while 30-min bilirubin represents total bilirubin. The quantity of free (indirect-reacting) bilirubin is the difference between the total (30-min) and direct (1-min) values.
b. Qualitative method
(1) Direct reaction
(a) Place 1 ml of nonhemolyzed serum from a fasting animal in a graduated centrifuge tube.
(b) Allow 0.5 ml of Ehrlich's diazo reagent to run down the side of the tube so that it will overlay the serum. Ehrlich's diazo reagent must be freshly prepared each day by mixing 10 ml of solution A with 0.3 ml of solution B (kept in brown bottle in refrigerator).

Solution A:	
Sulfanilic acid	1 g
Concentrated hydrochloric acid	15 ml
Distilled water q.s. to make	1000 ml
Solution B:	
Sodium nitrite	0.5 g
Distilled water	100 ml

(c) The contact zone between the serum and the reagent is examined against a good background for the development of a reddish-purple ring in 30 sec, which indicates a positive immediate direct reaction. If the color develops after 30 sec, it is a delayed direct reaction and has the same significance as an indirect reaction.

(2) Indirect reaction

(a) After the determination of the direct reaction, shake the tube containing the serum and diazo reagent, add 3 ml of 95% alcohol, and mix.

(b) If a definite pinkish color fails to appear in 15 min, and only a white turbidity occurs, the reaction is recorded as negative. If a definite pink color develops, or if the color already present from a positive direct test deepens upon the addition of alcohol, the reaction is recorded as positive for the indirect test.

c. Quantitative method

(1) Add 2 ml of nonhemolyzed serum to 18 ml of distilled water to make a 1:10 dilution, and mix well.

(2) Prepare the diazo reagent by adding 10 ml of solution A to 0.3 ml of solution B just before using.

(3) To prepare the standard, place 10 mg of bilirubin in a 100-ml volumetric flask and dilute to 100 ml with chloroform. Transfer 10 ml of the stock standard to a 100-ml volumetric flask and dilute to 100 ml with methyl alcohol.

(a) The dilute standard contains 0.01 mg bilirubin/ml and is prepared just prior to use.

(4) Into 4 colorimeter tubes measure:

	Tube 1 Direct blank	Tube 2 Direct test	Tube 3 Total blank	Tube 4 Total test
Distilled water, ml	5	5	...	...
Absolute methyl alcohol, ml	...	...	5	5
HCl (1.5%), ml	1	...	1	...
Diazo reagent, ml	...	1	...	1
1:10 dilution serum, ml	4	4	4	4
Stopper, shake, let stand (min)	1	1	30	30

(5) For direct bilirubin, set the direct blank (tube 1) at zero optical density at a wavelength of 540 nm, so that the optical density of direct bilirubin (tube 2) can be read exactly 1 min after the addition of the diluted serum.

(6) For total bilirubin, read the optical density of the unknown (tube 4) after it stands 30 min, with the total blank (tube 3) set at zero optical density.

(7) To determine the standard, place 4 ml of dilute standard in a colorimeter tube, add 5 ml of methyl alcohol and 1 ml of diazo reagent. Mix. Set total blank (tube 3) at zero optical density, remove, and after 30 min read the optical density (OD) of the standard.

(8) Calculation

(a) Direct reaction:

$$\frac{\text{OD of direct test}}{\text{OD of standard}} \times 0.04 \times \frac{10}{4} \times 100 = \text{mg direct-reacting bilirubin/dl serum}$$

(b) Total bilirubin:

$$\frac{\text{OD of total test}}{\text{OD of standard}} \times 0.04 \times \frac{10}{4} \times 100 = \text{mg direct-reacting bilirubin/dl serum}$$

(c) Indirect bilirubin:

Total bilirubin (mg/dl) − direct-reacting bilirubin (mg/dl) = indirect bilirubin (mg/dl)

d. Comparison of conjugated and unconjugated bilirubin

Factor	Conjugated	Unconjugated
Reaction with diazo reagent	Direct	Indirect
Structure	Bilirubin diglucuronide	Bilirubin
Solubility (water)	+	−
Type of compound	Polar	Nonpolar
Presence in urine	+	−
Hemolytic jaundice	± to +	+ +
Hepatocellular and obstructive jaundice	+ + +	+
Affinity for the central nervous system (lipid soluble and can enter cells of CNS)	−	+

e. Interpretation

(1) Normal values

	Total bilirubin (mg/dl)		Conjugated bilirubin (mg/dl)	
Species	Range	Mean	Range	Mean
Dog	0.07–0.61	0.25±0.1	0.06–0.12	0.14
Cat	0.15–0.20			
Horse	0.2–2.0	1.0	0–0.4	0.1
	0.2–6.2	2.7	0–0.4	0.1
Cattle	0.01–0.47	0.21	0.04–0.44	0.18
Sheep	0–0.39	0.19	0–0.27	0.12
Goat	0–0.1			
Pig	0–0.6	0.2±0.2	0–0.3	0.1±0. 1
Rabbit	0.7±0.06			
Rat	0.35±0.02			
White-tailed deer	0.4±0.1			
Baboon	0.33±0.16			
Chimpanzee	0.17±0.11			
Gorilla	0.22±0.14			
Monkey (African green)	0.27±0.13			
Monkey (rhesus)	0.38±0.28			
Monkey (squirrel)		0.50		
Orangutan	0.34±0.17 (male) 0.75±0.80 (female)			
Marmoset		0.102		
Armadillo	0.10±0.02			
Dolphin (bottle-nosed)		13.4		

(2) Increased bilirubin values
  (a) Prehepatic
    [1] Excessive hemolysis—initially will have more unconjugated bilirubin, but will be followed in 3 to 4 days by an increase in conjugated bilirubin, which is probably due to the insult of the hepatic excretory system by anemic hypoxia; decreased PCV
  (b) Cholestasis—if 50% or more of the bilirubin is conjugated, cholestasis is the most likely cause of the hyperbilirubinemia.
    [1] Intrahepatic cholestasis (regurgitation jaundice)
      [a] Hepatocellular injury—increase in both conjugated and unconjugated bilirubin due to the continuity of the biliary canaliculi being compromised or obstructed as a result of damage to the hepatic cells, as well as a decreased uptake of unconjugated bilirubin by the impaired hepatic cells; will be accompanied by greater increases in transaminase than alkaline phosphatase
      [b] Bile duct injury
    [2] Posthepatic or extrahepatic cholestasis—bilirubin and alkaline phosphatase will be very high
      [a] Inflammation
      [b] Neoplastic
      [c] Parasites
      [d] Congenital atresia
(3) Species variations in bilirubin metabolism
  (a) Horse
    [1] Normal ranges
      [a] Total—0.2 to 6.2 (2.7)
      [b] Conjugated—0 to 0.4 (0.1)
    [2] Most of the bilirubin excreted by the horse will be in the unconjugated form in both hepatic disease and hemolytic conditions and occasionally in other conditions.
      [a] Primary hepatic disorders—majority over 20 mg with conjugated form under 2 mg
      [b] Equine infectious anemia—25 to 75 mg
      [c] Other hemolytic anemias—up to 80 mg
      [d] Colic-constipation syndrome—usually markedly elevated
      [e] Pneumonia and other infectious diseases—10 to 50 mg
      [f] Cardiac insufficiency—2.76 to 6.27 mg
  (b) Cattle
    [1] In generalized liver disease the maximum will not exceed 3.5 mg, due to the large functional reserve of the bovine liver for excretion of bilirubin.
      [a] Hepatocellular and obstructive jaundice will have elevations of unconjugated bilirubin.
  (c) Dog
    [1] May be useful in the differential diagnosis of jaundice, but not a sensitive index of liver function
      [a] In autoimmune hemolytic anemia, there is usually about an equal amount of conjugated and unconjugated bilirubin.
  (d) Sheep
    [1] Dubin-Johnson syndrome in Corriedale breed
      [a] Congenital defect in hepatic excretion—autosomal recessive
      [b] Conjugated bilirubin increased, but clinical icterus not present
    [2] Gilbert's syndrome in Southdown breed
      [a] Congenital defect in hepatic uptake of unconjugated bilirubin—autosomal recessive
      [b] Unconjugated bilirubin increased, but clinical icterus not present

C. Urine bilirubin—azopigment conjugate of glucuronic acid
  1. Method—Ictotest (Ames Co.) is the test of choice
  2. Normal
    a. No reaction—in most animals

b. Small amounts
  (1) Dog
    (a) Healthy dogs may have a trace to 1+.
    (b) A small amount of glucuronyl transferase is located in the renal tubular epithelial cells of the canine kidney and has the ability to conjugate and excrete free bilirubin in limited quantities.
    (c) When serum bilirubin is greater than 0.4 mg, bilirubinuria can result.
  (2) Cat
    (a) As with the dog, the renal threshold is low.
  (3) Cattle
    (a) Although glucuronyl transferase has not been detected in renal epithelial cells of cattle, a small amount of bilirubinuria may occasionally be seen in healthy animals.
c. Hemolytic jaundice—theoretically, free bilirubin will not pass into the urine, as it is water insoluble; but since most cases of hemolysis are eventually associated with liver disease, due in part to the hypoxia that results, a positive reaction can sometimes be seen.

3. Increased
  a. Small amounts
    (1) Any febrile reaction in the dog and cat
    (2) When the liver disturbance is not sufficiently severe to cause clinical jaundice
  b. Moderate to marked reaction
    (1) Obstructive and hepatocellular jaundice—often the first test to become positive and frequently precedes measurable values for serum bilirubin
    (2) Acute enteritis
    (3) Intestinal obstruction

D. Urine urobilinogen
  1. Normal
    a. Urine of the dog and cat will have a color production in dilutions up to 1:32 and occasionally up to 1:64.
  2. Decreased amount or absence of urine urobilinogen
    a. Biliary obstruction
      (1) In animals with complete biliary obstruction, bilirubin glucuronide does not reach the intestinal tract and is not formed.
    b. Decreased destruction of erythrocytes
    c. Impaired intestinal absorption
    d. Polyuria associated with renal disease results in a dilution of the urine urobilinogen.
    e. Administration of antibiotics may inhibit intestinal bacteria and interfere with urobilinogen formation.
    f. Any delay in running the test can result in a loss of urobilinogen.
  3. Increased amounts
    a. Hepatocellular damage—urobilinogen cannot be effectively removed from the circulation because of the damaged liver cells
    b. Hemolytic jaundice—excessive hemolysis of erythrocytes results in an increased amount of bilirubin, an increase in the production of urobilinogen in the intestine, and an increased amount of urobilinogen excreted in the urine

E. Fecal urobilin (stercobilin)
  1. Chemical tests are not necessary because the color and character of the stool is usually sufficient for ascertaining the presence or absence of urobilin, a product of urobilinogen decomposition.
  2. Interpretation
    a. Increased amount—feces are usually dark orange in color
      (1) Hemolytic jaundice
    b. Decreased amount
      (1) Biliary obstruction—clay-colored feces may indicate total biliary obstruction

SERUM ENZYME LEVELS

Enzyme	Dog	Cat	Horse	Cattle	Sheep	Goat	Pig	Reference
Alkaline phosphatase								
IU/L	3-16	2-7	11-31	0-38	5-30	7-30	9-31	(14)
mU/ml (SMA 12/60)	20-150	10-44	80-216	28-227			119-175	(28)
			155.16 ± 49.11	52-400				(27)
IU (Hycel)	22.9 ± 8.9	8.34 ± 4.84	57.6 ± 11	25.4 ± 15.8				(18)
microM/ml							1.5-1.8	(24)
Bodansky units	3-6	0-7.1	6-22					(2)
	< 4							(23)
King-Armstrong	< 8							(11)
			5.1-12					(13)
				0.3-114.3	3-166.1			(1)
					14-427			(7)
Sigma units/ml	0.1-4.4							(26)
		0.8 ± 0.36						(15)
				0.9 ± 0.3				(19)
Arginase								
IU/L	0-4.7		0-70	1-30	0-4.5			(14)
microM/hr/ml (arginase units/ml)	0-0.28		0-4.2	0.08-1.77	0-2.68			(5)
Glutamic dehydrogenase								
IU/L			0-11.8					(14)
mU/ml (BMC)	0-2		0-2	0-3				(6)
IU/microM/min^{-1}/L			0-2					(8)
Sigma units			30-75					(9)
Isocitric dehydrogenase								
microM/hr/ml (W-WA)	0.027-0.437	0.118-0.703	0.291-1.075	0.565-1.314	0.026-0.482			(14)
W-WA units/ml	27-437	118-703	291-1075	565-1314	26-528			(4)
IU/L	0.4-7.3	2.0-11.7	4.8-18	9.4-21.9	0.4-8.0			(14)
Lactic dehydrogenase								
IU/L	10-35	16-69	41-104	176-365	60-111	31-99	96-160	(14)
IU (Hycel)	58.3 ± 27.8	151.8 ± 143.3		400 +				(18)
mU/ml (SMA 12/60)	90-400							(21)
				19-320				(27)
	50-495	75-490	142-354	486-903			565-690	(28)
mU/ml (BMC)	0-131		29-242	217-517				(6)
BBU	< 550	< 550	< 1000	< 2000	< 1800		< 1000	(25)
	260		150-1000	< 3500	< 2000			(16)
				1834.3 ± 56.2				(19)
Wacker units			179 ± 49					(29)
Ornithine carbamyl transferase								
IU/L	2.7 ± 0.7	3.8 ± 1.0	3.3 ± 4.2	4.7 ± 0.3				(14)
IU/L								(10)
Citrulline synthesis				0-44.7	0-31.6			
Citrulline arsenolysis				0-1.66	0-1.15			
microM/hr/min	0.157 ± .035	0.230 ± 0.058	0.20 ± 0.25	0.284 ± 0.20				(14)
Sigma units	< 500	< 500	< 500	< 500	< 500		< 500	(25)
OCT units/ml (Reichard)				2.1				(12)

SERUM ENZYME LEVELS *(continued)*

Enzyme	Dog	Cat	Horse	Cattle	Sheep	Goat	Pig	Reference
Sorbitol dehydrogenase								
IL/L	2.9-8.2	3.9-7.7	1.9-5.8	4.3-15.3	5.8-27.9	14-23.6	1.0-5.8	(14)
Sigma units			75-150					(9)
mU/ml (BMC)	0-3		0-3	0-4				(6)
IU (microM/min^{-1}/L)			0-2					(8)
Transaminase (SGOT)								
IU/L	6.2 ± 13	6.7-11	58-94	20-34	79 ± 11	43-132	8.2-21.6	(14)
IU (Hycel)	78.7 ± 60.9	160 ± 141	400.4 ± 101.6	178.2 ± 55.8				(18)
mU/ml (BMC)	0-16		47-185	13-40				(6)
Sigma-Frankel units	13-27	14-24	121-195	42-70	164 ± 23	90-275	17-45	(14)
	10-40		60-240	36-95				(6)
	22.7 ± 5.4	19 ± 4.8	165 ± 33.8	43.8 ± 5.7			31.1 ± 14	(4)
	3-80							(26)
				135.8 ± 91.7				(19)
					< 81			(17)
Transaminase (SGPT)								
IU/L	4.8-24	1.7-14	1-6.7	4-11	11 ± 1	7-24	9-17	(14)
IU (Hycel)	72.7 ± 43.4	76 ± 70.2		75 ± 9.7				(18)
IU (SMA 12/60)			5-30					(28)
Sigma-Frankel units	10-50	3.5-30	2-14	8-24	23 ± 2	15-50	19-35	(14)
	21 ± 11	15.6 ± 9.9	8 ± 6	16 ± 8			27 ± 8	(4)
mU/ml (BMC)	1.44							(6)

III. Tests based upon serum enzyme activity (See table of serum enzyme levels.)

A. Serum glutamic pyruvic transaminase (SGPT)

1. General considerations

a. The transaminases catalyze the transfer of an amino (NH_2) group from an alpha-amino acid to an alpha-keto acid, forming a new amino acid and a new keto acid.

(1) GPT catalyzes the transfer of the alpha-amino group of alanine to alpha-ketoglutaric acid, resulting in the formation of pyruvic and glutamic acids respectively.

$$\text{Alpha-ketoglutaric acid} + \text{alanine} \xrightarrow{\text{transaminase}} \text{pyruvic acid} + \text{glutamic acid}$$

b. The term, alanine aminotransferase, has been proposed for SGPT, but the older term is well entrenched in clinical usage.

2. Major sources of GPT

a. The greatest amounts are found in hepatocytes in the liver of dogs, cats, and primates, providing an enzyme that is specific for hepatocellular damage in these species.

(1) Little GPT is present in the hepatic tissues of the horse, cattle, sheep, and the pig, so its use in these species is not indicated.

b. Very low concentrations of GPT are found in other tissues.

3. Interpretation of increased values of SGPT

a. Hepatic cell damage

(1) Hepatic necrosis is not necessary for the elevation of SGPT, since an alteration in cell membrane permeability is all that is required to leak this cytoplasmic enzyme into the blood.

(a) There is poor correlation between hepatic cell necrosis and SGPT elevation.

(2) Normal to moderate SGPT elevations will be seen in:

(a) Passive congestion of the liver

(b) Fatty metamorphosis

(3) Hepatocellular necrosis will produce moderate to marked elevations.
  (a) Hepatotoxins—marked elevation because of the extensive liver cell damage
  (b) Individual circumscribed nodules or tumors may not involve a large number of cells at any given time, and the SGPT will be proportionately lower.
(4) Specific diseases produce elevated levels.
  (a) Leptospirosis
  (b) Infectious canine hepatitis
  (c) Feline infectious peritonitis
  (d) Fatty liver changes
    [1] Diabetes mellitus
    [2] Hypothyroidism
    [3] Hypoxia
  (e) Liver neoplasia
(5) Drugs
  (a) Corticosteroids, estrogens, androgens
  (b) Antibiotics—chloramphenicol, Ampicillin, Gentamycin, Lincomycin, Erythromycin
  (c) Dilantin, Primidone
  (d) Salicylates

4. Collection of the specimen
  a. Stability under various conditions of storage
    (1) Room temperature—2 days
    (2) Refrigerator temperature—1 wk
    (3) Frozen (−25° C)—unstable
  b. Both hemolysis and lipemia will invalidate the results
5. Conversion factor (unit x factor = IU)
  a. Sigma-Frankel—0.48
  b. Reitman-Frankel—0.48
  c. Worblewski-LaDue—0.48

B. Serum glutamic oxaloacetic transaminase (SGOT)
1. General considerations
  a. GOT catalyzes the transfer of the alpha-amino group of aspartic acid to alpha-ketoglutaric acid, resulting in the formation of oxaloacetic acid and glutamic acid respectively.

$$\text{Alpha-ketoglutaric acid} + \text{aspartic acid} \xrightarrow{\text{transaminase}} \text{oxaloacetic acid} + \text{glutamic acid}$$

  b. The term, aspartate aminotransferase, has been proposed for GOT.
  c. GOT is present in markedly different forms in the mitochondria and the cytoplasm.
2. Major sources of GOT
  a. The highest concentrations are located in the muscle cells, with slightly lesser amounts in the liver and heart muscle. GOT is not organ-specific.
  b. Small amounts are found in many other body cells.
    (1) Kidney
    (2) Pancreas
    (3) Brain
    (4) Erythrocytes—concentration varies with the species
3. Interpretation of increased values of SGOT
  a. Horse
    (1) Skeletal muscle system dominates the serum levels
      (a) Exercise—increases values to 150 IU from a normal range of 50 to 110 IU; hard-working horses may show values up to 300 IU
      (b) Muscular damage—increase from 200 to 2000 IU or above
        [1] Azoturia
        [2] "Tying-up" syndrome

(2) Liver damage
(a) In acute liver damage, levels increase from 200 to 1000 IU.
(b) Levels are never as high as those seen with extensive muscle damage.
(3) Myocardial infarction
(4) Intestinal complications
(5) Septicemia
b. Cattle and sheep
(1) Muscle necrosis
(a) Downer animals—values over 1000 IU would suggest a serious problem
(b) White muscle disease
(c) Blackleg
(2) Hepatic damage
(a) Liver necrosis—primary or secondary to traumatic reticulitis, metritis
(b) Ketosis
(c) Passive congestion
(d) Liver abscesses
c. Dogs and cats
(1) Myopathies
(2) Liver necrosis
(a) Primary and metastatic tumors
(3) Myocardial degeneration or necrosis—minor elevations
(4) Cardiac insufficiency—minor elevations
d. Drugs responsible for increases in SGOT
(1) Salicylates
(2) Corticosteroids
(3) Estrogens
(4) Androgens
(5) Antibiotics—Erythromycin, Lincomycin, Gentamycin
(6) Phenothiazine
(7) Anesthetic agents capable of causing liver damage
4. Collection of the specimen
a. Stability under various conditions of storage
(1) Room temperature (25°C)—3 days
(2) Refrigerator temperature—1 wk
(3) Frozen (−25°C)—1 mo
b. Both lipemia and hemolysis will result in erroneous values
5. Conversion factor (unit x factor = IU)
a. Sigma-Frankel—0.48
b. Reitman-Frankel—0.48
c. Karmen—0.48

C. Serum alkaline phosphatase (SAP)
1. General considerations
a. The alkaline phosphatases constitute a group of enzymes that are involved in the hydrolysis of phosphate monoesters at an alkaline pH (about 9).
b. Alkaline phosphatases are important in the transport of sugar and phosphate in the intestinal mucosa, kidney tubule, bone, and placenta.
(1) All the cells in the body utilizing glucose for energy contain phosphatase.
2. Major sources of alkaline phosphatase
a. Since alkaline phosphatase is present in nearly all tissues, it is in the group with low specificity.
b. Tissues that demonstrate the highest concentration of alkaline phosphatase activity include:
(1) Osteoblasts and chondroblasts
(2) Hepatobiliary system
(3) Gastrointestinal mucosa

(4) Renal tubules
(5) Placenta
(6) Spleen

c. Alkaline phosphatase is a microsomal enzyme, with its principal activity being intracellular, except in the case of osteoblasts, where it acts mainly in an extracellular location.

3. Methods
   a. Alkaline Phosphatabs (Warner-Chilcott)—one of the few simple kits for enzymes; useful for the dog and the cat, but not for the horse and cattle because of its limited range
      (1) Principle
         (a) A buffered phenolphthalein phosphate substrate remains colorless until decomposed by the phosphatase enzyme in the serum. The amount of phenolphthalein liberated is determined by a color change and is a measure of alkaline phosphatase activity.
      (2) Procedure
         (a) Place one Phosphatab tablet in a small tube provided in the kit.
         (b) Add 4 drops of serum or plasma.
            [1] If plasma is used, any anticoagulant may be used except EDTA.
            [2] Hemolysis will give false readings.
         (c) Crush the tablet with the applicator stick.
         (d) Allow mixture to stand 12 to 30 min, the time being determined by consulting the room temperature incubation table.
         (e) Add one drop of color developer.
         (f) Compare the color in the tube with the color chart.
   b. Methods using the colorimeter are available in kit form and are recommended for high concentrations in the serum.
   c. Alkaline phosphatase methods are available for the Accu-Stat and the Ames/BMI blood analyzer systems.
4. Interpretation of increased values
   a. Bone apposition or resorption—osteoblasts secrete alkaline phosphatase into the osteoid matrix in the form of calcinous bone
      (1) Normally elevated during periods of rapid bone growth in young animals
      (2) Healing fractures
      (3) During pregnancy because of the contributions of the fetal bones and placenta
         (a) The level does not seem to be correlated with the stage of pregnancy in cattle.
      (4) Osteomalacia
      (5) Osteogenic sarcoma—inconsistent
      (6) Hyperparathyroidism—primary and secondary (nutritional and renal)
   b. Hepatobiliary conditions
      (1) Two mechanisms have been suggested to explain the elevated SAP.
         (a) The enzyme cannot be excreted because of intrahepatic or extrahepatic obstruction and is therefore retained.
         (b) The increased amount of enzyme in hepatobiliary disease is in response to increased pressure within the biliary system.
            [1] This is the overproduction or regurgitation theory and evidence seems to favor this hypothesis.
            [2] It is not known whether it is the hepatocytes or the biliary tree epithelium that produce the most alkaline phosphatase, but it appears that the hepatocytes are the major contributors.
      (2) Biliary obstruction—intrahepatic and extrahepatic cholestasis results in marked SAP elevation
         (a) Secondary biliary obstruction, as with high intestinal obstruction, causes marked elevation.
      (3) Liver necrosis—moderate elevation
      (4) Fatty metamorphosis of the liver—normal to moderate
         (a) Diabetes mellitus
         (b) Hypothyroidism
         (c) Hyperadrenocorticism
      (5) Passive congestion—normal to moderate elevation

(6) Infiltrative lesions of the liver
(a) Tumors
(b) Amyloidosis
(c) Granulomatous diseases
c. Renal disease—inconsistent
d. Gastrointestinal lesions
e. Diseases of the spleen
f. Hemolysis
g. Administrations of drugs
(1) Corticosteroids
(2) Estrogens
(3) Androgens
(4) Antibiotics—erythromycin
(5) Phenothiazine

5. Collection of the specimen
a. Stability under various conditions
(1) Room temperature (25°C)—2 to 3 days (activity may increase)
(2) Refrigeration (0° to +4°C)—2 to 3 days
(3) Frozen (−25°C)—1 mo
b. Inhibited by EDTA
c. Hemolysis will interfere with the final color in some methods

6. Conversion factor (unit x factor = IU)
a. Bodansky—5.4
b. King-Armstrong—7.1

D. Lactic dehydrogenase (LDH)

1. General considerations
a. LDH catalyzes the following reaction:

$$\text{Lactate} + \text{NAD}^+ \rightleftharpoons \text{pyruvate} + \text{NADH} + \text{H}^+$$

b. LDH is located in body tissues that utilize glucose for energy.
c. Because of its high concentration in many tissues, it is not organ-specific unless isoenzyme analysis is employed.

2. Isoenzymes of LDH—five can be separated by electrophoresis (Fig. 21.2).

3. Sources of LDH isoenzyme fractions
a. LDH-1, LDH-2—heart, erythrocytes, kidney, brain

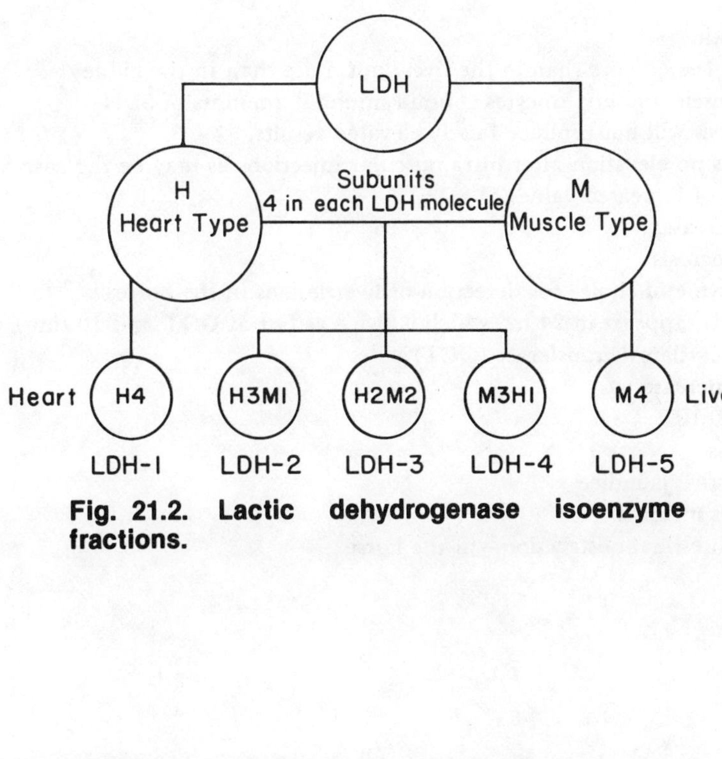

Fig. 21.2. Lactic dehydrogenase isoenzyme fractions.

b. LDH-3—lung, pancreas, adrenals, spleen, thymus, thyroid, lymph nodes, leukocytes
c. LDH-4, LDH-5—myocardium, skeletal muscle, brain

4. Interpretation of increased LDH levels
   a. LDH may be elevated in many processes in which there is cell necrosis, but because of the ubiquitous distribution of the enzyme, it cannot be considered specific for any tissue or pathognomonic for any specific condition. Tissue-specific isoenzymes are helpful in identifying the tissue of origin.
      (1) Hepatocellular necrosis
      (2) Muscle necrosis
      (3) Renal necrosis
      (4) Pancreatic necrosis
      (5) Pulmonary necrosis
      (6) Myocardial damage
      (7) Malignant neoplasms and leukemia
         (a) LDH elevation often occurs in lymphosarcoma, especially in cattle, and is probably associated with necrosis of the neoplasm or secondary necrosis of affected tissues.
   b. Hemolysis
5. Collection of the specimen
   a. Storage
      (1) Room temperature (25°C)—stable for 1 wk
      (2) Refrigeration (0° to 4°C)—1 to 3 days, depending upon the isoenzyme pattern in the serum
      (3) Frozen (−25°C)—1 to 3 days, depending upon the isoenzyme pattern in the serum; freezing alters the isoenzymes and is not recommended
   b. Avoid hemolysis, as the RBC/plasma LDH ratio is extremely high.
   c. LDH is inhibited by oxalate used as an anticoagulant.

E. Sorbitol dehydrogenase (SDH)
1. General considerations
   a. Sorbitol is a polyhydric alcohol derived from glucose. Its conversion to glucose takes place in the liver, and it is catalyzed by sorbitol dehydrogenase.
2. Major sources of SDH
   a. SDH is relatively liver-specific in most species.
      (1) It has been reported in high concentration in the livers of man; the dog, cat, horse, pig, rabbit, mouse, guinea pig, and frog; and in cattle and sheep.
   b. Kidneys—in lower concentrations
      (1) Pig—activity of the kidney is roughly 50% that of the liver
      (2) Man
      (3) Sheep
   c. Small intestine
      (1) Horse—less enzyme than in the liver, but more than in the kidney
   d. Skeletal muscle and erythrocytes contain minimal amounts of SDH.
      (1) Hemolysis will not produce falsely elevated results.
      (2) There is no elevation after intramuscular injections as may be the case for GOT and CPK.
3. Interpretation of increased values of SDH
   a. Marked increase
      (1) Liver necrosis
         (a) Enzyme of choice for detection of liver lesions in the horse
            [1] Disappears in 24 hr, which is twice as fast as GOT and 10 times as fast as ornithine carbamyl transferase (OCT)
   b. Moderate increase
      (1) Pancreatitis
      (2) Cirrhosis
      (3) Obstructive jaundice
      (4) Diabetes mellitus
      (5) Acute intestinal obstruction—in the horse

(6) Acute enteritis—in the horse
(7) Grass sickness—in the horse
c. Mild increase
(1) Severe azoturia—after a few days
(2) Influenza
(3) Arteritis
(4) Prolonged corticosteroid administration
4. Collection of the specimen
a. Immediate determination is necessary, as there is a rapid deterioration at room and refrigerator temperatures.
(1) After 24 hr at room temperature—1.4% of original value
(2) After 24 hr at −25°C—88% of original value
b. Hemolysis will not interfere with the test.

F. Glutamic dehydrogenase (GLDH)
1. Sources
a. GLDH is quite liver-specific and is mainly localized in the mitochondria.
b. Other organs such as muscle may contain a certain amount of this enzyme but do not appear to influence the serum level in a way that has clinical significance.
2. Interpretation of increased values
a. Liver disease—an elevation of its serum activity may indicate a more severe cellular lesion than an elevation of sorbitol dehydrogenase or transamine, especially in cattle
(1) It is probably the liver enzyme of choice for cattle, as it is much more sensitive than transaminase.
3. Limitation: Commercial kits are no longer available, which limits the use for testing in many laboratories.

G. Arginase
1. General considerations
a. Arginase is liver-specific for the horse, and values increase in the serum following liver damage.
b. Arginase is found in significant concentrations within the livers of:
(1) Horse
(2) Dog
(3) Cattle
(4) Sheep
(5) Rat
(6) Man
c. Method is by gel filtration, which limits its widespread use.

H. Ornithine carbamyl transferase (OCT)
1. OCT is liver-specific, but does not provide any more information than SGPT, except in large animals.
2. Method—cumbersome and requires several hours for results, so easier tests are usually preferred

IV. Bromsulphalein (BSP, sulfobromophthalein) excretion test

A. Principle
1. After the injection of BSP intravenously, the dye is bound to plasma albumin.
2. It is mainly confined in the vascular compartment except in the liver, where it readily moves across the sinusoidal endothelium and results in an accumulation within the hepatocytes.
a. Unlike capillaries in other tissues of the body, the sinusoids are freely permeable to proteins.
b. At the cell boundary of the hepatocyte, the dye dissociates from the plasma albumin, moves across the cell membranes, then associates again on the other side with proteins of the cytoplasm.
3. Within the hepatocytes much of the BSP is conjugated with glutathione.
4. Both conjugated BSP and unconjugated BSP are excreted into the canaliculi and the bile.

B. Summary of the significant variables concerned with the test.

1. The amount of dye injected and the time interval of the testing period
    a. Most of the dye is removed from the plasma relatively early, with the remaining amount becoming progressively less as time passes.
2. Hepatic blood flow
3. Ability of the hepatic parenchymal cell mass to remove the dye
4. Bile duct patency through which the excreted products pass to the intestine

C. Methods

1. Clearance method—for large animals (Fig. 21.3)
    a. First obtain a 5-ml sample of heparinized blood.
    b. Administer 1 g of BSP (20 ml ampoule of 5% solution) to any animal weighing between 181.5 to 544.3 kg (400 to 1200 lb).

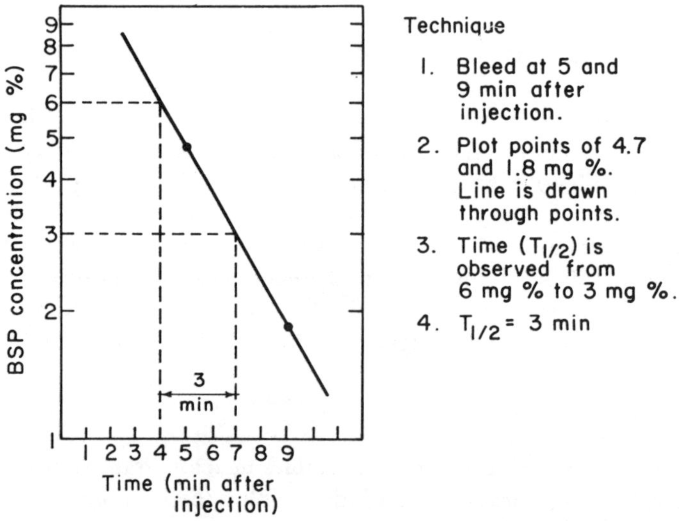

Fig. Fig. 21.3. Bromsulphalein clearance in the horse.

   c. Wait 5 min, then take 2 heparinized blood samples before 12 min have elapsed, preferably at 4 min intervals, such as 5 and 9 min, or 7 and 11 min.
      (1) Record the exact time of the collection on the respective tubes.
   d. Obtain plasma by centrifuging the samples.
   e. Place 2 ml of the respective plasmas into colorimeter tubes.
      (1) Tube 1 (blank)—presample plasma
      (2) Tube 2—1st postinjection sample
      (3) Tube 3—2nd postinjection sample
   f. Add 1 ml of distilled water and 3 ml of 0.1 N hydrochloric acid to tube 1 (blank).
   g. Add 3.0 ml of 0.1 N sodium hydroxide to each of the three tubes. Mix.
   h. Read the percent transmission of tubes 2 and 3 against the blank in a spectrophotometer with a wavelength set at 565 nm.
   i. A standard curve for BSP can be made with instructions supplied in the box of ampoules (Hynson, Westcott & Dunning, Inc.).
   j. The two BSP serum concentrations are plotted on semilog paper on the vertical axis, with time in minutes on the horizontal axis. The half-time ($T_{1/2}$) is the time required for the serum concentration to be halved.
2. Retention method—for small animals
   a. Weigh the animal and calculate the dosage of BSP on a basis of mg/kg body weight.
      (1) The body weight in pounds divided by 22 will give the amount of dye in milliliters.
   b. Inject into the cephalic vein slowly, taking 1 min and avoiding infiltration of the dye outside the vein.
      (1) If the dye is allowed to infiltrate outside the vein, it will cause necrosis of tissue.
      (2) Never inject the dye into an artery.

c. 30 min after injection, withdraw 4 to 5 ml of blood from the cephalic vein in the opposite limb.
   (1) Hemolysis can be avoided by:
      (a) Using heparin as an anticoagulant
      (b) Using a dry disposable syringe, needle, and tube
d. If an anticoagulant has not been used, allow the blood to clot, then centrifuge and collect the clear serum or plasma.
e. Two clean test tubes are marked "test" and "blank."
f. To each tube add 1 ml of clear serum or plasma.
g. To the "test" tube add 4.0 ml of 0.1 N sodium hydroxide and mix by gentle inversion.
h. To the "blank" tube add exactly 4.0 ml of 0.1 N hydrochloric acid and mix by gentle inversion.
   (1) The full reddish violet color develops in the alkaline solution, and the dye is colorless in acid solution.
i. Read the optical density (OD) of the "test" tube at 575 nm, setting the zero with the "blank" tube.
j. Refer the OD reading to the calibration curve to obtain the percentage of the dye remaining in the blood after the 30-min interval.

D. Interpretation
1. Normal
   a. Dog—less than 5% retention at 30 min is considered to be within normal limits
   b. Horse—the normal average $T_{1/2}$ value is 2.8 ± 0.5 min, with a range of 2 to 3.7 min.
   c. Cattle
      (1) Mature dairy cow—3.1 ± 0.6 min with a range of 2.5 to 4 min
      (2) Yearling feeder steers—average $T_{1/2}$ value of 4.5 ± 0.32 min
   d. Sheep—the normal $T_{1/2}$ value is 2 ± 0.3 min
2. Increased
   a. Parenchymal hepatic disease
      (1) Fatty metamorphosis—mild increase
      (2) Cirrhosis
         (a) Averaged 28% retention in the dog
      (3) Toxic hepatic injury
      (4) Hepatic necrosis, especially if acute and diffuse
   b. Biliary tract disease
      (1) Bile duct obstruction
   c. Extrahepatic disease
      (1) Circulation
         (a) Congestive heart failure
         (b) Shock
         (c) Fever—increases hepatic blood flow, but decreases BSP extraction
         (d) Hepatic vein occlusion
         (e) Spinal cord injury
      (2) Infiltrative lesions of the liver from systemic disease
         (a) Metastatic neoplasms
         (b) Granulomatous disease
            [1] Histoplasmosis
         (c) Amyloidosis
   d. Relative increases in canine liver disease

Condition	SGOT	SGPT	AP	BSP
Passive congestion	±	+	+	+
Fatty degeneration	+	+	+	+
Necrosis	+ +	+ + +	+ +	+ + +
Biliary obstruction	+	+ +	+ + +	+ + +

3. Contraindications
   a. Increased bilirubin levels in the blood—especially if over 4 mg/dl
      (1) The BSP will almost always be elevated due to competition for conjugation with free bilirubin.
   b. Drugs that compete for conjugation with BSP or interfere by sharing transport steps
      (1) Cholate
      (2) Telepaque
      (3) Phenolsulfonphthalein
      (4) Iodine

V. Cholesterol

A. General considerations
1. Cholesterol is a steroid alcohol with lipidlike solubility.
2. It is produced by almost every cell in the body, with the following tissues being especially active in its synthesis:
   a. Liver
   b. Adrenal cortex
   c. Ovaries and testes
   d. Intestinal epithelium
3. Besides the manufacture of cholesterol, the liver also:
   a. Esterifies it, chiefly with linoleic acid
   b. Converts a portion of it to cholic acid
   c. Excretes it in the bile

B. Interpretation
1. Normal values (in mg/dl)
   a. Dog—125 to 250
   b. Cat—95 to 130
   c. Horse—75 to 150
   d. Cattle—80 to 120
   e. Sheep—52 to 76
   f. Goat—80 to 130
   g. Pig—36 to 54
   h. Rabbit—30 to 70
   i. Guinea pig—43.91
   j. Rat—49.9 ± 11.7
   k. Baboon—89 ± 19
   l. Chimpanzee—270 ± 33.7
   m. Gorilla—332.3 ± 52.2
   n. Orangutan—208.9 ± 48.2
2. Increased (hypercholesterolemia)
   a. Intrahepatic and posthepatic cholestasis
      (1) The rate of cholesterol synthesis by the liver appears to be related inversely to the amount of chylomicron cholesterol reaching the liver. With cholestasis there is reduction of both chylomicron formation and cholesterol absorption, and as a result, hepatic synthesis of cholesterol is increased.
      (2) An increase in serum cholesterol esters occurs in obstructive jaundice with a reflux of cholesterol esters into the blood from the liver. Biliary obstruction stimulates hepatic cell membrane synthesis of cholesterol esters.
   b. Severe liver disease decreases cholesterol esters due to a decreased release of liver enzymes that influence esterification.
      (1) The use of the ratio of free to esterified cholesterol as an index of liver failure is no longer considered reliable and is of little diagnostic value.
   c. Nonhepatic causes to be considered in differential diagnosis
      (1) Diabetes mellitus
      (2) Hyperadrenocorticism
      (3) Hypothyroidism
      (4) Nephrotic syndrome
      (5) Pregnancy

VI. Tests based upon the activity of the liver in protein metabolism

A. General considerations (See table for normal values of serum protein.)
1. Albumin, alpha globulin, beta globulin, and fibrinogen are synthesized in the liver from amino acids.
2. Gamma globulin (immunoglobulin) is produced by the lymphoreticular system from amino acids.

NORMAL VALUES FOR SERUM PROTEIN

Serum protein	Dog	Cat	Horse	Cattle	Sheep	Goat	Pig
Total protein (serum) (g/dl)	5.40-7.10	5.40-7.30	5.70-7.80	6.74-7.46	6.00-7.90	6.40-7.90	7.90-8.90
Albumin (g/dl)	2.30-3.20	2.10-3.30	2.33-3.85	3.03-3.55	2.70-3.90	2.70-3.90	1.80-3.30
Globulin (g/dl)	2.70-4.40	2.60-5.10	2.62-4.04	3.00-3.48	3.50-5.70	2.70-4.10	5.29-6.43
Alpha-1	0.20-0.50	0.20-1.10	0.06-0.70	0.75-0.83	0.30-0.60	0.50-0.70	0.32-0.44
Alpha-2	0.30-1.10	0.40-0.90	0.31-1.31				1.23-1.54
Beta-1	0.60-1.20	0.30-0.90	0.40-1.58	0.80-1.12	0.70-1.20	0.70-1.20	0.13-0.33
Beta-2		0.60-1.00	0.29-0.89		0.40-1.40	0.30-0.60	1.26-1.68
Gamma-1	0.50-1.30	0.30-2.50	0.55-1.90		0.70-2.20	0.90-3.00	2.24-2.46
Gamma-2	0.40-0.90	1.40-1.90		1.69-2.25	0.20-1.10		
Albumin: globulin ratio	0.59-1.11	0.45-1.19	0.62-1.46	0.84-0.94	0.42-0.76	0.63-1.26	0.37-0.51

Source: J. J. Kaneko, Standard values in domestic animals, Univ. Calif., Davis.

B. Total serum protein
1. The normal range for most animals will vary between 5 and 8 g/dl.
   a. Young animals will usually fall below this range for adults.
2. The total serum protein concentration is usually of little value in the assessment of liver function or disease.
   a. The albumin fraction can be diminished and the globulin fraction increased; the sum of the two fractions may yield a wide range of values, from low to high, in the presence of hepatic disease.
   b. It is more reliable to consider the significance of abnormalities in albumin and in globulin separately, although a significant hypoproteinemia is usually going to be the result of a hypoalbuminemia.

C. Albumin
1. Methods
   a. Chemical—salt, alcohol, or isoelectric precipitation
   b. Physical—electrophoresis, chromatography, or ultracentrifuge
   c. HABA dye
      (1) This is the method used in many automated clinical chemistry instruments such as the SMA 12 of Technicon and blood analyzer systems such as the Ames/BMI.
      (2) It produces consistently lower albumin values for animals than for man when compared to chemical or electrophoretic methods, as different species have different dye-binding activities.
      (3) In the dog, the ratio of the electrophoretic albumin values to the HABA dye method values is not too consistent, the average ratio being 1.56.
2. Hypoalbuminemia
   a. Chronic diffuse liver disease, especially cirrhosis
      (1) Failure of hepatic parenchymal synthesis of serum albumin is not an early alteration.
         (a) The normal half-life of canine albumin varies from 7 to 10 days, so that alterations in serum albumin are not seen in acute hepatic failure.

(2) In portal cirrhosis the characteristic finding is a decrease in serum albumin and an increase in gamma globulin.

b. Nonhepatic causes
  (1) Renal disease—glomerulonephritis, amyloidosis, nephrotic syndrome
  (2) Inadequate intake or absorption
    (a) Inadequate diet
    (b) Malabsorption
    (c) Pancreatic hypoplasia or atrophy
    (d) Protein-losing gastroenteropathy
    (e) Gastrointestinal parasitism
    (f) Increased protein need—pregnancy, lactation
  (3) Excessive loss of protein
    (a) Renal disease—with albuminuria
    (b) Draining wounds
    (c) Burns
    (d) Internal losses—acute intestinal obstruction, pancreatitis, acute peritonitis
    (e) Increased protein breakdown for gluconeogenesis—fever, diabetes mellitus, hyperadrenocorticism

c. When used in conjunction with other tests, albumin is helpful in the differential diagnosis of cirrhosis and hepatocellular damage:

Substance	Cirrhosis	Hepatocellular
Transaminase	Normal to increased	Elevated
Bromsulphalein	Increased	Increased
Serum albumin	Low	Normal

D. Globulins
  1. Hyperglobulinemia—in liver disease the change is usually polyclonal
    a. Alpha globulins—in general, are elevated in trauma, fever, and certain malignancies
      (1) Alpha-1 is not affected in liver disease.
      (2) Alpha-2 will have a relative increase in cirrhosis and hepatitis.
    b. Beta globulins—increased in hepatitis and cirrhosis
    c. Gamma globulins—Kupffer cell proliferation and increased numbers of plasma cells in the bone marrow may represent the sources for increased production and elevation
      (1) Consistent elevations are seen in hepatitis, carcinoma of the liver, and cirrhosis.

E. Albumin: globulin ratio (A/G)
  1. Normal species variation in the A/G ratio
    a. Albumin tends to predominate over globulin in:
      (1) Dog
      (2) Horse
      (3) Sheep
      (4) Goat
      (5) Man
    b. Relative amounts of albumin and globulin are nearly equal or globulin tends to be in excess of albumin in:
      (1) Cattle
      (2) Pig
      (3) Cat
  2. Low A/G ratio
    a. Either a relative or absolute increase in globulin and/or a decrease in albumin

(1) Chronic inflammation
(2) Antigenic stimulation

3. Elevated A/G ratio
   a. Usually the result of decreased globulin, as increases in albumin are not likely to occur
      (1) Newborn animal before nursing
4. Flocculation or turbidity tests based upon the alteration of the A/G ratio
   a. Usually unreliable in animals, since the tests are based upon the A/G ratio for human serum, which does not correspond to the A/G ratios in many animals, so false positive reactions occur
   b. Examples of these tests include:
      (1) Cephalin-cholesterol flocculation
      (2) Thymol turbidity
      (3) Takata-Ara
      (4) Zinc sulfate—sometimes used to determine if colostrum has been ingested
      (5) Formol-gel

F. Prothrombin

1. Principle—the liver converts vitamin K into prothrombin
2. Method
   a. The capillary coagulation time can be used as a screening test to detect prothrombin deficiencies. If the capillary coagulation time is prolonged, then the longer procedure for prothrombin time can be conducted.
   b. Prothrombin time determination is best performed by a commercial laboratory or a technologist experienced in running the test.
3. Interpretation
   a. Decreased prothrombin levels (increased prothrombin time)
      (1) Two types of liver disturbance
         (a) Inability to synthesize prothrombin from vitamin K due to a reduction of functional hepatic mass
         (b) Fat-soluble vitamin K cannot be absorbed from the intestine with an inadequate amount of bile.
            [1] If obstruction of the bile duct occurs, an injection of 50 mg of vitamin K may decrease coagulation time.
            [2] Lack of response to parenteral vitamin K injection suggests diffuse parenchymal insufficiency.
      (2) The value of this test varies with the species
         (a) Dog
            [1] Acute hepatic failure, as clotting factors have shorter half-lives than albumin
            [2] Rather insensitive indicator, except during the acute phase; not as sensitive as the BSP or alkaline phosphatase elevation in detecting liver injury
            [3] Should be a screening test for coagulation problems before performing a liver biopsy
         (b) Horse
            [1] Helpful in prognosis, as the severity of the liver damage is related to the prolongation of prothrombin time
            [2] Levels of prothrombin significantly reduced in acute and subacute hepatitis, hepatic necrosis with regeneration, and diffuse fibrosis

G. Urea or urea nitrogen

1. Principle—urea is produced in the liver from the catabolism of protein in the ornithine, citrulline, arginine cycle
2. Interpretation
   a. Urea or urea nitrogen is quite insensitive as an indicator of liver damage.
   b. In advanced liver damage, there is a tendency for the blood urea nitrogen to be low, if there is not concomitant renal damage resulting in impaired excretion.

H. Blood ammonia

1. Principle—ammonia is produced in the gastrointestinal tract and reaches the liver through the portal circulation. The ammonia is produced by bacterial action.
2. Hepatic cell damage
    a. Removal of ammonia is incomplete and can be aggravated by large amounts of protein in the diet.
        (1) Hepatic coma is usually associated with elevated blood and cerebrospinal fluid ammonia concentrations.
3. Patent ductus venosus—the laboratory test of choice for confirmation of this diagnosis

I. Uric acid

1. General considerations
    a. In most mammals, purines are metabolized to uric acid and then to allantoin.
        (1) Exceptions include man, monkey, and the Dalmatian breed of dog.
            (a) In the Dalmatian, only about one-third of the uric acid is converted to allantoin, while in other breeds of dogs it is nearly complete.
    b. The site of conversion of uric acid to allantoin is in the liver, and this is accomplished by the enzyme uricase.
2. Interpretation
    a. Increased—in liver cell damage, as the conversion of uric acid to allantoin is incomplete; as a result the amount of uric acid in the blood and urine is elevated
        (1) The practical value of uric acid as a liver function test is questionable, as the enzymes and other newer tests are more sensitive indicators of liver damage.

22 PANCREATIC FUNCTION TESTS

I. Pancreatic cell damage—acute pancreatic necrosis, chronic recurring pancreatitis, abscessation, or trauma

A. Serum amylase
1. Major sources of serum amylase
a. Pancreas
(1) However, normal serum levels of amylase are maintained in the dog after total removal of the pancreas.
b. Intestinal mucosa
c. Liver
d. Salivary gland
2. Methods of analysis—two general methods
a. Saccharogenic—measures the amount of reducing sugars released or increased by the action of serum amylase on starch
(1) Old method—measured the number of fragments or rate of appearance of reducing groups
(a) Not recommended for canine serum because the high maltase in serum produces high amylase values
(2) New method—serum amylase hydrolyzes a dyed starch substrate into alcohol-soluble fragments
(a) The unhydrolyzed starch substrate and serum proteins are precipitated with the dyed fragments in solution and measured by absorbance.
(b) The size of the fragments is of little importance when they are smaller than a critical size, which is where the new method differs from the original techniques.
(c) The method can be adapted for canine and feline serum by making a higher dilution, as these sera have much higher normal amylase activity than human serum.
[1] When submitting canine serum samples to a commercial laboratory, technicians should be alerted to the fact that normal values are 5 to 10 times higher in the dog than in human serum.
[2] Cat serum has 7 to 10 times more amylase activity than that in human serum.
(d) Commercial kits available include:
[1] Dy Amyl—General Diagnostics Inc.
[2] Amylochrome—Roache Diagnostics
(e) Advantage—easier to perform than the amyloclastic technique
b. Amyloclastic—measures the hydrolysis or breakdown of starch and its disappearance
(1) Harding's modification of the Somogyi method—one of the recommended methods
(a) Incubate for 5 min at 37° C:
[1] Sodium chloride solution (0.9%)—0.5 ml
[2] Amylase solution (1.7%)—4 ml
(b) Add 0.5 ml of patient's serum and mix.
(c) At 30-sec intervals add 0.5 ml of the mixture to 0.002 N dilute iodine solution in a 2% solution of potassium iodide.
(d) The end point is the last time a blue-black color persists.
(e) Divide 6400 by the time in minutes required to digest the amylase solution, to obtain the amylase value expressed as Harding units.
3. Interpretation—normal values
a. Dog
(1) Modified Caraway units (amyloclastic)—under 1000
(2) Harding units (amyloclastic)—under 3200
(3) Gomori (amyloclastic)—0 to 800
(4) Dy Amyl (new saccharogenic)—under 3200

(5) IU/L—185 to 700
(6) Somogyi units—100 to 400

b. Cat
(1) Harding units—0 to 2700
(2) Dy Amyl (new saccharogenic)—0 to 2600 units

4. Interpretation of increased serum amylase activity
a. Pancreatic necrosis
(1) Amylase activity increases within the first 12 hr after an insult and usually attains its maximum value within 24 hr. When the insult does not persist, serum levels return to normal in 2 to 6 days.
(a) Provided several days have elapsed since the onset of clinical signs, a normal amylase value does not rule out a healing pancreatic process.
(2) Amylase activity should be at least double that of the normal mean for consideration of a diagnosis of acute pancreatic disease.
(a) With acute pancreatic necrosis (acute pancreatitis), amylase may be 4 to 10 times that seen in the serum of the normal dog.
b. Intestinal obstruction
c. Renal insufficiency—both serum amylase and BUN will increase
(1) Amylase is eliminated in the urine, so very high values (2 to 3 times the normal limit) are seen in the serum due to impaired excretion.
(2) Increases due to prerenal uremia, where the associated shock reduces renal perfusion, will have a urine specific gravity greater than 1.027. A fixed specific gravity (1.010) suggests that the high amylase level in the serum is due to renal impairment without pancreatic involvement.
d. Some forms of stress, corticosteroids, and ACTH will lead to a 30 to 40% increase in serum amylase values, so that the magnitude of the increase is helpful in differentiation from pancreatic problems.
(1) Significant elevations were not reported in routine ovariohysterectomy operations.
e. Parotid gland disease

B. Serum lipase
1. Major sources of serum lipase—lipase is present in fewer tissues than amylase, so that elevations of lipase are more specifically related to pancreatic disease.
a. Pancreas—major source
b. Intestinal mucosa
2. Methods—lipase catalyzes the hydrolysis of triglycerides to fatty acids and glycerol, the substrates that can be utilized are olive oil, coconut oil, and tributyrin
a. Cherry-Crandall method—serum is incubated for 24 hr with a buffered olive oil emulsion, and the fatty acids produced are titrated with an alkaline reagent
(1) The long incubation period is the main objection, so modifications requiring shorter incubation times have been devised.
(a) A technique using a 6-hr incubation period has been found to be sensitive and is in common use (Sigma Chemical Co.).
b. Roe-Byler method—1 hr incubation period with olive oil as a substrate and the end point achieved by titration with sodium hydroxide
c. Turbidimetric measurement of loss of turbidity of a dilute olive oil emulsion, with the incubation time as little as 20 min
d. Tietz modification titrates to a constant end point of pH 10.5, using a pH meter to improve accuracy.
3. Normal values for serum lipase
a. Dog
(1) Sigma-Tietz units (6-hr incubation)—0 to 1
(2) Roe-Byler units—0.8 to 12, with a mean of 5.6
(3) International units—13 to 200
b. Cat
(1) International units—0 to 83
(2) Roe-Byler units—0 to 5
4. Interpretation of increased serum lipase activity
a. Pancreatitis necrosis

(1) Elevation occurs shortly after necrosis and persists in a parallel manner to serum amylase.

b. Intestinal obstruction

c. Renal insufficiency—produces the highest elevations

(1) Lipase is excreted by the kidneys; if there is oliguria or anuria, serum lipase will increase.

5. Collection of the serum specimen

a. Stability under various conditions of storage

(1) Room temperature—7 days

(2) Refrigerator (4° C)—3 wk

b. Avoid hemolysis—a hemoglobin concentration of 500 mg/dl inhibits enzyme activity by 50%

6. Conversion factor (unit x factor = IU)

a. Roe-Byler—16.7

C. Blood and urine glucose—hyperglycemia and glycosuria are frequent findings

1. Although diabetes mellitus is a potential sequel to pancreatitis, its incidence is probably low except when the disease progresses to the chronic form, where an incidence of 50% has been reported in the dog.

D. Serum glutamic pyruvic transaminase—normal to increased (100 to 500 units)

1. Fatty changes in the liver are thought to be the cause of elevations.

E. Serum alkaline phosphatase—elevated with concurrent liver involvement

F. Serum cholesterol—marked increases may occur during hyperlipemic conditions, with increases varying from 400 to 800 mg/dl

1. May be related to altered liver metabolism or endogenous lipids

2. Hypercholesterolemia often characterizes diabetes mellitus.

G. Serum calcium—marked hypocalcemia may occur due to the formation of insoluble calcium soap in areas of fat necrosis around the pancreas

H. Hematologic alterations include:

1. Total leukocyte count—degree of leukocytosis dependent upon the amount of necrosis, inflammation, and duration of the condition

a. Mild case—may have no alteration

b. Early stage—leukocytosis with mature neutrophils, eosinopenia, and a lymphopenia

c. 2 to 3 days after onset, a leukocytosis of the magnitude of 20,000 to 35,000 can develop, with a neutrophilia and a shift to the left, as well as an increasing monocytosis.

d. In the terminal stage a degenerative shift to the left may be detected, with a normal to depressed leukocyte count.

2. Hematocrit

a. Packed cell volume—usually increased due to loss of fluids by vomiting and reduced fluid intake

b. Lipemia—frequently seen with acute pancreatitis

II. Pancreatic insufficiency (juvenile atrophy or fibrosis)

A. Examination of feces for pancreatic enzyme deficiency

1. Gross examination

a. Undigested food

b. Bulky

c. Semisolid or soft in consistency

d. Pale in color—yellow to clay-colored

e. Steatorrhea (fat)—neutral fat may glisten

f. Foul, rancid odor

2. Microscopic examination

a. Fat (steatorrhea)

(1) Mix a small portion of feces with water or saline solution on a slide and combine with equal parts of Sudan III (equal parts of 70% alcohol and acetone with an excess of Sudan III stain) or Sudan IV stain.

(a) It may be helpful to counterstain with new methylene blue stain.
(2) Examine under the low power objective (x10) after placing a coverglass on the mixture.
(3) Neutral fat will appear as orange or red globules, which vary in size and shape and indicate a deficiency of pancreatic lipase.

b. Striated muscle—after a meal of uncooked muscle (creatorrhea)
(1) In a diluted sample of feces note muscle fibers, which will be light yellow in color.
(2) Examine the muscle fibers for the presence of cross-striations, which indicate a deficiency of trypsin or increased peristalsis, as in diarrhea.

c. Starch (amylorrhea)
(1) Mix feces with Lugol's solution, which stains the starch a blackish blue color.
(2) Little significance in pancreatic disease

3. Test for proteolytic activity employing gelatin digestion (for use in small animals only).

a. Film test
(1) Bring 9 ml of 5% sodium bicarbonate to 10 ml total volume by adding feces. Mix well.
(2) Place ½ to ¾ in. of the mixture in a vial or test tube and place a narrow strip of radiographic film in the vial so that the lower portion is submerged in the mixture.
(a) Unprocessed film will work better than processed film, as it will be easier to detect digestion of the gelatin in the emulsion.
(3) Incubate at 37° C for ½ hr.
(4) Wash film under a gentle stream of tap water.
(a) A cleared area on the submerged portion of the film indicates the presence of trypsin.
(b) With a deficiency of trypsin, the emulsion will only be water-marked or partially removed.
(5) Consistently negative results may indicate:
(a) Pancreatic enzyme deficiency
(b) Retention of feces—trypsin is not very stable and is autodigestible
(c) Trypsin inhibitors
(d) Intestinal disease
(e) Enterokinase deficiency
(6) Consistently positive results may indicate:
(a) Presence of fecal trypsin
(b) Presence of proteolytic enzymes (proteases) from the intestine—only weakly proteolytic
(7) Lack of consistency in results can be explained by:
(a) Differences in diet
(b) Amount of food consumed
(c) Variation in absorption
(d) Transit time
(e) Cyclic release of enzymes into the intestinal tract
(f) Only a small amount of enzyme is required to digest the emulsion.
(g) Relying on only one test—the test should be repeated several times

b. Tube test of gelatin—more sensitive than the film test method
(1) Warm two tubes, each containing 2 ml of 7.5% gelatin, to 37° C to liquefy.
(a) Knox gelatin can be used.
(2) Add 2 ml of the feces mixture as described above to one gelatin tube.
(3) Add 2 ml of 5% sodium bicarbonate to the other gelatin tube for the control. Mix well.
(4) Incubate both tubes at 37° C for 1 hr.
(5) Refrigerate or place in cold water (4° C) for 20 min.
(6) The results are read as follows:
(a) Failure to gel indicates the presence of trypsin, which has digested the gelatin.
(b) Gel formation indicates the absence of trypsin and a pancreatic insufficiency if tests are repeatedly deficient.

B. Fat absorption

1. A baseline blood sample is drawn, following which the patient is given material of a fatty nature by the l route.

a. Heavy cream, half-and-half cream and milk, corn oil, or Lipomul may be given.

(1) 3 ml/kg of body weight is the amount of Lipomul to be fed to a fasting patient.

2. At hourly intervals afterward additional blood samples are obtained.
   a. Usually 2 to 3 hr will be the maximum time required for lipemia to appear in the serum or plasma.
3. The blood samples are centrifuged, and the sera or plasma are compared for lipemia.
4. Results
   a. A normal dog should exhibit an increase in fat in the serum.
   b. A dog with a deficiency of pancreatic lipase or one having malabsorption will show no lipemia in the serum or plasma.
      (1) The inclusion of commercial pancreatic enzymes with a fatty meal may help to differentiate pancreatic lipase deficiency from malabsorption.
         (a) Pancreatic lipase deficiency—lipemia produced when enzymes are added
         (b) Malabsorption—in spite of additional enzymes supplied, lipemia does not occur because of intestinal block, which interferes with absorption
   c. This test will not work in the horse.

III. Diabetes mellitus

A. Pathophysiology

1. Diabetes mellitus is a chronic metabolic disorder characterized by disturbances in carbohydrate, lipid, and protein metabolism.
2. Causes
   a. A relative or absolute deficiency of insulin for the requirements of the tissues
      (1) Insulin deficiency is usually due to beta cell destruction in the islets of Langerhans in the pancreas.
         (a) Frequently accompanies acute pancreatitis
      (2) Antagonists to insulin may develop—antiinsulin antibodies
   b. Excess of corticosteroids, ACTH, or growth hormone has a diabetogenic influence.
   c. Miscellaneous influences
      (1) Pregnancy
      (2) Stress reactions
3. Pathogenesis:

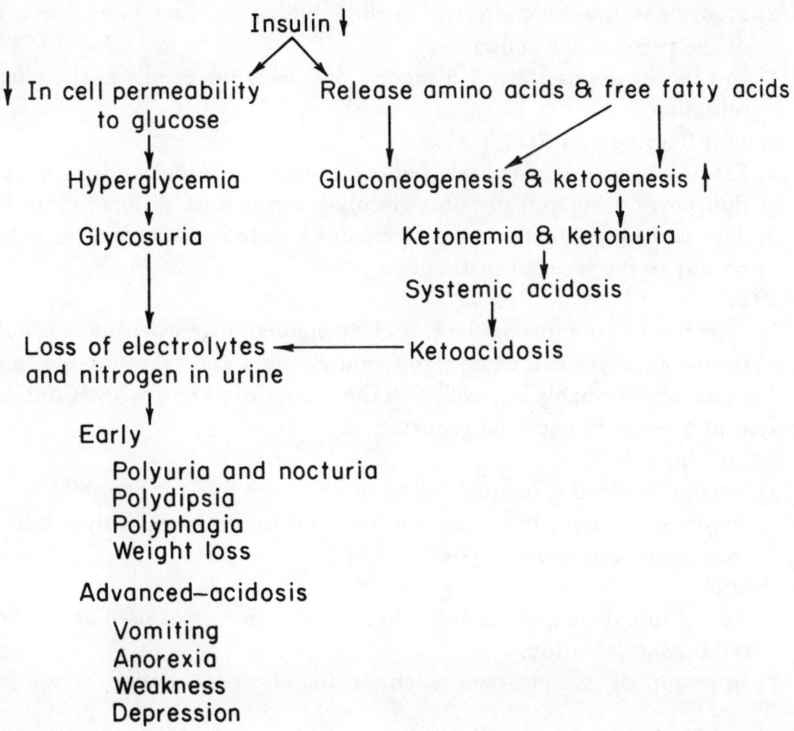

B. Laboratory findings
1. Blood glucose
a. Specimen collection and preservation
(1) General rules for collection
(a) Blood specimen should be obtained after an overnight fast (usually 12 hr), as food intake influences blood glucose levels.
(b) All collection equipment must be sterile or contain insignificant numbers of organisms and must be chemically clean.
(2) Choice of specimen
(a) Serum
[1] Whenever practical, serum is the sample of choice for the determination of glucose.
[2] Every effort should be made to obtain nonhemolyzed serum and to separate the clot as soon as possible. Glycolysis, the utilization of glucose by enzymes in the erythrocytes, takes place while serum remains in contact with the cells. The longer the contact, the greater the loss of glucose. The time elapsed from obtaining the blood to removal of serum from the clot should not exceed 30 min.
(b) Plasma
[1] Plasma should be separated from the erythrocytes by centrifugation immediately after obtaining the blood.
[2] Plasma is almost equal to serum as the sample of choice and has some advantages over serum; for example, no delay is necessary to obtain plasma by centrifugation of whole blood, and a greater volume of plasma is obtained from a given volume of blood.
(c) Whole blood
[1] Satisfactory if it can be assayed without delay
[2] Usually susceptible to contamination and errors in sample measurement
[3] Values usually about 15 to 20 mg lower than serum or plasma values in most glucose procedures
[4] Used in the Dextrostix method
(3) Anticoagulants
(a) Sodium fluoride
[1] Acts effectively to preserve glucose when used in the concentration range between 5 and 10 mg/ml
[2] Fluoride is especially effective in the inhibition of certain enzymes, a possible explanation of the preservative action.
[3] In concentrations above 7.5 mg/ml, it affects the results of the glucose oxidase determination.
(b) Sodium fluoride and EDTA
[1] EDTA (1 mg/ml) effectively removes the calcium ions and prevents coagulation; sodium fluoride (2.5 mg/ml) prevents glycolysis for at least 48 hr at room temperature.
[2] This is the combination of choice from a technical standpoint, as it has no obvious effects on any of the selected methods.
(c) EDTA
[1] Effective as an anticoagulant; a clear nonhemolyzed plasma is usually obtained
(4) Preservation—glycolysis can cause significant changes and takes place as a result of many factors; two that can be reasonably controlled in the laboratory are glycolysis due to enzymatic action and glycolysis as a result of bacterial growth
(a) Sodium fluoride
[1] Generally effective for prevention of glycolysis due to the inhibitory action on glycolytic enzymes, but not sufficiently antibacterial to prevent glycolysis due to bacterial growth if the specimen is contaminated
(b) Thymol
[1] Added to anticoagulants and other preservatives, it is used as a precaution against bacterial contamination.
[2] In serum, thymol possesses an enhancing effect (false high values) in the ferricyanide

glucose method (about 5% error) and an inhibiting effect on the reaction in the glucose oxidase method (about 10%).

(c) Temperature effect

[1] Room temperature—ideal for enzymatic and bacterial action, so samples should not be left at room temperature any longer than absolutely necessary

[2] Refrigerator temperature—the lower the temperature, the greater the stability of the glucose specimen; microbial growth is considerably lessened at 4° C

[3] Frozen state—microbial growth greatly inhibited in the frozen state; analysis should be performed within 2 or 3 hr after removal from the freezer; some damage to enzymes results from freezing, but enzymatic as well as bacterial activity is usually resumed at room temperature; freezing and thawing may denature constituents and cause them to act as impurities, so freezing and thawing should not be permitted more than once before analysis

b. Methods for glucose determination

(1) Specific methods

(a) Glucose oxidase—absolute specificity

[1] The assay of glucose based on the enzymatic reaction of glucose oxidase is essentially specific for glucose; other sugars are oxidized also, but at a slower rate than glucose.

[2] Enzyme activators or inhibitors may be introduced with the sample or the reagents—sodium fluoride and thymol inhibit the reaction of enzymes and must be removed or decreased to a compatible concentration in the preparation of a protein-free filtrate; uric acid, ascorbic acid, glutathione, cysteine, and bilirubin are reducing agents that interfere

[3] Results that approach the true glucose value are possible if strict control over variation due to laboratory techniques is maintained.

[4] The Ames/BMI blood analyzer system utilizes this method.

(b) Ortho-toluidine—specific for aldohexoses

[1] Of the aldohexoses present in blood, glucose is predominantly abundant. Galactose and mannose react also but are usually insignificant in concentration compared to glucose, so the procedure becomes relatively specific for glucose.

[2] With respect to reliability, it gives values similar to those of the Nelson-Somogyi method.

[3] Advantages are its simplicity and economy, stability of reagents and final color development, and relative rapidity of analysis.

[4] The Hycel Mark X and XVII as well as the Clay-Adams Accu-Stat utilize this method.

(2) Nonspecific methods

(a) Nelson-Somogyi—approaches "true" glucose

[1] Since most of the nonglucose-interfering substances are removed by precipitation, it gives relative specificity.

[2] Results are slightly above those of the glucose oxidase method.

(b) Ferricyanide—approaches "true" glucose

[1] The bulk of the interfering substances are removed by passing whole blood or serum through a dialyzing membrane, so specificity is about the same as the Nelson-Somogyi method.

[2] The Technicon Auto Analyzer and SMA 12/60 utilize this method.

(c) Folin-Wu—total reducing

[1] Serum or plasma glucose results, compared to the glucose oxidase method, tend to approach the true level.

[2] Blood glucose levels are about 5 mg/dl more than the level by the glucose oxidase method.

[3] Specificity for glucose is less than desired, since the presence of other reducing substances in the filtrate react to give false high results.

(3) Screening method

(a) Dextrostix (Ames Co.)—semiquantitative

[1] This method is only reliable when the Eyetone Reflectance meter is used to evaluate the color reaction on the strip.

[2] Visual comparison to the color chart is useful only when there is a marked hyperglycemia.

[3] Glucose oxidase is present on the strip and is used only with whole blood.

c. Interpretation

(1) Normal ranges—in mg/dl: (36)

Species	Serum or plasma	Whole blood
Dog	70-110	55-90
Cat	70-110	60-100
Horse	75-115	60-100
Cattle	45-75	35-55
Sheep	50-80	35-60
Goat	50-75	45-60
Pig		
Baby		75-150
Adult	85-150	65-95

(2) Diabetic

(a) A fasting blood glucose over 200 mg/dl is generally considered diagnostic for the dog and cat.

(b) Values under 200 mg but consistently over the normal range would recommend a glucose tolerance test for confirmation of diabetes mellitus.

[1] Seldom necessary

(3) Conditions other than diabetes mellitus that can be associated with a hyperglycemia:

(a) Postprandial—for up to 4 hr after a meal

(b) Epinephrine release—from excitement, pain, or injection

[1] Mobilizes stored carbohydrate in the liver

[2] Usually transient

(c) Stress, with increase in glucocorticoid and catecholamine secretion

[1] Stimulates glycogenolysis and gluconeogenesis

[2] Transient hyperglycemia due to stress is common in the cat—returns to normal within 6 to 24 hr

(d) Pancreatitis—often associated with disturbed carbohydrate utilization; although there may be no disturbance in islet cell function, in many of the advanced cases diabetes mellitus may follow

(e) Cushing's disease or administration of corticosteroids

[1] Increases hepatic gluconeogenesis

(f) Convulsions—of epilepsy, tetany, eclampsia, and intracranial trauma

(g) Administration of drugs

[1] After general anesthetics

[2] Morphine

[3] Strychnine

[4] Thyroid preparations

[5] Glucose infusions

(h) Liver disease—in some cases

(i) Moribund state

2. Urine glucose—marked reaction (++++) when hyperglycemia exceeds the renal absorption of glucose in the proximal convoluted tubules

a. Renal threshold

(1) Dog—175 to 220 mg/dl

(2) Horse and cat—180 to 200 mg/dl

(3) Cattle—100 mg/dl

(4) Sheep—160 to 200 mg/dl

b. Reagents

(1) Clinitest tablets (Ames)—recommended, as they are quantitative for reducing substances even though not specific for glucose

(2) Clinistix—reaction for glucose is inhibited by ascorbic acid, which is commonly excreted in large quantities by the diabetic animal

(3) Diastix

3. Urine ketones—marked reaction in the ketoacidotic state
   a. Reagent
      (1) Acetest tablets (Ames)—more sensitive than Ketostix
      (2) Measures acetoacetic acid and acetone, but not beta-hydroxybutyric acid
4. Serum ketones
   a. Reagent—crush Acetest tablet and mix with serial dilutions of serum or plasma and saline or control serum such as 1:2, 1:4, 1:8, 1:16, 1:32
   b. Record the highest dilution at which a reaction is observed.
5. Serum cholesterol—usually high due to increased fat mobilization
   a. Serum from a diabetic animal is often lipemic and may be the first clue that would lead one to suspect diabetes.
6. Liver enzymes—usually elevated
7. Blood urea nitrogen—often elevated due to renal failure
   a. Important to establish for prognostic purposes
8. Glucose tolerance test
   a. Fast for 24 hr
   b. Intravenous glucose tolerance
      (1) Give 0.5 g of glucose per kilogram of body weight as a 50% solution after obtaining a preinjection blood sample.
      (2) Take blood samples at 30-min intervals for 3 hr.
      (3) Interpretation
         (a) Normal animal—blood glucose returns to fasting level in 60 to 90 min
         (b) Diabetic animal—takes more than 90 min to return to the fasting level
   c. Oral glucose tolerance
      (1) Give 1 g of glucose per pound of body weight after obtaining a preinjection blood sample.
      (2) Blood samples are taken at 30 min, 1 hr, 2 hr, 3 hr, and sometimes 4 hr.
         (a) A single blood sample at 2 hr as a screening test can be used in animals where obtaining multiple samples is difficult.
      (3) Interpretation
         (a) Normal—blood glucose returns to the fasting level in 2 hr
         (b) Diabetic animal—blood glucose level has not returned to the fasting level in 2 hr

IV. Hypoglycemia

A. Causes

1. Hyperinsulinism
   a. Functional beta cell tumor
   b. Insulin overdose
2. Glycogen storage disease—glycogen accumulates in the liver
   a. von Gierke-like disease—due to a deficiency of glucose-6-phosphatase
      (1) Seen in toy breeds of dogs
3. Functional hypoglycemia
   a. Seen in small breeds of dogs under stress and in hunting dogs
4. Adrenocortical insufficiency
5. Hypothyroidism—occasionally
6. Starvation
7. Malabsorption—occasionally
8. Hepatic disease in the terminal stages
9. Bovine and ovine ketosis—primary or nervous forms
10. Hypoglycemia of baby pigs

B. Clinical signs
  1. Extreme weakness
  2. Convulsions
  3. Mental confusion
  4. Ataxia

C. Laboratory findings
  1. Blood glucose—under 40 mg/dl
    a. If the level is over 40 mg/dl, fasting and/or exercise should precipitate a drop to the significant level.
  2. Glucagon tolerance test
    a. Principle
      (1) Glucagon is a hormone that causes hyperglycemia from glycogenolysis when administered intravenously.
      (2) Glucagon directly stimulates insulin release from the beta cells.
    b. Method
      (1) Fast patient for 12 hr.
      (2) Inject 0.03 mg/kg of glucagon intravenously after taking a preinjection blood sample.
      (3) Draw additional blood samples at 3, 5, 15, 30, 60, and 120 min and assay for glucose levels.
    c. Interpretation
      (1) Normal animal—blood glucose will increase 20 to 60 mg/dl and will return slowly to fasting levels in 3 or 4 hr
      (2) Functional beta-cell tumor (insulinoma)
        (a) Blood glucose of less than 50 mg/dl 60 to 90 min after injection—highly diagnostic
        (b) Peak blood glucose is under 135 mg/dl.
        (c) Plasma immunoreactive insulin (IRI) at 1 min after injection is over 50 microunits/ml—diagnostic of insulinoma
      (3) von Gierke-like disease
        (a) Little or no blood glucose response
  3. Epinephrine tolerance test
  4. Tolbutamide response test
  5. Radioimmunoassay for insulin
    a. Normal for dog (fasting)—around 20 microunits/dl
    b. Insulinoma—50 microunits/dl or more 1 min after glucagon injection

23 CARDIOVASCULAR DISEASE TESTS

I. Blood picture in specific conditions

A. Dog

1. Acute bacterial endocarditis
   a. The usual picture is one of a neutrophilic leukocytosis, but a leukopenia may occur in the presence of an overwhelming septicemia.
   b. There is a marked shift to the left with many young forms of granulocytes such as myelocytes and even myeloblasts. Toxic neutrophils are abundant.
   c. Thrombocytes are usually normal in number, sometimes giant in form, but in an occasional case there may be a thrombocytopenia.
2. Heartworms
   a. A neutrophilia and eosinophilia are seen. It is not unusual to find basophils associated with the eosinophils; when this combination is seen in the dog, it should indicate an examination for microfilaria.

B. Cattle

1. Traumatic pericarditis
   a. The total leukocyte count is usually increased early in the course of the disease, but later may drop rapidly.
   b. A neutrophilia with a marked shift to the left is characteristic. The neutrophils will appear to be toxic.
2. Lymphosarcoma—involvement of the myocardium is a frequent finding in the adult form of lymphosarcoma
   a. In a rare case, the count may be leukemic with a total leukocyte count exceeding 100,000/microliters.
   b. A persistent lymphocytosis and/or immature forms of lymphocytes may be seen, but these findings are not consistent.
3. High mountain disease
   a. The total erythrocyte count is variable and may be high, normal, or low.
   b. Hemoglobin values are usually normal to elevated, but occasionally are reduced.
   c. Variations in the total leukocyte counts are seen, but they are usually high.
      (1) High total leukocyte counts coinciding with temperature elevations are believed to indicate secondary infection.
   d. Neutrophilia, eosinopenia, and lymphopenia are usually reported, but occasionally lymphocytosis and eosinophilia are seen.

C. Horse

1. Viral arteritis
   a. Leukopenia is a constant finding, usually evident by the 2nd day after exposure and persisting up to 13 days.
   b. Lymphopenia is more severe than neutropenia.

II. Secondary polycythemia—increased stimulation of erythrocyte production, characterized by an absolute erythrocytosis; erythropoietin released in response to tissue hypoxia; arterial oxygen saturation decreased

A. Congenital heart disease—polycythemia usually seen

1. Right-to-left shunt
2. Pulmonic stenosis
3. Patent ductus arteriosus

B. Acquired heart disease—erythrocytosis seldom occurs, but nucleated erythrocytes may be seen in the peripheral blood

III. Protein

A. Plasma protein decreases rapidly with retention of sodium and water in congestive heart failure.
B. Average protein concentration in gm/dl in various conditions:

Condition	Plasma	Ascitic fluid
Heart failure	4.8	3.0
Mitral insufficiency		
Myocardial disease		
Heartworm disease	6.0	3.8
Cirrhosis of the liver	3–5	<0.5
Peritonitis or neoplasia	...	>3.0

IV. Serum enzymes—certain enzymes present in cardiac muscle are released when tissue necrosis (myocardial infarction) or increased cell permeability occurs

A. Serum glutamic oxaloacetic transaminase (SGOT)
1. The blood levels have a rough correlation with the extent of the infarct and may be only transiently and minimally abnormal.
2. SGOT may be elevated due to acute damage to the parenchymal cells of other organs.
   a. Liver cell necrosis—common in congestive heart failure
   b. Skeletal muscle damage—can occur if animal is down in the cage or stall for long periods
3. Normal values—in IU/L (7)
   a. Dog—6.2 ± 13
   b. Cat—6.7 to 11
   c. Horse—58 to 94
   d. Cattle—20 to 34
   e. Sheep—79 ± 11
   f. Goat—43 to 132
   g. Pig—8.2 to 21.6

B. Creatine phosphokinase (CPK)
1. This enzyme is found primarily in the skeletal muscle, cardiac muscle, and brain. It is absent in the liver.
2. CPK may be elevated in:
   a. Acute myocardial infarction—occurs in the serum within 12 hr, reaches a peak within 24 to 36 hr, and returns to normal within 4 days
   b. Skeletal muscle damage—greatest increase
   c. Pulmonary embolism—minimal increase
      (1) To differentiate between acute myocardial infarction and pulmonary embolism, it is necessary to compare increases in CPK and LDH.
         (a) Myocardial infarction—both enzymes are increased in the serum
         (b) Pulmonary embolism—LDH is prominently elevated
3. CPK is not elevated in:
   a. Liver congestion due to congestive heart failure
      (1) SGOT elevation may occur in congestive heart failure, as this enzyme is found in hepatic cells. The comparison of increases of CPK and SGOT may be helpful if one also takes into consideration the variation of time for the duration of the elevation of the two enzymes.

4. Normal values

Species	IU/L(3)	mU/ml(4)
Dog		
Male	0.2-2.6	0-69
Female	0-1.8	0-82
Cat		
Male	0.4-3.4	...
Female	0-4.5	...
Horse		
Unexercised, 3 to 12 yr	0-3.6	...
Mares	...	0-65
Geldings	...	8-58
Cattle		
Dairy	...	0-17
Feedlot	...	3-50
Sheep		
Male	0-2.9	...
Female	0-0.9	...
Goat, female	0-2.5	...

C. Lactic dehydrogenase (LDH)

1. Total LDH—has limited usefulness in diagnosis, although the results are usually available in the profile of tests supplied by automated chemical analysis procedures
   a. It is widely distributed throughout the body.

Species	IU/L(7)	mU/ml(4)
Dog	10-35	...
Male	...	0-124
Female	...	0-131
Cat	16-69	...
Horse	41-104	...
Mare		48-242
Gelding	...	29-172
Cattle	176-365	...
Dairy	...	217-420
Feedlot	...	326-517
Sheep	60-111	...
Goat	31-99	...
Pig	96-160	...

(1). Since LDH is an intracellular enzyme, elevations occur when there is cellular death and leakage of the enzyme from a variety of cell types.
(2) Serum LDH will also be elevated when there is increased production as neoplastic cells proliferate.
(3) Strenuous exercise or muscle exertion during labor may increase serum LDH due to leakage from skeletal muscle.

b. It has a wide range of normal values (see table).

2. LDH isoenzymes—LDH can be separated into 5 major fractions by electrophoresis
   a. LDH-1—found mainly in cardiac muscle, along with smaller amounts of LDH-2
      (1) Is of value in the diagnosis of cardiac muscle damage
   b. LDH-3—found mainly in the lung
   c. LDH-5—mainly from the liver, with smaller amounts in skeletal muscle

D. Comparison of enzyme elevations

Condition	SGOT	SGPT	CPK	LDH	Isoenzymes
Myocardial infarction	Increased	N	Increased	Increased	1,2
Congestive heart failure (liver congestion)	Increased	Increased	N	Increased	4,5
Muscle necrosis	Increased	N	Increased	Increased	4,5
Lung embolism	N	N	Minimal increase	Increased	2,3

V. Blood cultures—indicated in bacterial endocarditis

A. Should be obtained before starting therapy
B. Request both aerobic and anaerobic cultures, as well as sensitivity tests
   1. Organisms most frequently incriminated in dogs:
      a. Nonhemolytic *Streptococcus*—most common
      b. Hemolytic *Streptococcus*
      c. *Staphylococcus*
      d. *Pseudomonas aeruginosa*
      e. *Escherichia coli*

VI. Serum electrolytes—alterations of serum electrolyte levels produce a secondary effect upon the heart.

A. Potassium
   1. Hyperkalemia
      a. Renal shutdown
      b. Hypoadrenocorticism
      c. Diabetes mellitus
   2. Hypokalemia
      a. Prolonged corticosteroid or ACTH therapy
      b. Renal loss—diuretics
      c. Potassium-free fluids administered intravenously
      d. Insulin administration
      e. Protracted vomiting or diarrhea

B. Calcium
 1. Secondary renal hyperparathyroidism
 2. Secondary nutritional hyperparathyroidism
 3. Puerperal tetany
 4. Therapy with calcium solutions intravenously

VII. Examination of pericardial or pleural effusion

A. Types of pericardial effusion
 1. Transudate
  a. Hypoalbuminemia
 2. Modified transudate
  a. Neoplasia
  b. Congestive heart failure
 3. Exudate
  a. Sterile
   (1) Neoplasia—heart base tumor, metastatic tumors
   (2) Idiopathic
  b. Septic
   (1) Infectious pericarditis
    (a) Bacterial
    (b) Mycotic
 4. Hemorrhage
  a. Hemostatic disorder
  b. Trauma
  c. Neoplasia—hemangiosarcoma

B. Differential characteristics of pericardial effusions

Characteristic	Transudate	Modified transudate	Exudate	Hemorrhage
Color	Clear to light yellow	Clear to serosanguineous	Pink to wine color	Red
Specific gravity	< 1.017	1.017-1.022	> 1.022	> 1.030
Protein (gm/dl)	< 2.0	2-3	> 3.0	> 4.5
Coagulation	. . .	. . .	±	±
Microorganisms	. . .	. . .	±	. . .

24 CALCIUM, PHOSPHORUS, AND METABOLIC BONE DISORDERS

I. Osteopenia — too little bone

A. Insufficient formation of bone

1. Osteoporosis — osteoblastic insufficiency with decreased formation of matrix, characterized by a quantitative decrease in qualitatively normal bone
   a. Causes
      (1) Malnutrition
         (a) Protein deficiency
            [1] Primary — restricted protein-calorie intake
            [2] Secondary — gastrointestinal disorders
         (b) Deficiency of calcium or high phosphorus — in these cases osteoporosis may be a stage in the progression to osteodystrophia fibrosa
      (2) Hormonal alterations
         (a) Pituitary insufficiency
         (b) Hyperadrenocorticism
         (c) Hypothyroidism
         (d) Senile metabolic decline
      (3) Poisoning
         (a) Excess lead
      (4) Disuse or immobilization — may be local following application of a cast or due to paralysis
   b. Clinical signs — seldom seen
      (1) Increased fragility increases susceptibility to fractures
      (2) May be localized to a single bone, group of bones, or may involve the entire skeleton
   c. Radiographic findings
      (1) Decreased skeletal mass — matrix and mineral alike
   d. Laboratory findings — the presence of normal chemical and histologic findings may be helpful in excluding other skeletal disorders with the same clinical and radiographic picture
      (1) Serum calcium — normal
      (2) Serum inorganic phosphate — normal
      (3) Serum alkaline phosphatase — normal
      (4) Urine calcium — normal or even low normal
2. Insufficient mineralization of bone
   a. Rickets — in young animals there is a failure of mineralization of osteoid and cartilaginous matrix and may be an excess of both types of matrix
      (1) Causes
         (a) Low calcium or phosphorus
            [1] Dietary deficiency
            [2] Interference with absorption from the gastrointestinal tract
         (b) Vitamin D deficiency
            [1] Lack of sunlight
            [2] Green forage with much carotene that antagonizes vitamin D
            [3] Defective absorption from the gut
      (2) Clinical signs and radiographic findings
         (a) Enlarged joints of limbs — epiphyses of long bones and costochondral junctions are enlarged
         (b) Bowing deformities — the bone is soft and not resistant to bearing weight
         (c) Fractures occasionally seen
         (d) Decreased density of all bones

(e) Resorption due to osteoclastic activity need not be seen, as osteoid is produced in greater amounts than in adult bones and is more resistant to resorption.

(f) All bones do not discontinue growth at the same time, so rickets and osteomalacia may be seen together.

[1] Rickets is seen in bones that are growing.

[2] Osteomalacia is seen in bones that have stopped growing.

(3) Laboratory findings

(a) Low-calcium rickets

[1] Serum calcium—low

[2] Serum inorganic phosphate—normal or low

[3] Serum alkaline phosphatase—high

(b) Low-phosphorus rickets

[1] Serum calcium—normal or low

[2] Serum inorganic phosphate—low

[3] Serum alkaline phosphatase—high

b. Osteomalacia—in adult animals bone growth has stopped, and this condition is characterized by an increased amount of matrix in the bone, but failure of osteoid to be mineralized

(1) Stages—failure to have normal mineralization of bone may occur in any of the three steps

(a) Deposition of matrix by osteoblasts

(b) Maturation or ripening of the matrix by the osteoblasts

(c) Mineralization of the matrix

(2) Causes

(a) Vitamin D deficiency

(b) Error in metabolism of vitamin D

(c) Mineral deficiency, especially phosphorus

(d) Intoxification by elements such as fluoride or strontium interferes with the action of the osteoblasts, so that they are incapable of ripening or maturing the matrix adequately.

(3) Clinical signs and radiographic finding

(a) Increased susceptibility to fractures

(b) Pseudofractures

(c) Softening, fragility, deformities

(d) Shifting lameness that is transient

(4) Laboratory findings

(a) Serum calcium—normal to low

(b) Serum phosphate—low

(c) Serum alkaline phosphatase—high

(d) Urine calcium

[1] Low—vitamin D deficiency

[2] Normal—other osteomalacias

B. Excessive bone resorption—generalized osteodystrophia fibrosa, i.e., hyperparathyroidism

1. Primary hyperparathyroidism

a. Cause—parathyroid hormone excreted in excess amounts

(1) Parathyroid neoplasia—usually an adenoma in the cervical region, near the thyroid gland, or near the base of the heart; derived from ectopic parathyroid; can be carcinoma

(2) Parathyroid hyperplasia

b. Occurrence—rare

c. Radiographic finding—generalized osteodystrophia fibrosa

(1) Areas of subperiosteal cortical resorption

(2) Loss of lamina dura about the teeth

(3) Soft tissue mineralization

(4) Bone cysts

(5) Generalized decrease in bone density

(6) Fractures in advanced cases

d. Laboratory findings
  (1) Serum calcium—high; most consistent finding
    (a) Results from accelerated release of calcium from bones
    (b) In the dog, calcium values consistently exceed 11.5 mg/dl of blood (normal is near 10 mg). Usually will range from 12 to 20 mg or greater.
  (2) Serum phosphorus—low or in low normal range
    (a) Due to inhibition of renal tubular reabsorption of phosphate
  (3) Alkaline phosphatase—may be elevated
    (a) Enzyme involved in both apposition and resorption of bone
    (b) Increased activity due to compensatory increase in osteoblasts along trabeculae as a response to mechanical stress in bones weakened by excessive resorption
  (4) Urine calcium and phosphorus—excretion increased
    (a) May result in nephrocalcinosis and urolithiasis
e. Differential diagnosis
  (1) Vitamin D intoxication
    (a) The hypercalcemia is usually accompanied by a hyperphosphatemia and normal alkaline phosphatase activity.
      [1] Increased concentration of calcium and phosphorus are due to augmented intestinal absorption rather than bone resorption.
  (2) Malignant neoplasms with osseous metastases
    (a) Moderate hypercalcemia—due to release of calcium and phosphorus into the blood from areas of bone destruction faster than they can be cleared by kidney and intestine
    (b) Hypercalciuria
    (c) Alkaline phosphatase—normal or slightly elevated
    (d) Serum phosphate—normal or slightly elevated

2. Secondary hyperparathyroidism
  a. Nutritional
    (1) Cause—nutritional imbalance produces increased secretion of parathyroid hormone as a compensatory mechanism directed against a disturbance in mineral homeostasis
    (2) Occurrence
      (a) Dog
      (b) Cat
      (c) Primates—cage paralysis, simian bone disease
      (d) Fox
      (e) Laboratory animals—ground squirrel, green iguana
      (f) Farm animals
      (g) Lions and tigers
      (h) Birds—domestic and wild
    (3) Pathophysiologic mechanism
      (a) Dietary mineral imbalances
        [1] Low calcium and/or excessive phosphate
          [a] Hyperphosphatemia does not stimulate the parathyroid gland directly, but does so indirectly by virtue of its ability to decrease blood calcium according to the mass-law equation when the serum becomes saturated with these two ions.
          [b] Hypocalcemia results in parathyroid stimulation.
        [2] Inadequate amounts of vitamin D_3 (even with normal vitamin D_2)
          [a] Causes diminished intestinal calcium absorption and hypocalcemia in certain New World monkeys
    (4) Compensatory actions
      (a) Since renal function is normal, the increased amount of parathyroid hormone results in compensatory activity in returning blood levels toward normal.
        [1] Diminished renal tubular reabsorption of phosphate
        [2] Increased renal tubular reabsorption of calcium
      (b) Bone resorption is accelerated.
        [1] Release of calcium elevates blood calcium to the low normal range.

[2] Resorption of bone proceeds at a faster rate than repair by fibrous connective tissue proliferation, resulting in decreased bone volume (hypostotic fibrous osteodystrophy).

(5) Clinical signs
- (a) Kittens—fed mostly beef, beef heart, or liver
  - [1] Disturbance in locomotion
  - [2] Posterior lameness
  - [3] Incoordinated gait
  - [4] Sudden onset of lameness due to fracture
  - [5] Appear well-nourished and have good hair coat due to high content of digestible protein and fat
  - [6] Vertebral fractures with compression of spinal cord
- (b) Dogs
  - [1] Bone loss sites are, in order:
    - [a] Alveolar bone
    - [b] Vertebrae
    - [c] Long bones—last
  - [2] Lameness in growing dogs—slight limp to complete immobility
  - [3] Bones painful on palpation
  - [4] Fractures of long bones and vertebrae
  - [5] Resorption of jaw bones in adult dogs
  - [6] Resorption of alveolar socket—loosening of teeth and recession of gingivae
  - [7] Diarrhea caused by the high phosphorus content in meat
  - [8] Retarded growth
- (c) Monkeys
  - [1] Inactive
  - [2] Difficulty chewing
  - [3] Maxillary hyperostosis—in advanced stage
  - [4] Joint pain
  - [5] Distortion of limbs
- (d) Young horses—fed excessive bran or large amounts of grain
  - [1] Epiphysitis
  - [2] Insidious shifting lameness

(6) Radiographic findings
- (a) General skeletal demineralization
- (b) Loss of lamina dura
- (c) Subperiosteal cortical bone resorption
- (d) Bowing deformities
- (e) Multiple fractures of long bones

(7) Laboratory findings
- (a) Renal function—normal
- (b) Compensatory mechanisms are complex so that results of a single determination are sometimes misleading
  - [1] The blood parameters can be normal in spite of progressive bone loss.
- (c) The dietary imbalance is a deficiency of calcium or vitamin D_3 with adequate phosphorus
  - [1] Mild hypocalcemia (8.0 to 9.5 mg) or isocalcemia (10 to 11 mg)
  - [2] Normal or slightly reduced serum phosphorus
- (d) Diet of excess phosphorus but normal calcium
  - [1] Serum phosphorus—either normal or increased
  - [2] Serum calcium—normal or slightly decreased
- (e) Alkaline phosphatase—increased in overt bone disease
- (f) Urine—calcium decreased, phosphate increased

b. Renal

(1) Cause
- (a) Renal disease—long-standing progressive
  - [1] Older dogs

[a] Interstitial nephritis
[b] Glomerulonephritis
[c] Nephrosclerosis
[d] Amyloidosis
[2] Young dogs—congenital anomalies
[a] Cortical hypoplasia
[b] Polycystic kidneys
[c] Bilateral hydronephrosis

(2) Pathophysiology
(a) Reduction in glomerular filtration rate
(b) Phosphorus is retained—progressive hyperphosphatemia
(c) As phosphorus concentration increases, blood calcium decreases reciprocally, according to the mass-law equation.
(d) The calcium ion controls the secretory activity of the parathyroid gland by a linear inversely proportional relationship.
(e) Impaired intestinal absorption of calcium because of an acquired defect in vitamin D—may contribute

(3) Clinical signs
(a) Signs relating to renal insufficiency and uremia
[1] Vomiting
[2] Dehydration
[3] Depression
[4] Polydipsia
(b) Skeletal lesions
[1] Range from minor change to severe fibrous osteodystrophy
[2] Volume of affected bones—normal in adult
[3] Hyperostotic bone lesions
[a] Facial swellings in younger dogs—with repair by proliferation of fibrous connective tissue; deposition of osteoid far exceeds the resorption
[4] Resorption of alveolar socket bone and loss of lamina dura occur early and result in loose teeth.
[5] Cancellous bones of maxilla and mandible
[6] Bones become softened and readily pliable due to accelerated resorption—"rubber jaw"
[7] Lameness and stiff gait
[8] Fractures

(4) Radiographic findings
(a) General skeletal demineralization
(b) Loss of lamina dura about the teeth

(5) Laboratory findings
(a) Blood urea nitrogen—increased
(b) Creatinine—increased
(c) Glomerular filtration rate (GFR)—decreased
(d) Variation in calcium and phosphorus depending on the stage of disease and compensatory mechanism
[1] Serum phosphorus—increased from retention of phosphate by damaged kidneys
[a] 6 mg or more in older dogs
[b] More in young dogs
[2] Serum calcium—usually near normal or low normal because of mobilization by skeletal reserves
(e) Alkaline phosphatase—increased in overt bone disease
(f) Urine calcium and phosphorus—decreased

DIFFERENTIAL LABORATORY FINDINGS

Condition	Serum calcium	Serum phosphorus	Alkaline phosphatase	Urine
Osteoporosis	Normal	Normal	Normal	Ca usually normal or even low normal
Rickets, low Ca	Low	Normal or low	High	. . .
Rickets, low P	Normal or low	Low	High	. . .
Osteomalacia	Normal to low	Low	High	Ca low in vitamin D deficiency Ca normal in others
Hyperparathyroidism				
Primary	High	Low	High	High Ca and P
Secondary				
Renal	Low	High	High	Low Ca and P
Nutritional	Low	High	High	Increased P and decreased Ca
Ca or vitamin D_3 deficiency with adequate P	Mild decrease or normal	Normal or slightly decreased	Increase in overt bone disease	. . .
Excess P and normal Ca	Normal or slightly decreased	Normal or increased	Increase in overt bone disease	. . .
Vitamin D intoxication	High	High	Normal	. . .
Malignant neoplasm with osseous metastasis	Moderately high	Normal or slightly increased	Normal or slightly increased	Increased Ca

25 CEREBROSPINAL FLUID EXAMINATION

I. General considerations

A. Formation

1. The process of origin is not entirely known but is probably a combination of active transport and ultrafiltration.
    a. The process is not entirely that of filtration from the blood plasma through a selective permeable membrane, for even though the cerebrospinal fluid (CSF) contains only constituents present in the blood, they are not necessarily present in the same concentration.
        (1) Lower in the CSF than in the plasma of most animals
            (a) Glucose
            (b) Calcium
            (c) Phosphorus
            (d) Bicarbonate
            (e) Potassium
            (f) Sulfate
            (g) Cholesterol—considerably lower
        (2) Higher in the CSF than in the plasma
            (a) Sodium
            (b) Chloride
2. The CSF also represents a secretion of the choroid plexus and ependymal cells, in addition to some selective reabsorption.

B. Circulation

1. Fluid formed within the lateral ventricles flows through the interventricular foramina (Monro) to the 3rd ventricle, and then through the narrow aqueduct of Sylvius to the 4th ventricle. The CSF reaches the subarachnoid space from the 4th ventricle by two lateral foramina (Luschka). The 4th ventricle also opens to the central canal of the spinal cord.
2. The CSF circulates upward over the cerebral hemispheres as well as down over the spinal cord and nerve roots in the subarachnoid space that lies between the pia and the arachnoid.
    a. The subarachnoid space enlarges at some sites such as the cisternal magna, which is used as a location for puncture to obtain CSF for examination.
3. The CSF is returned to the blood through the arachnoid villi in the dural sinuses.

C. Functions of CSF

1. Protection—cushion for the brain and spinal cord, as it acts as a fluid buffer
2. Volume regulation—space-compensating mechanism in regulating the contents of the cranium by shifting the amounts of fluid and blood
3. Metabolic
    a. The blood-CSF barrier reflects the diffusion of different solutes at different rates between the blood and the CSF.
        (1) The lining cells of the capillaries of the choroid plexus prevent certain substances from crossing into the CSF.
        (2) Normally, free bilirubin and many drugs, e.g., penicillin and streptomycin, do not cross.
            (a) Conjugated bilirubin will cross.
        (3) Pathologic conditions, especially inflammatory processes, interrupt the vital action of the lining cells, and the blood-brain barrier is destroyed.
    b. The CSF is an agent in the exchange of metabolites between blood and brain.
        (1) The fluid might assist in nourishing the brain during embryonal and early postgestational periods.

(2) It serves as a medium for transfer of metabolic waste products, such as nitrogenous excretions, from the brain to the bloodstream.

D. Indications for collection of cerebrospinal fluid
1. Diagnostic
a. When clinical signs of central nervous system disease are displayed, examination of CSF may aid in ascertaining the cause.
(1) A CSF examination should be done routinely if there have been seizures for less than 3 mo, as there is a good possibility of finding an intracranial condition such as encephalitis or neoplasia.
(2) Animals with seizures recurring for 3 to 6 mo should have a CSF examination if there is other neurologic evidence of intracranial disease.
(3) If seizures have occurred for more than 6 mo, there is little probability of finding an underlying lesion by means of a CSF examination and the risk of a tap is usually not warranted.
b. The routine examination of CSF should include:
(1) Color
(2) Turbidity
(3) Coagulation
(4) Total protein and Pandy or Nonne-Apelt tests for globulin
(5) Total cell count
(6) Differential cell count—when total count is elevated
c. Estimation of intracranial pressure using a manometer
d. Introduction of material for radiographic examination
2. Relief of abnormally high pressure and drainage of blood or exudate

II. Collection of cerebrospinal fluid

A. Amount—collect a minimum of 1 ml in a sterile syringe
B. Have at least 3 test tubes ready to receive the CSF.
1. If the first few drops contain blood from the puncture, it can be used for microbiological culture only, for even the slightest amount of blood invalidates cell counts and chemical tests.
2. Attach a second sterile syringe to the needle and withdraw additional fluid, for it is often clear after the initial sample is removed.
a. If it is a traumatic tap, less blood should appear in the second or third tube, as the bleeding decreases.
b. With previous CSF bleeding, the erythrocytes should be distributed equally throughout the CSF and show equal numbers of erythrocytes in each tube.

C. The cell count (total and differential) and examinations for glucose and bacteria should be performed at once, while other tests may be delayed if the specimen is refrigerated.

III. Macroscopic examination

A. Color
1. Clear and colorless as distilled water
a. Normal
b. In encephalitis and meningitis associated with viral infections, the fluid may remain clear and colorless, for there may be a moderate increase in the number of cells before the gross appearance of the fluid is altered.
2. Bright red
a. Fresh blood from a blood vessel puncture while inserting the needle
(1) After centrifugation, the supernatant will be clear, in contrast to the yellow supernatant of an old hemorrhage.
3. Dull red or brown—depending upon the age of the lesion
a. Hemorrhage
(1) Intracranial hemorrhages

(2) Fracture of the cranium
(3) Chronic hemorrhagic pachymeningitis
(4) Generalized hemorrhages from coagulation problems

4. Yellow (xanthochromic)—due to free bilirubin resulting from disintegration of erythrocytes within the subarachnoid space from an old hemorrhage, or may be due to altered permeability of the lining membranes to free bilirubin in the plasma; conjugated bilirubin can pass through the normal membrane if present in increased amounts in the plasma
   a. Hemorrhage—after 2 days; may persist up to 40 days
      (1) Subarachnoid hemorrhage
      (2) Extradural and subpial hematoma
   b. Spinal block
   c. Neoplasms
   d. Abscesses
   e. Acute inflammation
   f. Toxoplasmosis
   g. Severe jaundice
5. Gray to green
   a. Suppurative conditions

B. Turbidity
1. Turbidity is due to the presence of cells but becomes evident only if there are 500 or more/microliter.
   a. Acute bacterial meningitis—slight turbidity to opacity of almost straight pus
   b. Hemorrhage

C. Coagulation
1. Normal CSF does not clot.
2. Abnormal
   a. An increase in proteins, including fibrinogen, causes clotting.
   b. Acute suppurative meningitis produces a heavy coagulum and sediment.

D. Specific gravity—1.003 to 1.008
E. Reaction—alkaline, similar to blood

IV. Chemical examination

A. Protein
1. General considerations
   a. The amount of normal protein is very small and consists almost entirely of albumin.
      (1) Only the smaller albumin molecules pass into the CSF, while the larger globulin molecules are excluded.
   b. Globulin is the protein of chief interest since it is increased in pathological conditions.
      (1) Tests for globulin cannot be applied to fluid containing blood, due to the presence of serum globulin.
2. Total protein
   a. Foam test
      (1) Shake the tube of CSF.
      (2) Normally the foam is slight and disappears after a few minutes.
      (3) When protein is increased, there is more foam and it will remain for 5 min or more.
   b. Sulfosalicylic acid
      (1) Add 3 ml of 3% sulfosalicylic acid to 1 ml of cerebrospinal fluid.
      (2) Mix and allow to stand for 5 min.
      (3) The turbidity is noted visually or can be compared in a colorimeter to a standard.
   c. Biuret modifications
3. Globulin
   a. Nonne-Apelt (same as Ross-Jones) test
      (1) Place 1 ml of ammonium sulfate solution in a small test tube and overlay carefully with 1 ml of CSF.

(a) Reagent—dissolve 85 g of ammonium sulfate in 100 ml of hot distilled water; after several hours at room temperature, filter

(2) Allow to stand for 3 min.

(3) No ring forms in normal CSF, while a white to gray ring at the zone of contact indicates the presence of globulin in increased amounts.

(a) Report positive tests as + to ++++.

b. Pandy's test

(1) To 1 ml of a saturated solution of phenol in a test tube, add one or more drops of CSF.

(a) Pandy's reagent—dissolve 10 g of pure phenol in 150 ml of distilled water; when solution is discolored, discard

(2) Abnormal CSF produces a definite white cloud or a turbidity after shaking.

(3) Pandy's test is slightly more sensitive than the Nonne-Apelt test for globulin, but has the disadvantage of turbidity forming in the reagent.

c. Electrophoresis

4. Interpretation of protein or globulin in CSF

a. Normal—10 to 40 mg, which is mainly albumin

b. Increased

(1) Inflammation—increased permeability of capillaries allows direct passage of blood proteins into the CSF, or there is production of antibodies in the subarachnoid space

(a) Encephalitis

[1] Viral—in canine distemper, the protein may vary from 40 mg to as high as 500 mg, with the globulin fraction almost always elevated

[2] Bacterial—over 100 mg

(b) Meningitis

[1] Viral—50 to 100 mg

[2] Bacterial—over 100 mg

(2) Neoplasia—mild increase

(3) Hemorrhage—approximately 1 mg/dl of protein for every 1000 erythrocytes

(4) Blockage—increase in protein within a confined area probably due to transudation from local vessels

(a) Hydrocephalus

[1] Clear specimens—normal total protein

[2] Xanthochromic specimens—50 to 100 mg

(5) Tissue destruction—the result of edema, congestion, or hemorrhage caused by the lesion, rather than disintegration of tissue protein

(6) Uremic or convulsive states—small amounts

B. Glucose

1. Method—similar to method for blood glucose

2. Interpretation

a. The level is dependent upon three factors

(1) Blood glucose level

(a) In many animals the normal values are about half that of the blood; the dog is the exception.

(2) Selective permeability of the blood-CSF barrier

(3) Presence of pyogenic organisms that utilize glucose in their metabolism

b. Decreased glucose level

(1) Acute pyogenic meningitis—chief indication for test

(2) Hypoglycemia

(3) Metastatic carcinoma to the meninges

(4) Subarachnoid hemorrhage—probably due to glycolytic enzymes in erythrocytes

c. Increased glucose level

(1) Hyperglycemia

d. Normal or slightly increased

(1) Viral encephalitis or meningitis

(2) Brain tumor

(3) Brain abscess

NORMAL CEREBROSPINAL FLUID

Substance	Dog	Cat	Horse	Cattle	Sheep	Goat	Pig	Ref.
Cells per microliter	0–8(2)	0–1	1–7(4)	0–3	0–5	1	0–7	(4)
	5–8	1–5	1–5	2–10	2–9	2–9		(5)
Protein, total, mg/dl	11–55(27.5)	0–20	28.75–71.75(47.58)	23.3–30	8–70	12	24–29	(4)
	15–20	8–16	29.7–40	11.5–33	20–25	20–25		(5)
Albumin, mg/dl	16.5–37.5(27)		22.62–67.94(38.64)	10–22			17–24	(4)
Globulin, mg/dl	5.5–16.5(9.0)		3.37–18.37(9.34)	2–8			5–10	(4)
Nonne-Apelt	− to ±	−	± to +	−	−	−	−	(4)
Pandy	− to +	−	+ to +++(++)	−	−	−	−	(4)
Pressure, mm H_2O	24–172(86.5)	100	272–490(379)	Below 200	60–270		80–145	(4)
Specific gravity	1.0033–1.0125 (1.0056)		1.004–1.008 (1.006)	1.005–1.008	1.004–1.008 (1.007)			(4)
	1.006–1.0069	1.005–1.007	1.000–1.007	1.006–1.008	1.004–1.008	1.004–1.008		(5)
Glucose, mg/dl	61–116(74)	85	40–78(57.2)	35–70	48–109	70	45–87	(4)
pH		Slightly alkaline	7.13–7.36(7.25)		7.3–7.4			(4)
	7.4–7.6	74–7.6	7.4–7.6	7.4–7.6	7.3–7.4	7.3–7.4		(5)
Cholesterol, mg/dl			0.25–0.65 (0.36–0.55)			0.51		
Transaminase (GOT)								
Units	9–46(20.1)							(6)
Units/ml/min	2.04 ± 0.23							(7)
Sigma-Frankel units	32							(3)
Transaminase (GPT)								
Units	2–32(13.7)							(6)
Lactic dehydrogenase								
Units/ml/min	4.46 ± 1.77							(7)

NORMAL CEREBROSPINAL FLUID

Substance	Dog	Cat	Horse	Cattle	Sheep	Goat	Pig	Ref.
Alkali reserve, vol %	48.5-68.6		41-67					(4)
	(55.25)		(55.6)					
	42-50		50-57	9.6-53	49-52.6			(5)
Bicarbonate, mEq/L	23.5 ± 0.19							(1)
Calcium, mg/dl	5.13-7.40	5.2	5.55-6.98	5.1-6.3	5.77			(4)
	(6.56)		(6.26)					
	6.2 ± 1.22							
Chloride, mg/dl	761-883	670-723	690-792	650-725	750-868			(4)
	(808)		(737)					
mEq/L	125.5 ± 6.24							(9)
Magnesium, mg/dl	2.58-3.81		1.06-2.95	2.17	2.86			(4)
	(3.09)		(1.98)					
Phosphorus, mg/dl	2.82-3.47		0.87-2.20	2.15-4.06				(4)
	(3.09)		(1.44)	(3.2)				
	1.1 ± 0.25							(9)
Potassium, mg/dl	10.5-11.8		10.65-14.20	11.2-13.8				(4)
			(12.66)					
mEq/L	3.1 ± 0.17							(9)
Sodium								
mg/dl			620-760					(2)
mEq/L	156.3 ± 7.17	162						(9)
Urea, mg/dl	6-10		2.3-3.1	4.6-6.5	5-6.2	5-6.2		(5)

C. Sodium
  1. Normal—slightly higher in CSF than in blood
  2. Increased
    a. Salt poisoning in swine

D. Chlorides
  1. Methods—similar to methods for blood chloride
    a. Cotlove chloridometer
    b. Schales and Schales mercuric nitrate method
  2. Interpretation
    a. Normally higher in CSF than in serum
    b. Reduced
      (1) Pyogenic meningitis—seldom has important differential value because its chief use is in the differential diagnosis of meningitis, which can be accomplished with simpler procedures
      (2) Hypochloremia

E. Calcium
  1. Normally the calcium is lower in CSF than in serum.
  2. Increased level of protein-bound calcium in CSF indicates a disturbance in the blood-brain barrier.

F. Cholesterol
  1. Normal levels of cholesterol in CSF are very low and difficult to assay on the standard curves used for blood cholesterol.
    a. Horse—0.36 to 0.55 mg/dl
    b. Goat—0.51 mg/dl
  2. Increased
    a. Hemorrhage involving the central nervous system
    b. Tumor
    c. Meningitis
    d. Brain abscess

G. Enzymes
  1. Lactic dehydrogenase (LDH)
    a. Increased
      (1) Bacterial meningitis
      (2) Metastatic carcinoma
      (3) Lymphoid tumor
      (4) Subarachnoid hemorrhage
      (5) Cerebral infarction
  2. Transaminase
    a. Normal levels in CSF of dogs
      (1) GOT—20.1 (9 to 46) units
      (2) GPT—13.7 (2 to 32) units
    b. Elevated
      (1) Canine distemper—20 to 260 units (GOT); 14 to 44 units (GPT)
      (2) Purulent meningitis—result of brain injury
      (3) Cerebral infarction—marked increase
  3. Creatine phosphokinase (CPK)
    a. Normal levels—high levels in human brain extracts suggest it may be useful in the diagnosis of neurological conditions
      (1) Compared to levels in skeletal and cardiac muscle, brain levels of CPK are about half.
    b. Elevated
      (1) Marked elevations in CSF due entirely to brain isoenzyme have been reported in neurological conditions.

(a) The elevation will be short lived, as the half-life of canine brain CPK is approximately 1.5 hr.

(2) Elevation of serum CPK may be from skeletal muscle in diseases of the central nervous system that involve motor function.

(a) It is possible that agents, such as the virus of canine distemper, may alter membrane permeability in the brain to allow the leakage of brain CPK into the blood, for brain CPK cannot usually pass the blood-brain barrier.

(3) Quantitative and isoenzyme analysis of CPK in CSF should result in a more definite indicator of central nervous system lesions than the analysis of serum CPK levels.

V. Cytology

A. Cell count—must be performed within 20 min after collection of CSF, as the cells disintegrate upon standing

1. Methods

a. Undiluted—for total cell count, including both erythrocytes and leukocytes

(1) Place CSF on one chamber of the hemocytometer and count the cells in all 9 squares.

(2) The number of cells is multiplied by 1.1 to determine the total cell count per microliter.

b. Diluted for leukocyte count

(1) Draw the diluting fluid in a leukocyte diluting pipette up to the 1 mark and fill to the 11 mark with CSF.

(a) Diluting fluid—aids in the differentiation of cells

Glacial acetic acid	10 ml
Distilled water	90 ml
Crystal violet	0.1 g

2 or 3 drops of 5% phenol as preservative

(2) Mix thoroughly, and discard 2 or 3 drops.

(3) Fill each side of a standard hemocytometer in the same manner as for blood counts, and wait 2 min for the cells to settle.

(4) Count all the cells within the entire ruled areas on both sides of the counting chamber (18 one-mm squares) and multiply by 0.6 to obtain the number of cells per microliter.

2. Interpretation

a. The normal cell count is under 20/microliter in all species.

b. Increased (pleocytosis)

(1) Inflammatory lesion or irritation of the brain, spinal cord, or meninges

(a) Marked increase

[1] Acute pyogenic meningitis—100 to 500 or more per microliter

[2] Brain or spinal cord abscess—normal to increased, depending upon location

(b) Moderate increase

[1] Encephalitis

(c) Mild increase

[1] Neoplasia—under 50/microliter

[2] Viral infections—10 to 100/microliter; except for rabies, where it may be up to 500/microliter

[3] Degenerative disease

(2) Subarachnoid hemorrhage or traumatic tap

(a) Approximately one leukocyte is added for every 1000 erythrocytes

(3) Hydrocephalus—normal to elevated

B. Differential count—indicated when the total count is elevated

1. Centrifugation—if total cell count is under 500/microliter

a. After centrifugation, pour off supernatant, add a drop or two of serum, and make a smear of the sediment.

CEREBROSPINAL FLUID FINDINGS IN DISEASE

Disease	Appearance	Cell count	Cell type	Protein
Encephalitis				
Pyogenic	Turbid; gray or green	Increased, > 100	Neutrophils	Increased, > 100 mg
Virus	Clear to slightly turbid	Increased, 10-100	Lymphocytes Mononuclears	Increased, 30-500 mg
Meningitis				
Pyogenic	Slight to marked turbidity	Increased, 1000's	Neutrophils	Marked increase 100-50
Virus	Milky to yellow color	Increased, 50-500	Lymphocytes	Increased, 50-100 mg
Brain abscess	Clear to slightly turbid; xanthochromic	Normal to increased	Neutrophils or monocytes (usually)	Increased to normal
Toxoplasmosis	Xanthochromic	Increased	Lymphocytes	Increased
Brain tumor	Clear to slightly turbid; xanthochromic	Usually normal or mild increase, < 50	Lymphocytes (mainly)	Normal or mild increase, 50-100 mg
Subarachnoid hemorrhage	Turbid; dull red, brown, or xanthochromic	Increased	RBC Neutrophils	Increased
Cerebral thrombosis	Clear	Normal		
Degeneration encephalomalacia	Clear	Normal to slightly increased	Lymphocytes Mononuclears	Increased
Spinal cord compression	Clear or xanthochromic	Normal to slightly increased	Lymphocytes	Increased, 50-2000 mg

b. Dry in air without heat and stain with new methylene blue, Wright's, or Giemsa stain as for a blood smear.

c. Count and tabulate 100 cells, if present.

2. Membrane filtration technique for cytologic evaluation—even small numbers of cells can be examined and identified with this method
   a. CSF samples are collected into premeasured fixative to allow a semiquantitative evaluation of the cell population.
   b. Cell morphology was clear even after specimens had remained in 40% ethanol for up to 120 hr prior to membrane filtration and staining.
3. Interpretation
   a. Normally only small lymphocytes and an occasional large mononuclear cell, polygonal ependymal cell, or histiocyte will be found.
   b. Neutrophils
      (1) Not normally found in CSF, unless the tap has been traumatic.
      (2) Usually indicates a pyogenic or bacterial infection
         (a) Bacterial encephalitis
         (b) Bacterial meningitis
         (c) Abscess—some nearly always present
      (3) Hemorrhage—blood may cause moderate meningeal irritation with an increase in neutrophils
   c. Lymphocytes increased
      (1) Viral infection
         (a) Also accompanied by degenerate, small, mononuclear cells, probably of mesothelial origin
      (2) Abscess—mononuclear types generally predominate
      (3) Fungal infections
         (a) *Cryptococcus neoformans* produces pleocytosis that is predominantly mononuclear.

(4) Postvaccinal inflammation
(5) Chronic infections
(6) Toxic conditions

d. Neoplastic cells—quite large and arranged in clusters when there is meningeal involvement

VI. Examination for microorganisms—especially when total cell count is high and protein is present

A. Direct smear of sediment

1. When *Cryptococcus neoformans* is suspected, a new methylene blue or india ink preparation should be made to demonstrate the capsule of the organism.
2. *Toxoplasma* organisms—sometimes detected in stained smears
3. Trypanosomes
4. Bacteria

B. Culture—depends upon direct smear results and suspected cause

1. Aerobic and anaerobic cultures indicated
2. Virus isolation

26 SERUM BIOCHEMISTRY ABNORMALITIES

I. Blood urea nitrogen

A. Increased
1. Prerenal disease
a. Reduced renal blood flow
(1) Heart failure
(2) Shock
b. Decreased glomerular filtration pressure
(1) Hypotension
(a) Heart failure—some
(b) Adrenocortical insufficiency
(c) Shock
(2) Increased protein osmotic pressure
(a) Severe dehydration
2. Renal disease
3. Postrenal disease
a. Urinary tract obstruction
b. Urinary tract perforation
4. Secondary renal hyperparathyroidism
5. Pseudohyperparathyroidism (neoplasia)
6. High protein ration—nonfasting sample

B. Decreased
1. Hepatic insufficiency
2. Low protein ration
3. Malabsorption
4. Overhydration with fluids

II. Creatinine

A. Increased
1. In the same conditions as in BUN, except is not affected by:
a. Protein diet or catabolism
b. Exercise

B. Decreased
1. No significance

III. Blood glucose

A. Increased
1. Diabetes mellitus
2. Pancreatitis, acute and chronic
3. Excitement, convulsions, exercise—transitory
4. Hyperadrenocorticism—mild increase
5. Corticosteroid or ACTH administration

6. Glucose infusions
7. Chronic hepatic disease
8. Hyperthyroidism
9. Hyperpituitarism
10. Recent high-carbohydrate meal

B. Decreased
1. Hyperinsulinism
a. Pancreatic tumor—insuloma
b. Insulin injection
2. Functional hypoglycemia
3. Glycogen storage disease
a. Von Gierke-like syndrome
b. Cori's disease
4. Hypoadrenocorticism
5. Hypothyroidism
6. Hypopituitarism
7. Hepatic insufficiency—marked
8. Serum not removed from clot rapidly
9. Pregnancy toxemia
10. Malnutrition

IV. Serum amylase

A. Increased
1. Acute pancreatitis
2. Renal insufficiency
3. ACTH or corticosteroids
4. Hyperadrenocorticism
5. Salivary duct occlusion or suppuration
6. Opiate administration

V. Serum lipase

A. Increased
1. Acute pancreatitis
2. Chronic pancreatitis
3. Renal shutdown
4. Intestinal obstruction
5. Opiate administration

VI. Serum bilirubin

A. Increased
1. Hemolysis
2. Liver disease
a. Hepatocellular disease
(1) Infection
(2) Neoplasia
b. Biliary obstruction

B. Decreased
1. Bone marrow depression anemia

VII. Total serum cholesterol

A. Increased
1. Hypothyroidism
2. Diabetes mellitus
3. Pancreatitis
4. Liver disease
a. Hepatocellular disease
b. Biliary obstruction
5. Renal disease
a. Nephrosis
b. Nephritis—occasionally
6. Hyperadrenocorticism
a. Corticosteroid or ACTH administration
7. Pregnancy

B. Decreased
1. Hyperthyroidism—sometimes
2. Low saturated-fat diet

VIII. Total protein (TP)

A. Increased
1. Polycythemia
a. Relative—in proportion to water lost
b. Transient—only slight increase
2. Increased gamma globulin production
a. Response to antigens
(1) Infections
(2) Aging
b. Gammopathies
(1) Lymphosarcoma
(2) Multiple myeloma
(3) Liver disease
(4) Infection—feline infectious peritonitis

B. Decreased
1. Inadequate production
a. Age—in young animals
b. Malnutrition
c. Hepatopathy
d. Neoplasia
e. Pregnancy and lactation
2. Loss of body protein
a. Acute blood loss
b. Chronic blood or protein loss
3. Loss of blood or protein into body cavities

IX. Serum glutamic oxaloacetic transaminase

A. Increased
1. Hepatocellular disease
2. Skeletal muscle necrosis or degeneration
3. Cardiac muscle necrosis or degeneration

X. Serum glutamic pyruvic transaminase

A. Increased
1. Hepatocellular disease

XI. Alkaline phosphatase

A. Increased
1. Increased osteoblastic activity—mild increase
a. Young animals
b. Rickets
c. Osteomalacia
d. Hyperparathyroidism—primary and secondary
e. Bone tumors—mild increase
2. Liver disease
a. Extrahepatic obstruction
b. Intrahepatic obstruction
(1) Neoplasia
(2) Hepatitis
(3) Cirrhosis
(4) Amyloidosis
3. Intestinal mucosal disorders
4. Renal disease
5. Pregnancy
6. Hyperadrenocorticism
7. At room temperature serum may increase 5 to 30% in 12 hr

XII. Lactic dehydrogenase

A. Increased
1. Necrosis of any cell—need isoenzymes to establish source
2. Hemolysis of blood serum

XIII. Creatine phosphokinase

A. Increased
1. Skeletal or cardiac muscle necrosis or degeneration
2. Encephalopathy—occasionally

XIV. Calcium

A. Increased
1. Primary hyperparathyroidism—rare
2. Pseudohyperparathyroidism
a. Usually lymphosarcoma
3. Vitamin D intoxication
4. Malignant neoplasm with osseous metastasis—moderately high
5. Neoplasms of bone—lytic
a. Multiple myeloma

B. Decreased
1. Blood collected in anticoagulant
2. Secondary renal hyperparathyroidism
3. Secondary nutritional hyperparathyroidism

4. Hypoparathyroidism
5. Osteomalacia—low to normal
6. Low-calcium rickets
7. Low-phosphorus rickets—low to normal
8. Acute pancreatitis—with fat necrosis
9. Renal insufficiency
10. Tetany
11. Hypoproteinemia
12. Pregnancy and lactation
13. Malabsorption syndrome
14. Eclampsia or parturient paresis
15. Oxalate poisoning

XV. Inorganic phosphorus

A. Increased
1. Renal insufficiency
2. Vitamin D intoxication
3. Hemolysis of blood sample
4. Hypoparathyroidism
5. Normal in young animals
6. High-phosphorus and low-calcium ration
7. Secondary hyperparathyroidism

B. Decreased
1. Low-phosphorus rickets
2. Osteomalacia
3. Primary hyperparathyroidism
4. Low-phosphorus ration with high calcium:phosphorus ratio
5. Hyperinsulinism

XVI. Sodium

A. Increased
1. Excessive salt intake with water restricted
2. Dehydration
3. Hyperadrenocorticism—rarely

B. Decreased
1. Hypoadrenocorticism
2. Renal disease
3. Diuretics (osmotic)
4. Prolonged treatment with sodium-deficient fluids
5. Water intoxication
6. Prolonged diarrhea

XVII. Potassium

A. Increased
1. Renal disease
2. Hypoadrenocorticism
3. Acidosis
4. Shock
5. Circulatory failure

B. Decreased
  1. Diuretics
  2. Administration of potassium-deficient solutions over a long period
  3. Metabolic alkalosis
  4. Prolonged vomiting and/or diarrhea
  5. Insulin injections
  6. Hyperadrenocorticism
  7. Corticosteroid or ACTH injections

XVIII. Chlorides

A. Increased
  1. Metabolic acidosis
  2. Respiratory alkalosis
     a. Hyperventilation
  3. Decreased excretion
     a. Urinary tract obstruction
     b. Nephrosis
  4. Excessive intake of salt
  5. Water intake limited
  6. Hyperadrenocorticism

B. Decreased
  1. Metabolic alkalosis
  2. Respiratory acidosis
     a. Hypoventilation
  3. Persistent vomiting
  4. Intestinal obstruction (high)
  5. Renal disease, chronic
  6. Hypoadrenocorticism

27 THYROID FUNCTION

I. Anatomy

A. Size—0.1 g/kg body weight in mature domestic animals
B. Locations
1. Dog
a. Two elongated symmetrical lobes lateral to the first 5 to 8 tracheal rings
b. Isthmus in brachycephalic breeds
c. Accessory thyroid tissue in association with periaortic or abdominal fat bodies
2. Cat
a. Two flattened elongated lateral lobes
b. May have an isthmus
3. Cattle
a. Pale, flattened, irregularly triangular lateral lobes
b. Isthmus broad and glandular
4. Horse
a. Firm, rounded, dark red lobes
b. Narrow isthmus

II. Physiology

A. Iodide absorption
1. Absorbed by gastrointestinal tract
a. In ruminants 70% to 80% is absorbed by the rumen and 10% by the omasum.
b. In other species it is primarily absorbed by the small intestine; small amounts are absorbed by the stomach.

B. Iodide utilization
1. About ⅔ of the absorbed iodide is excreted in the urine; the remainder is concentrated by thyroid gland cells.
2. In ruminants a significant amount is excreted in the feces.
3. Iodide enters thyroid follicular cells by diffusion and active transport and also becomes available for hormone synthesis by deiodination of organic iodide-containing compounds in the thyroid gland.
a. Active transport is the most important mechanism for concentration.
4. Iodide is trapped by the thyroid gland under the influence of the thyroid-stimulating hormone (TSH) and oxidized to free iodine (I_2).

C. Thyroid hormone synthesis
1. Active iodine is bound to the 3 position of tyrosine molecules attached to thyroglobulin.
2. Monoiodotyrosine (MIT) is iodinated in the 5 position to form diiodotyrosine (DIT).
3. Two DIT molecules condense, liberating alanine and forming thyroxine (T_4), which is the principal circulating hormone of most domestic animals.
4. Triiodothyronine (T_3) is formed by condensation of MIT and DIT.

D. Secretion
1. The hormone is secreted into circulation or stored in follicles bound to thyroglobulin.
2. Peptide bonds between T_3 and T_4 and thyroglobulin are broken by proteases in lysozymes.
3. T_3 and T_4 are secreted into capillaries by thyroid cells.

This chapter was written by Dr. Joseph S. Spano, Associate Professor, Pathology and Parasitology, Auburn University, Auburn, Ala.

E. Effects of TSH on the thyroid
1. Stimulates iodide uptake
2. MIT, DIT, and T_4 synthesis is increased.
3. More T_3 and T_4 is secreted.
4. Continued stimulation leads to hypertrophy of cells.
5. Thyroglobulin synthesis is increased.

F. Nature and affinity of T_3 and T_4 for plasma proteins
1. T_3 and T_4 are carried in plasma bound to protein in a reversible equilibrium. Little is known about these proteins in domestic animals.
   a. In cattle, swine, and horses T_4 is bound to an alpha globulin.
   b. In the dog albumin and three globulin fractions are important carriers for T_3 and T_4.
2. There is variation in activity of T_3 and T_4, some of which depends on the strength with which the respective hormone is bound.
   a. Only free hormone is a physiologically active form, and it is found in very low levels.
   b. T_3 is biologically more potent than T_4.
   c. Evidence exists that there is conversion of T_4 to T_3 in peripheral tissues by monodeiodination.
   d. T_4 is the major circulating hormone, and only the free form is able to diffuse into the cell to exert its effect.

G. Effects of thyroid hormones
1. Calorigenic action
   a. Increases oxygen consumption of almost all metabolically active tissues
   b. Depresses oxygen consumption of anterior pituitary, possibly because it inhibits TSH secretion
   c. Effects secondary to calorigenesis
      (1) Nitrogen excretion is increased.
         (a) If food intake is not increased, fat and protein stores are catabolized.
         (b) The skin contains a variety of proteins combined with hyaluronic acid, polysaccharides, and chondroitin sulfuric acid; in hypothyroidism these accumulate, causing puffiness of skin in man.
         (c) Moderate anemia exists in hypothyroidism due to decreased bone marrow metabolism and poor absorption of B_{12} from the gut.
   d. Effects on the nervous system
      (1) In hypothyroidism lethargy and dull mental attitude is seen.
      (2) In hyperthyroidism irritability and restlessness is seen.
   e. Effects on carbohydrate metabolism
      (1) Thyroxine increases the rate of absorption of carbohydrate from the gastrointestinal tract.
      (2) However, increased catabolism prevents storage in the liver.
   f. Effects on cholesterol metabolism
      (1) Thyroxine stimulates cholesterol synthesis.
      (2) T_4 stimulates cholesterol removal from the circulation by the liver.
   g. Effects on the reproductive system
      (1) Lack of the thyroid hormone results in decreased libido in males and irregular estrous cycles and poor conception in females.

H. Regulation of thyroid secretion
1. Stimuli that alter thyroid secretion
   a. Circulating level of pituitary TSH
      (1) TSH secretion is inhibited by a rise in circulating free thyroxine and is stimulated when the free T_4 level drops.
      (2) TSH secretion is increased by exposure to cold and is depressed by heat and trauma.
2. Control mechanisms
   a. Thyrotropin-releasing factor (TRF), which stimulates TSH, has been extracted from the hypothalamus.
   b. Day-to-day maintenance of thyroid secretion depends on feedback interplay between TSH and thyroxine.

c. Feedback is exerted at the pituitary and hypothalamic level.
d. The hypothalamus adjusts TSH secretion, especially in heat and cold situations.

3. Effect of stress
   a. Stress inhibits thyroid secretion.
      (1) Stress-induced vasoconstriction of thyroid blood vessels probably decreases thyroid hormone release.
      (2) Iodide uptake is decreased because glucocorticoids increase urinary iodide excretion.

I. Mechanism of action of thyroid hormones
1. Uncouples phosphorylation from oxidation in the mitochondria
2. Thyroxine stimulates mitochondrial respiration and phosphorylation and activity of respiratory and other enzymes.

J. Antithyroid compounds
1. Thiocarbamides—thiouracil, propylthiouracil
   a. Act by blocking oxidation of iodide to iodine
   b. Used in treatment of certain thyroid diseases
2. Aminobenzene derivatives—*p*-aminobenzoic acid, sulfanilamide
   a. Act by inhibiting conversion of iodide to iodine
   b. Doses used in treatment of infections have little effect.
3. Iodine
   a. In the hyperthyroid state, large doses of iodide inhibit hormone secretion.
   b. No effect on euthyroid state
4. Naturally occurring goitrogens
   a. Vegetables of Brassicacae family—rutabagas, cabbage, turnips
   b. In normal or mixed diets these are usually not harmful.
5. Mode of action of antithyroid compounds
   a. Interference with thyroid hormone production by these compounds causes increased secretion of TSH.
   b. Increased TSH secretion causes enlargement of the thyroid gland without increased production of thyroid hormones.

III. Disease of the thyroid

A. Simple goiter—nonneoplastic enlargement of the thyroid gland, either diffuse or nodular
1. Etiology
   a. Initially, a decreased hormone production stimulates TSH secretion, which causes thyroid hyperplasia and hypertrophy in an attempt to maintain normal hormone levels.
      (1) Iodide deficiency
      (2) Action of goitrogenic compounds
      (3) Dyshormonogenesis—defective synthesis of thyroid hormone
   b. If adequate compensation is not achieved, some degree of hypothyroidism may occur.
2. Clinical signs
   a. Enlargement of the thyroid gland
      (1) Lobes may not be equally affected.
      (2) Gland feels firm to spongy.
      (3) In long-standing cases, nodules may be felt.
3. Occurrence
   a. In the dog goiter occurs in iodine-deficient areas due to low intake of iodide. This is rare, since dog food is now supplemented.
   b. In the lamb goiter may be congenital due to goitrogens in feed.
   c. In adult sheep goiter may be due to several factors.
      (1) Goitrogens in feed
      (2) Substances such as cottonseed meal and walnuts, which prevent reabsorption of T_4 excreted in bile
      (3) In Merinos may be due to an inborn defect in hormone synthesis
   d. In cattle goiter may be due to goitrogens in feed or an inborn defect in hormone synthesis, as described in African cattle.

e. The goat, horse, and pig are susceptible to congenital goiter because of iodine-deficient areas or goitrogens.
   (1) Enlarged thyroid may or may not be seen in these animals.
   (2) Hairlessness or extreme weakness at birth may be seen.

B. Hypothyroidism in adult animals

1. Definition—develops when there is a deficiency in the supply of thyroid hormone to tissue
2. Occurrence—rarely reported in adult animals other than the dog
3. Classified according to causes—iodine deficiency, goitrogens, defect in hormone synthesis, thyroiditis, lack of function of thyroid tissue, pituitary insufficiency
   a. Dietary iodine deficiency is probably the most common cause in domestic animals; it is rare, however, in the dog.
   b. Goitrogens—development of hypothyroidism depends on completeness and duration of antithyroid activity
   c. Dyshormonogenesis
      (1) Five biochemically distinct conditions causing hypothyroidism in man as a result of inborn errors of metabolism have been described.
      (2) There are reports of congenital and genetically determined hypothyroidism in cattle and sheep.
   d. Thyroiditis and thyroid atrophy
      (1) 16% incidence of thyroiditis has been reported in one group of 167 dogs of a certain family line.
      (2) Circulating antithyroglobulin antibodies have been described in Beagle dogs with thyroiditis.
      (3) 90% of the cases of hypothyroidism in the dog are due to thyroid atrophy where cell death and disappearance occurs.
      (4) The relationship between these two types of thyroid degeneration in the dog is unclear.
   e. Pituitary hypothyroidism
      (1) Failure of the pituitary to secrete TSH
      (2) Most commonly described in the dog due to compression of functional tissue by neoplastic growths
      (3) May be associated with adrenocortical and gonadal deficiencies in these cases
4. Clinical features—none pathognomonic, but finding of several positive signs is highly suggestive
   a. Lethargy and easy fatigability are the most prominent signs.
   b. Some intolerance to cold
   c. Bilaterally symmetrical alopecia and follicular and epidermal hyperkeratosis
   d. Disturbances of the reproductive cycle in intact females
   e. Reduction of libido and fertility in males
   f. Occasionally intermittent constipation and diarrhea
   g. Borderline normochromic normocytic anemia, slight to moderate leptocytosis
   h. Hypercholesterolemia in ½ to ⅔ of the cases
5. Diagnostic procedures
   a. Radioiodine uptake studies
      (1) Principle
         (a) Ability of thyroid gland to concentrate ^{131}I is the basis for these studies.
         (b) A scintillation detector is used to monitor the amount of an injected dose of ^{131}I taken up by the thyroid.
      (2) Interpretation
         (a) Decreased uptake is seen with high dietary intake of iodine, after antithyroid medication, with TSH deficiency, or with primary atrophy of the thyroid gland.
         (b) Increased uptake is seen with iodine deficiency and certain functional thyroid tumors (hyperthyroidism).
         (c) The normals below are expressed as a percentage of administered dose taken up by the thyroid.(7, 19, 20, 24, 30)
            [1] Dog: 10 to 30 microcurie dose i.v.—10 to 40% at 72 hr
            [2] Dog: 50 microcurie dose—14.2 ± 4% at 24 hr, 17.0 ± 4% at 48 hr, 17.4 ± 4.2% at 72 hr, 16.4-4.2% at 96 hr

[3] Dog: 10 to 100 microcurie dose i.v.—14.4% at 24 hr, 17.3% at 48 hr, 16.7% at 72 hr, 16.2% at 96 hr

[4] Dog: 7 to 37% at 72 hr

(3) Problems

(a) Because of the injection of radioactive materials into the animal's body and laws governing the use of these materials, this test is limited to research situations.

(b) The test is highly dependent on dietary intake of iodide.

(c) Any iodine-containing compound can interfere.

b. Serum protein-bound iodine (PBI) or PBI^{131}

(1) Principle

(a) A measure of the amount of iodide bound to serum proteins is a reflection of the amount of circulating hormone.

(b) A radioactive PBI^{131} estimates the amount of organically bound iodine concentrated and released by the thyroid gland after administration of ^{131}I.

(2) Interpretation

(a) An elevated PBI indicates increased levels of circulating hormone and will be seen in hyperthyroid conditions.

(b) A decreased PBI will be seen in hypothyroid states.

(c) Normals: (12, 16, 26)

[1] Horse—1.64 to 2.36 micrograms/dl

[2] Horse—mean of 1.86 micrograms/dl for 48 horses

[3] Dog—2.42 to 4.38 micrograms/dl

(3) Problems

(a) The test does not distinguish between dietary PBI and hormonal iodide and is unreliable in the dog.

(b) Any medications containing iodide affect PBI, causing a falsely elevated value. Sodium disophenol (DNP) and radiographic contrast media are examples.

c. T_4 by column chromatography

(1) Principle

(a) T_4 and T_3 can be separated from nonhormonal iodide by column chromatography.

(b) The resulting iodide thus separated then represents hormonal iodide.

(c) Since the majority of circulating hormonal iodide is T_4 iodide (T_4I) the test is designated T_4I by column.

(2) Interpretation

(a) Normal values should be established by the laboratory using the test.

(b) Lower than normal T_4I indicates a hypothyroid state.

(c) Elevated T_4I indicates increased levels of circulating thyroid hormones.

(d) Normals: (25, 31)

[1] Dog—0.9 to 2.3 micrograms/dl

[2] Horse—0.7 to 2.1 micrograms/dl

[3] Rat—1.3 to 1.9 micrograms/dl

[4] Monkey (rhesus)—1.8 to 4.0 micrograms/dl

(3) Problems

(a) The test as designed for man is not sufficiently sensitive for use in the dog.

(b) A modification of the test for specific use in animals renders it useful for the detection of hypothyroid states. The sensitivity of a standard curve must be increased to read the low values found in animals.

(c) Disophenol and radiographic dyes may interfere, giving falsely elevated values.

d. T_4 by competitive protein binding (CPB)

(1) Principle

(a) Radioactively labeled T_4 and the patient's T_4 compete for binding sites in an *in vitro* situation.

(b) The amount of radioactive T_4 that remains attached to the binding agent after equilibrium is established is dependent upon the quantity of the patient's T_4 present in the reaction mixture.

(c) A standard curve is constructed using known quantities of T_4; the patient's T_4 can be read from the curve.

(2) Interpretation
(a) Normal values should be established by the laboratory using the test.
(b) Low T_4 levels are indicative of hypothyroid states.
(c) Tetrasorb by Abbott Laboratories, which is a modified CPB method, has been a commonly used kit for the determination of T_4, but it must be modified for use in animals.
(d) Normals: (1, 16, 31)
[1] Dog—1.4 to 2.1 micrograms/dl
[2] Dog—1.5 to 3 micrograms/dl (normal, pre-TSH); 3 to 6 micrograms/dl (24 hr post-TSH)
[3] Dog—8 normal Beagles, 2.38 micrograms/dl
[4] Rat—1.8 to 2.7 micrograms/dl
[5] Cat—0.1 to 2.5 micrograms/dl (normal, pre-TSH); 2.5 to 5.1 micrograms/dl (24 hr post-TSH)
[6] Horse—2.57 ± 0.71 micrograms/dl
(e) Hypothyroid: (1, 3)
[1] Dog—0 to 1.7 micrograms (pre-TSH); 0 to 2 micrograms (post-TSH)
[2] Dog—12 thyroidectomized Beagles, 1.27 ± 3.6 micrograms/dl
[3] Cat—0 to 0.5 micrograms (pre-TSH); 0 to 0.6 micrograms (post-TSH)
(3) Problems
(a) The test procedure as used in man must be modified for animal use in order that low levels of T_4 can be determined from a standard curve.
(b) The test, when properly used, is reliable for the separation of hypothyroid from euthyroid dogs.

e. T_4 by radioimmunoassay (T_4 RIA)
(1) Principle
(a) This test is similar to the principle of T_4 by CPB except the T_4 binding agent is replaced by a specific T_4 antibody.
(b) The test is very sensitive for the detection of T_4 specifically.
(2) Interpretation
(a) Normal values should be established by the laboratory using the test. This is a promising test for the future.
(b) Low levels of T_4 RIA are indicative of low circulating levels of thyroxine.
(c) Although hyperthyroid states have not been reported using this procedure, the test would be reliable.
(d) Normals: (19, 20, 25)
[1] Dog—1.2 to 3 micrograms/dl
[2] Dog—1.14 ± 1.52 micrograms/dl
(3) Problems
(a) Low levels of the standard curve must be defined for accurate use in animals.
(b) The test currently available uses antihuman thyroxine antibody. Reliability of this procedure has not been documented in the literature, although preliminary reports look promising until a specific anticanine thyroxine can be obtained.

f. T_3 by resin sponge uptake
(1) T_3 by resin sponge uptake has not proved to be a reliable test for use in animals.
(2) The test has been designed for human use, and the resin used appears to be an active competitor with canine thyroid hormone-binding proteins.
(3) The T_7 (or free thyroxine index) obtained by multiplying T_4 times the percent of uptake as determined by the T_3 test therefore is also not reliable.

g. T_3 by radioimmunoassay (T_3 RIA)
(1) Principle
(a) Similar to the procedure for T_4 RIA except an antibody to T_3 is used
(2) Interpretation
(a) Normal values should be established by the laboratory using the test.
(b) T_3 RIA has not been used sufficiently in veterinary medicine for interpretation of results to become familiar. It is speculated, however, that with poor conversion of T_4 to T_3 an animal could be hypothyroid but have normal T_4 values. This may make T_3 RIA a valuable tool in the future in the diagnosis of hypothyroidism in animals.

(c) Normals: (19, 20)
[1] Dog—217 ± 45 micrograms/dl
(3) Problems
(a) More experience is needed to interpret the results obtained.
(b) Currently used methods use antihuman T_3, making results questionable until proved otherwise.
h. Thyroid-stimulating hormone (TSH) response test
(1) Principle
(a) The test has not been extensively used in the dog yet, but it appears promising.
(b) The test appears useful in differentiating primary hypothyroidism from secondary hypothyroidism.
(c) A control sample is drawn followed by an injection of TSH. A second sample is drawn at 12 hr, and appropriate thyroid function tests are done on the two samples and compared.
(2) Interpretation
(a) In the normal dog there is a given response to TSH as measured by thyroid function tests.
(b) In primary hypothyroidism no response is seen.
(c) In secondary hypothyroidism low response occurs, or it may take repeated injections of TSH to obtain a good response.
(d) Normals and abnormals: (3, 11, 25)
[1] Dog (normal): pre-TSH—1.5 to 3.5 micrograms/dl; 24 hr post-TSH—3 micrograms above control (using PBI and 5 to 10 units TSH)
Dog (primary hypothyroid): 24 hr post-TSH—0.5 micrograms above control
Dog (secondary hypothyroid): 24 hr post-TSH—1 microgram above control
[2] Dog (normal): pre-TSH—1.6 ± 0.7 micrograms/dl; 12 hr post-TSH—7.9 ± 1.84 micrograms/dl (using Tetrasorb and 1 IU TSH/lb)
[3] Dog (normal): pre-TSH—1.5 to 3 micrograms/dl; 24 hr post-TSH—3 to 6 micrograms/dl
Dog (hypothyroid): pre-TSH—0 to 1.7 micrograms/dl; 24 hr post-TSH—0 to 2.0 micrograms/dl
[4] Cat (normal): pre-TSH—0.1 to 2.5 micrograms/dl; 24 hr post-TSH—2.5 to 5.1 micrograms/dl
Cat (hypothyroid): pre-TSH—0 to 0.5 micrograms/dl; 24 hr post-TSH—0 to 0.6 micrograms/dl
(3) Problems
(a) Some controversy exists concerning the correct dose and route of administration (i.v. or i.m.) of TSH and the time at which the post-TSH sample is drawn.
(b) Studies indicate peak response to TSH is 10 to 12 hr postinjection.

C. Hyperthyroidism
1. Occurrence
a. Reported in the dog and cat but uncommon
b. Some indication that it may occur in the horse and cattle
2. Clinical features
a. Peculiar restlessness but tire easily
b. Appear thin and are hyperirritable
c. Muscular tremors and dyspnea
d. Often a palpable thyroid
e. Heart may be enlarged.
3. Diagnostic features
a. A peak ^{131}I uptake of greater than 40% is reported in the dog.
b. Other function tests, such as T_3 and T_4, have not been correlated because the condition is so uncommon.

Part three
CYTOLOGY

28 GENERAL CYTOLOGY

I. General considerations

A. Exfoliative cytology is the examination of "shed" or individual cells without regard to the general architectural structure of the tissue of origin. Collection of exfoliated cells is usually a bloodless type of biopsy, as the cells have desquamated from the surface of the linings of various body cavities and channels or from neoplasms.
B. Cytology should be an adjunct to and not a replacement for biopsy and histopathology.
C. Simple and rapid methods for the cytological examination of fluids and solid masses may be useful to any practitioner who has access to a centrifuge and a simple stain.
D. A positive test is highly significant; the absence of tumor cells does not exclude the presence of neoplasia and may be regarded as inconclusive.

II. Collection of the specimen

A. Effusions—pleural, peritoneal, pericardial
  1. Direct smear—for fluids of low viscosity
    a. Spread rapidly on the slide and leave a feathered edge where many cells tend to congregate.
    b. Centrifuge to concentrate and then smear.
  2. Squash technique—for thicker material or fluid with high viscosity
    a. Place material on a slide, crush with another slide on top, and spread with a wavy motion.

B. Scraping—for exposed lesions or excised biopsy material
  1. After cleaning off the surface, scrape slightly with a dull surgical blade or with the edge of a slide to yield a representative sample.
  2. Smear thinly over the slide.

C. Touch impression—for draining lesions, external lesions, or excised biopsies
  1. Remove superficial exudate, debris, or crusts.
  2. Blot excess blood or serum to provide contact with exterior cells on the surface of the lesion.
  3. Place the slide on the exposed or draining lesion.

D. Aspiration biopsy—for effusions, cysts, synovial fluid, cerebrospinal fluid, or solid masses such as tumors
  1. After introducing a small amount of air into the syringe, gently expel the sample onto the middle of the microscope slide.
  2. When there is marked contamination with blood, expel the sample into a Petri dish and select tissue fragments.
  3. Solid masses (tumors or lymph nodes)—blot with cleansing tissue or a paper towl and gently touch the cut surface with the slide; repeat the impression on the same slide only if the mass is small.

III. Fixation of the specimen

A. Air dry—for Romanowsky stains (Wright's or Giemsa) and new methylene blue
B. Fix while wet—for Pollak's trichrome or Papanicolaou's stains
1. Spraycyte
2. Equal amounts of ether and 95% ethyl alcohol

IV. Stains

A. Wright's—simple and readily available but does not show nuclear detail as well as some of the other stains
B. New methylene blue—only one color, not a permanent stain, nucleoli well demonstrated; good for a few tumors
C. Papanicolaou—cumbersome, excellent nuclear detail
D. Modified Pollak's trichrome stain

V. Examination of the cells

A. Erythrocytes—useful as a marker in measuring the size of other cells
1. Hemorrhage
a. Chronic hemorrhage—erythrophagocytosis and histiocytes containing hemoglobin pigment

B. Neutrophils
1. Sterile conditions—neutrophils are well preserved
2. Septic conditions—neutrophils are degenerating and may contain phagocytized microorganisms
a. Pyknotic
b. Karyorrhexis
c. Smudged
d. Vacuolated

C. Lymphocytes
D. Plasma cells
E. Histiocytes (macrophages)
1. Large—15 to 50 microns
2. Phagocytized particles in cytoplasm, which may contain vacuoles

F. Mesothelial cells
1. Large round cells that commonly travel to the feathered end of the slide
2. Can be phagocytic and may transform into macrophages
3. May be seen in clumps (2, 4, 8, 16, or 32)
4. Become reactive and are shed due to irritation of mesothelial lining
a. Clumps
b. Basophilic cytoplasm
c. Large nuclei
d. Can be multinucleated
e. Can contain mitotic figures
f. Nucleoli are generally small (3 microns)
g. May have a ciliated border—red "beard"
h. Easily confused with neoplastic cells

G. Eosinophils
H. Mast cells—metachromatic granules in the cytoplasm; normal tissue may have occasional mast cells
I. Liver and liverlike cells
1. Large round cells
2. May be in clumps
3. May be vacuolated

4. Normally have nucleoli
5. Nuclei small with large amount of cytoplasm

J. Squamous epithelial cells and cholesterol clefts—epidermal cysts
K. Neoplastic cells
1. Benign—cells usually uniform in size and shape
2. Malignant
a. Pleomorphic—vary in size and shape within cell clusters
b. Tend to be large cells
c. Large nuclei—often vary in size and shape
(1) High nuclear-cytoplasmic ratio
d. Nucleoli often large and bizarre in shape but tend to be round
(1) Often multiple
e. Many mitotic figures
f. Cytoplasm—basophilic; vacuoles may be present
(1) Signet-ring cell

VI. Steps in the evaluation of the cells in the smear

A. Are the cells normal or abnormal?
B. Is the process noninflammatory or inflammatory?
1. Noninflammatory conditions—fluids low in protein and cells
a. Sebaceous and epidermal cysts—contain cholesterol clefts
b. Salivary cysts—contain salivary cells
c. Transudates
2. Inflammatory conditions—contain neutrophils, plasma cells, and histiocytes
a. Septic
(1) Bacterial infections—toxic neutrophils, often degenerating and vacuolated; bacteria may be seen
(2) Mycotic infections—numerous macrophages and lymphocytes
b. Nonseptic
(1) Many healthy intact neutrophils
(2) Numerous lymphocytes and macrophages
(3) Allergic and parasitic conditions have abundant eosinophils.

C. Is there evidence of neoplasia?
1. Is it benign or malignant?

D. If malignant, is it carcinoma or sarcoma?
E. The cell type of the neoplasm is the last thing to determine and often is not possible to ascertain.

VII. Cytology of specific tissues

A. Lymph nodes
1. Normal
a. Small lymphocytes—75 to 95%; small amount of cytoplasm
b. Plasma cell—occasionally
2. Benign hyperplasia—enlarged lymph node
a. Increased number of plasma cells due to antigenic stimulation
3. Lymphosarcoma
a. Lymphoblasts—large percentage (usually all abnormal)
(1) Nucleoli—can see them well with new methylene blue; large, odd shapes
(2) Large cells
(3) Basophilic cytoplasm
(4) Mitotic figures—increased
(5) Pleomorphic

(6) Difficult to obtain a good stain—addition of serum to smear may help

4. Lymphadenitis (primary infection)
   a. Neutrophils
   b. Macrophages
   c. Microorganisms
5. Metastatic tumors

B. Tumors

1. Carcinoma
   a. Often in clumps
   b. Large nuclei
   c. Basophilic cytoplasm with vacuoles
2. Lipoma—soft fluctuating mass
   a. Appears as normal adipose tissue
   b. Occasional nucleus present
   c. Apply fat stain such as Sudan III or IV
3. Mastocytoma—button tumor of skin
   a. Metachromatic granules in cytoplasm
4. Melanoma
   a. Brown, grey, or black granules in cytoplasm
   b. Tendency of cells to clump
5. Histiocytoma—button tumor in skin of young dogs; tends to be ulcerated
   a. Large nondescript-appearing cell
   b. Moderate amount of cytoplasm
   c. Nucleus oval, round, or indented

29 TRANSUDATES AND EXUDATES

I. General considerations

A. Purpose of differentiating between transudates and exudates
  1. It is important to determine if an accumulation of extravascular fluid has resulted primarily from transudation or exudation, as there is a marked difference in the conditions that may be responsible for the two processes and their therapeutic responses.
  2. A typical transudate can usually be readily distinguished clinically from a typical exudate; but many extravascular fluids are modified transudates or modified exudates with some characteristics of both, so that recognition of the etiologic process may be difficult without a more complete examination of the fluid.

B. Transudate
  1. Noninflammatory in origin
     a. Hypoproteinemia
     b. Venous stasis
  2. Tends to recur unless the etiologic factor is removed
  3. Known under different terms, depending upon its location
     a. Hydrothorax—pleuritic effusion
     b. Hydroperitoneum—ascites
     c. Hydropericardium
     d. Hydroarthrosis

C. Exudate
  1. Inflammatory in origin
     a. Infections—bacterial, fungal, viral, parasitic
     b. Trauma—physical, chemical, or thermal injury
     c. Sterile inflammation—foreign bodies, pancreatic and intestinal secretions
     d. Neoplastic diseases—can produce transudates or exudates
  2. Removal often has a definitely beneficial influence on the etiologic disease process.
  3. The character of the exudate may determine the adjective used to describe it—serous, catarrhal, fibrinous, hemorrhagic, or purulent

II. Collection of the specimen

A. Whenever possible at least 10 ml of fluid should be aseptically obtained to provide an amount sufficient for determination of specific gravity and concentration for microscopic examination.
B. Since exudates coagulate and modified exudates may coagulate, it it advisable to collect a portion of the specimen in a tube containing an anticoagulant such as EDTA.
C. A sterile tube should be used for one portion to assure a satisfactory specimen in the event that a culture is indicated.

III. Physical examination

A. Color
  1. Serum or plasma—light to dark yellow, depending upon the amount of bilirubin present
  2. Erythrocytes—red, dark red, or reddish brown
  3. Leukocytes—white, cream, yellow, gray, or green

4. Chyle—milky white (after centrifugation), peach, or pink
5. Bilirubin—yellow, orange, red, brown

B. Turbidity—depends upon the number of suspended cells
1. Erythrocytes—grayish-red turbidity, red button in bottom of tube after centrifugation
2. Leukocytes (pus cells)—from light turbidity to thick, creamy pus
3. Fat droplets—milky turbidity
a. Confirm by dissolving in ether or applying Sudan III or IV stain to stain fat droplets an orange to red color.

C. Coagulation—depends upon the amount of fibrin present
1. Transudates—rarely show spontaneous complete or partial coagulation
2. Exudates—usually coagulate very quickly after removal from the serous cavity
a. In some purulent processes, exudates lose the ability to coagulate if fibrin is destroyed by cellular enzymes or bacteria.

D. Odor
1. Exudates and transudates are usually odorless unless combined with putrefactive change, so odor has little diagnostic significance.

E. Specific gravity—determined by a refractometer or a hydrometer similar to the one used in urinalysis
1. Transudate—under 1.017
2. Exudate—over 1.017

IV. Chemical examination

A. Protein
1. Method—refractometer
2. Results
a. Transudates—less than 3 g/dl
b. Exudates—more than 3 g/dl

B. Fibrinogen—difference in protein reading with the refractometer after heating the sample to remove the fibrinogen by precipitation
C. Urea nitrogen
1. Simultaneous determinations of urea nitrogen levels of the blood and of the unknown fluid are often of value in differentiating ascitic fluid from urine in the peritoneal cavity as the result of a ruptured bladder.
a. Ascitic fluid—urea nitrogen levels of the fluid and the blood are approximately the same, with an equilibrium established across the membranes
b. Urine in the peritoneal cavity—the urea nitrogen level of the fluid will be much higher than the blood level, due to the high urea content of the urine, which continues to accumulate

D. Occult blood—Hema-Combistix or Labstix
E. Glucose
1. Colorimetric methods
2. Tes-Tape, Clinistix, or Diastix

F. Bilirubin—Ictotest tablets

V. Cytological examination

A. Packed cell volume—microhematocrit
1. Will include both erythrocytes and leukocytes

B. Total nucleated cell count—hemocytometer or Coulter Counter
   1. Transudate—as few as 100 cells/dl
   2. Exudate—will vary but is usually over 50,000 cells/dl

C. Differential cell count
   1. Method
      a. Make a thin smear on a slide and stain with new methylene blue, Wright's, or Giemsa stain.
      b. If the fluid is thin and watery, centrifuge a portion and smear the sediment on a slide.
   2. Interpretation
      a. Purulent exudate—neutrophils predominate; macrophages and some mesothelial cells may be present
      b. Chronic exudative process—lymphocytes predominate
      c. Allergic or parasitic process—eosinophils predominate
      d. Transudate—endothelial cells from the lining of the large serous cavities, a few erythrocytes, and a few lymphocytes may be present
      e. Tumor cells—may be detected in some malignancies by examination of smears
         (1) A few may have to be confirmed by histologic section of formalinized sediment, biopsy, or other techniques.
         (2) The Papanicolaou stain may be used in conjunction with the information derived from the Romanowsky stains.
         (3) The Millipore filter technique for concentration may be useful when few cells are recovered.

VI. Microbiological examination

A. Direct examination
   1. Wet mount—plain or with new methylene blue stain
   2. Smear and stain
      a. Romanowsky stains (Wright's, Giemsa)—will demonstrate microorganisms; when present or when in doubt, should be followed by a Gram's stain.
      b. Gram's stain
      c. Special stains such as periodic acid Schiff (PAS)

B. Culture—method will probably be determined by results of direct smear
C. Animal inoculation—if indicated

VII. Summary of general differential characteristics of transudates and exudates

Characteristic	Transudate	Exudate
Appearance	Clear, serous, light yellow	Clear or cloudy
Coagulation	None	Clots spontaneously
Specific gravity	< 1.017	> 1.017
Protein (g/dl)	< 3.0	> 3.0
Cells	Few mesothelial cells, small lymphs, and erythrocytes	Neutrophils or lymphocytes, erythrocytes
Bacteria	Absent	Usually present

VIII. Paracentesis in the horse

A. Normal values for equine peritoneal fluid

Item	Bach and Ricketts (1)	McGrath (4)
Protein (g/dl)	0.1-3.4(1.1)	0.1-2.5
Specific gravity	1.000-1.093(1.001)	1.006-1.030
Clot	–	–
Nucleated cell count (microliters)	200-9,000(3,244)	50-4,600
Neutrophils (%)	36-78(59.5)	80-98
Mononuclears	3-50(30.4)	1-17
Lymphocytes	0-29(10)	1-11
Eosinophils	0-3(0.2)	0-7
Mast cells		Few
Fibrinogen (mg)		0-50
Bilirubin		–
pH		6.5-7.5

B. Alterations in equine peritoneal fluid

Item	Transudate	Modified transudate	Exudate
Specific gravity	< 1.020	> 1.020	1.029-1.035
Protein (g/dl)	< 1.6	> 1.6	4.3-5.1
Fibrinogen (mg)	< 50	> 50	100-400
Fibrin strands	– to few	Moderate	Numerous
Clot	–	–	+
Nucleated cell count	Low	360-2700	60,000-278,000
Neutrophils	Predominate	Increased	Markedly increased
Autolyzed	–	Significant number	Marked
Mononuclears	Low	Increased	Increased
Lymphocytes	Low	Increased	Increased
Eosinophils	Low	Increased	Increased
Reactive mesothelial cells	Occasional	Increased	
Glucose	– to +	+ + to + + + occasionally	– to + + +
Occult blood	– to +	– to + +	– to + + +

C. Summary of changes in equine peritoneal fluid in various abdominal conditions

Condition	Color	Protein	Cell count	Additional
Impaction	Pale yellow or yellow	2-2.5	Normal to slightly increased	Neutrophils Fibrinogen 50-300
Enteritis with diarrhea	Colorless	Normal	Normal	Neutrophils
Abdominal abscess				
Chronic fibrotic	Pale yellow	Normal	Normal	
Acute formative or ruptured	Yellow or white	++++	++++	Degenerating neutrophils Fibrinogen 100-400
Peritonitis, purulent	Yellow or yellow-brown	++++ (>4)	++++	Degenerating neutrophils Phagocytosis, marked Coagulation + Fibrinogen 100-400
Infarction	Amber and turbid		++	Neutrophils Erythrocytes Macrophages
Rupture, intestinal	Brown, turbid, granular	++++	++++	Neutrophils Macrophages Plant fibers
Neoplasia				
Carcinoma	Red-brown		++	Degenerating neutrophils Carcinoma cells Mononuclear cells
Lymphosarcoma	Yellow or white, turbid	+	+	Lymphoblasts
Melanoma, malignant	Slightly opalescent	+	+	Melanin in macrophages
Hepatic fibrosis	Yellow, orange, or red	+	+	Bilirubin ++++ Degenerating neutrophils Fibrinogen 100 Reactive mesothelial cells
Parasitic larval migration	Slightly amber	+	+	Eosinophils Neutrophils

30 VAGINAL SMEARS

I. Establishment of the optimum time for breeding the female dog should be based upon several factors.

A. History
1. Character and duration of vaginal discharge
2. Duration of previous estrous cycles

B. Character of vaginal discharge
C. Degree of vulval swelling
D. Attitude of female toward male dog
E. Vaginal smears
1. A series of smears will establish the stage of the estrous cycle with greater accuracy than a single vaginal smear.(4)

II. Methods

A. Obtain secretions from the vagina with a cotton swab, special wooden spatula, bulb pipette, or glass rod inserted well into the vagina.
B. Staining may be accomplished by either of the following techniques.
1. Place the secretions on a clean slide, allow to air dry, and stain with Wright's or Giemsa stain, using the same technique as for a blood smear.(1,4)
2. Mix 1 drop of vaginal secretion with 1 drop of 0.1 to 0.25% Toluidin Blue O stain, allow to stand for 3 to 5 min, apply a coverglass, remove excess fluid with a blotter, and examine immediately.(2,3)

III. Stages of the estrous cycle (1,2,3) (Fig. 30.1)

A. Anestrus
1. Duration—maximum of 2 mo
a. Period is shorter in animals submitted to pregnancy and lactation than in nonpregnant animals.
2. Clinical signs
a. Period from end of regression to next incidence of proestrus bleeding
3. Vaginal smear
a. Noncornified epithelial cells are present in varying numbers.
(1) Small circular or oval cells containing large nuclei with distinct chromatin granules
b. Leukocytes may be few in number or absent.
(1) Chiefly segmented neutrophils and a few lymphocytes

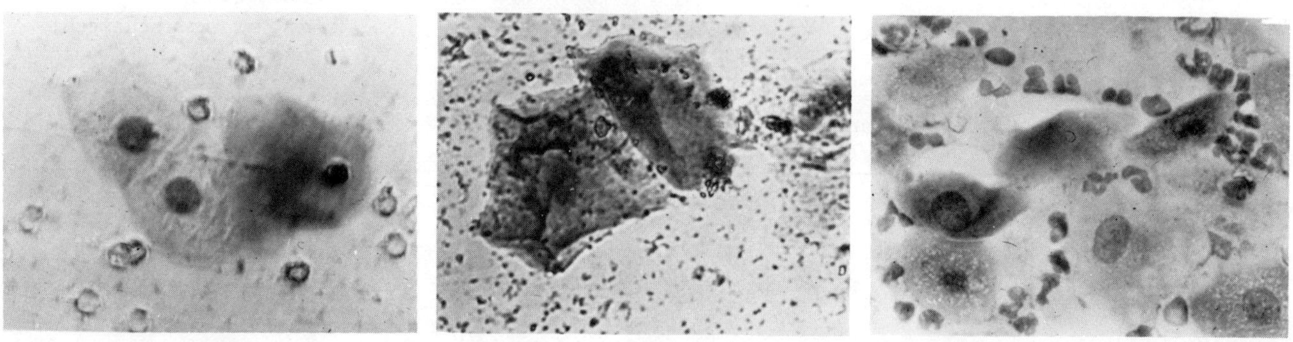

Proestrus — Estrus — Metestrus

Fig. 30.1. Vaginal smears.

B. Proestrus
   1. Duration—4 to 13 days, with an average of 9 days
   2. Clinical signs
      a. Period extending from the first appearance of blood-tinged discharge from vulva to time of first acceptance of the male
   3. Vaginal smear
      a. Epithelial cells
         (1) All noncornified epithelium disappears by the 4th or 5th day of proestrus.
         (2) Cornified epithelium appears almost immediately and constitutes a major fraction of all epithelial elements present in the smear by the 2nd or 3rd day.
      b. Erythrocytes are numerous and are the predominating cell type by the middle of proestrus.
      c. Leukocytes disappear by the last day or two of proestrus.

C. Estrus
   1. Duration—4 to 13 days, with an average of 9 days
   2. Clinical signs
      a. Period extending from first acceptance to the time of last acceptance of the male
      b. Yellowish rather than reddish discharge from the vulva
         (1) That estrus begins when bleeding ends is only approximately true, for external bleeding may last throughout estrus, and even into metestrus.
   3. Vaginal smear
      a. Epithelial cells are all of the cornified type.
         (1) Large, flat, angular cells that become wrinkled and irregular as estrus progresses
            (a) Nucleus becomes pyknotic, nucleolus disappears, and cytoplasm contains large numbers of bacteria.
      b. Erythrocytes may be detected microscopically throughout estrus, even though there is no evidence of gross bleeding.
      c. Leukocytes appear in the last day or two of estrus.
         (1) Segmented neutrophils are seen.
         (2) The appearance of large numbers of leukocytes denotes the end of estrus.

D. Metestrus
   1. Duration—approximately 3 mo
   2. Clinical signs
      a. The period is characterized by pregnancy or pseudopregnancy changes and then by a succeeding period of regression from these changes.
      b. Vaginal discharge has a puslike appearance.
   3. Vaginal smear
      a. Epithelial cells
         (1) Noncornified epithelial cells suddenly reappear.
         (2) Cornified epithelial cells disappear before the 10th day of metestrus.
      b. Leukocytes increase tremendously in number in the first few days of metestrus and reach a peak by the 3rd day, and then gradually decline in number so that they are practically absent between the 10th and 20th days of metestrus.
         (1) Most conspicuous characteristic of the vaginal smear at this period and impart the white, purulent appearance to the vaginal discharge

Part four
MYCOLOGY

31 MYCOTIC SKIN LESIONS

I. Dermatomycosis—refers to infections involving the keratinized cells of the stratum corneum, hair, and nails; in animals the hair is the usual site of infection

A. Organisms most commonly involved
1. Dog and cat—99% of the infections will involve one of the following:
   a. *Microsporum canis*—most common
   b. *Trichophyton mentagrophytes*—occasionally produces severe infections
   c. *Microsporum gypseum*—organism of the soil (geophilic) that varies in different geographic areas
2. Horse—*Trichophyton equinum*
3. Cattle—*Trichophkyton verrucosum*
4. Pig—*Microsporum nanum*
5. Rodents—*Trichophyton mentagrophytes*

B. Course of the condition—variable, as it may clear spontaneously in a few weeks, or it may persist for months
1. A number of factors will influence the duration of the lesions.
   a. Species of animal
      (1) In the cat there is minimal rejection, so that most lesions are mild or inapparent.
      (2) In the dog there is more reaction and the response includes more inflammation.
   b. Age of the animal—young animals more susceptible
      (1) The skin is thinner than in adult animals.
      (2) The chemistry of the skin changes at puberty.
2. Type of organism responsible for the lesion
   a. *Trichophyton mentagrophytes* produces infections that are much more severe and more difficult to treat than *Microsporum* infections.
3. Secondary bacterial infections

C. Clinical signs—vary with species of animal and fungus involved
1. Dog
   a. Circular lesions characterized by loss of hair or brittle, broken hairs and covered by scales or crusts, especially at the border of the lesion
   b. Usually located on the head, but may be on the body, extremities, or tail
   c. The degree of inflammation depends upon the host reaction and whether secondary bacterial invaders are present.
   d. Occasionally the lesion is completely depilated and free of scales, with a moist appearance suggestive of moist eczema.
2. Cat
   a. Lesions may vary from inapparent infections, with discoloration of the skin and shortened hairs, to circular areas free of hair and covered by scales.
   b. Lesions are usually located on the face or head.

3. Horse
   a. Circular or irregularly shaped lesions from coalescence of smaller ones, characterized by a loss of hair and light to heavy gray crusts
   b. Usually located in areas where the saddle or bridle contact the skin, or occasionally on the head
4. Cattle
   a. Hairless, circular lesions covered by thick, tan to gray crusts
   b. Usually located on the head or neck
   c. More likely to occur in calves or animals stabled in barns
5. Pig
   a. Circular lesions with discoloration of the skin, often undetected because of skin pigmentation or dirt on the skin
   b. Located on the head or body

D. Diagnosis
1. Fluorescence test
   a. Examine the animal in a darkened room with a Wood's light, which is an ultraviolet light with a special nickel oxide filter.
      (1) Several commercial models are available, some of which have a magnifying glass attached for improved examination.
   b. The infected hairs will glow with a bright yellow to yellow-green fluorescence. Also check the nails for fluorescence, especially in the cat.
   c. Limitations of the Wood's lamp
      (1) Its chief value is in the recognition of hairs infected with *Microsporum canis* (common in the dog and cat, but not in large animals), *Microsporum audouini,* or *Microsporum distortum* (both rare in animals), for only these three organisms consistently produce fluorescence.
      (2) The characteristic fluorescence may be masked or confused with the white or bluish white fluorescence from skin scales, mud, nails, substances with a petrolatum base, and some of the other common medications.
      (3) Even if no fluorescence is seen, the animal may still have a fungus infection.
         (a) Infection may be with one of the many dermatophytes that do not fluoresce.
         (b) Even when *Microsporum canis* infection is present, a large number of hairs will not fluoresce.
2. Microscopic examination
   a. The success of the microscopic examinations depends upon the care taken in selecting hairs and skin scrapings.
      (1) If fluorescing hairs are seen, pluck out with tweezers or a hemostat.
      (2) If no fluorescing hairs are detected, select the dull, broken hairs or those that show a grayish-white collarette at the base. Hairs near the periphery of the lesion will give better results than those in the center.
   b. Place hairs on a glass slide in a few drops of 10% potassium hydroxide.
   c. Apply a coverglass and apply gentle heat to the bottom of the slide by holding it over a flame for a few seconds or by placing it on the microscope lamp for a short time.
      (1) If heat is not used, allow the preparation to stand 20 to 30 min before examination.
      (2) An alternate clearing solution is potassium hydroxide/dimethyl sulfoxide, which eliminates the need for heat.
         (a) Formula:

Potassium hydroxide	20 gm
Dimethyl sulfoxide	40 ml
Water	60 ml

   d. Examine first under the low power (x10) of the microscope, looking for hairs that contain arthrospores.
      (1) Suspicious hairs should be examined with the high dry (x45) objective to see the details of the spores and hyphae on or in the hairs. Reduce the illumination.
         (a) Fungus arthrospores appear as small, refractile, spherical bodies, in chains or as a complete mosaic sheath around the infected hair. All fungi producing lesions in animals have arthrospores that are ectothrix in location on the hair.

(b) Pigment granules in the hair may be confusing, but they are brown and nonrefractile.

(c) Hyphae may be seen as filaments, sometimes fragmenting into arthrospores, on the infected hair, especially when the infected hairs are of equine or bovine origin.

e. The hairs may be stained with lactophenol cotton blue, writing ink, new methylene blue, or periodic acid Schiff; but this is not necessary for detection, as the spores and hyphae can readily be seen in subdued light when the hair has been cleared.

3. Culture

a. Identification of the causative fungus must be established by inoculation of culture media and study of morphologic characteristics of the growth.

b. Cleaning the lesion with 70% alcohol is helpful in reducing the contamination of cultures.

c. Large test tubes or bottles of the appropriate agar are inoculated by placing the hairs or skin scrapings on the surface of the medium and pushing partially into the agar.

d. Sabouraud's dextrose agar is the standard medium for the isolation of dermatophytes from clinical material; however, hair and skin scrapings are often heavily contaminated with saprophytic fungi and bacteria, which makes isolation difficult unless selective isolation media are used.

(1) Cycloheximide medium is a Sabouraud's dextrose agar to which several antibiotics have been added to inhibit the growth of both bacteria and saprophytic fungi without changing the character of the fungus growth.

(a) Mycosel Agar (Baltimore Biological Laboratory) or Mycobiotic Agar (Difco) are both complete commercial media that contain cycloheximide (Acti-dione), to inhibit the saprophytic fungi, and chloramphenicol, to inhibit bacterial growth.

(b) The addition of 0.01 mg of thiamine per milliliter of medium will facilitate isolation of *Trichophyton verrucosum,* the common cause of bovine dermatomycoses.

(c) Dermatophyte test medium (Fungassay DTM Agar is the trade name of the Pitman-Moore product) contains phenol red. Before inoculation, the agar is amber in color, but a characteristic of certain pathogenic fungi is the production of alkaline metabolites, which cause the phenol red indicator dye to turn red, sometimes before the colony growth is apparent. Saprophytic fungi will cause the indicator to turn red if the medium is held too long.

(2) Bacto-Trichophyton agars can be used to supply the special nutritional requirements of *Trichophyton verrucosum* and *Trichophyton equinum,* although *T. equinum* grows well on dermatophyte test medium.

(a) *Trichophyton verrucosum*—use Trichophyton Agar 3, which contains inositol and thiamine

(b) *Trichophyton equinum*—use Trichophyton Agar 5, which contains nicotinic acid

e. The inoculated slants should be incubated at room temperature (25° C) and examined every few days for evidence of growth.

(1) If the slants are in screw-capped containers, it is best to loosen the cap to allow air to enter, as growth and sporulation will be inhibited by tightly capped containers.

(2) The fungi commonly isolated have rapidly growing colonies that are white, tan, or cream in color.

(3) Some, however, are slow in producing growth. For this reason the tubes or bottles should be held for at least 3 to 4 wk before being reported as negative.

(4) Specimens from cattle should be incubated at 37° C, as *Trichophyton verrucosum* will grow better at this temperature than at room temperature.

f. A microscopic mount of the fungus growth will reveal identifying characteristics that will vary with the particular fungus isolated.

(1) Occasionally it is necessary to make a slide culture, using potato dextrose agar or wort agar, to produce characteristic macroconidia by which some of the dermatophytes may be identified.

(2) Lactophenol cotton blue may be used in preparing mounts for the study of morphological features.

(a) Place a drop or two of the stain on a slide and in it place a small portion of the filamentous growth from the culture, which can then be gently separated with teasing needles. Apply a coverglass and examine with the microscope for characteristic macroconidia.

4. Biopsy

a. Small sections of skin may be removed, from which tissue sections can be made for histopathological examination.

b. Equipment:

(1) Keyes cutaneous punch, 4 mm

DIFFERENTIAL CHARACTERISTICS OF THE TWO COMMON DERMATOPHYTES

	Miscrosporum canis	*Trichophyton mentagrophytes*
Hairs		
Fluorescence of hair	Yellow-green	None
Arthrospores on hair	Mosaic sheath of small (2 to 3 microns) arthrospores surround hair shaft	In parallel rows, appearing as chains of large (3 to 5 microns) arthrospores
	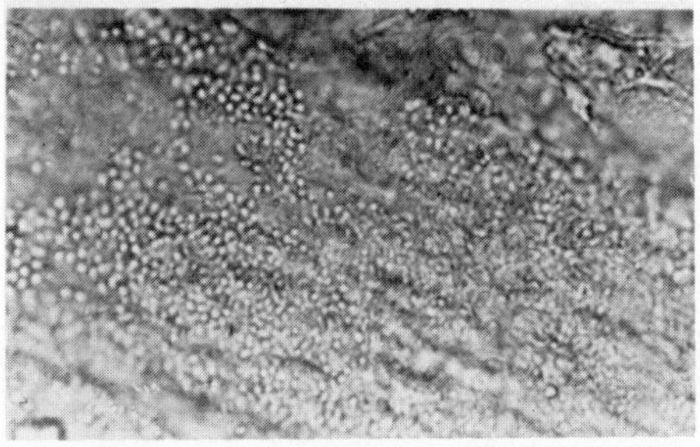	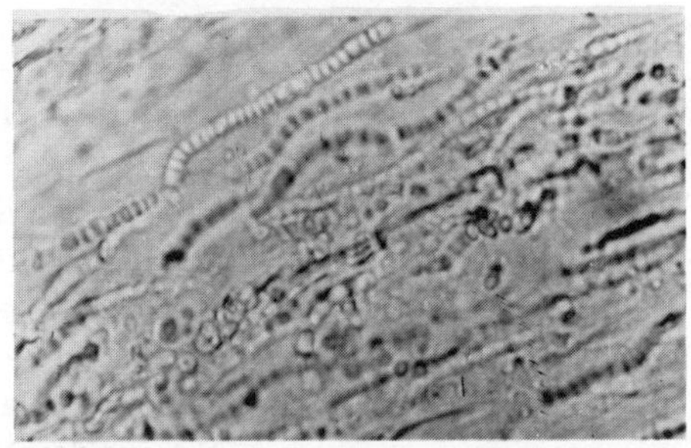
Cultural characteristics		
Rate of growth	Rapid—as early as 3 to 4 days	Fairly rapid—1 wk to 10 days
Surface texture	Flat, downy	Downy or granular
Color of colony	White—when very early may appear yellow	White, often turning tan with age
Reverse pigment	Yellow-orange	Often red
Microconidia	Few, if any—borne laterally	Numerous—no other pathogen produces as many; borne singly and in clusters
Macroconidia	Numerous Large Spindle shaped Multiseptate Knob at tip Thick walled	Rare—often require special sporulating agar to demonstrate Smaller than *Microsporum* Club shaped Multiseptate Thin walled
	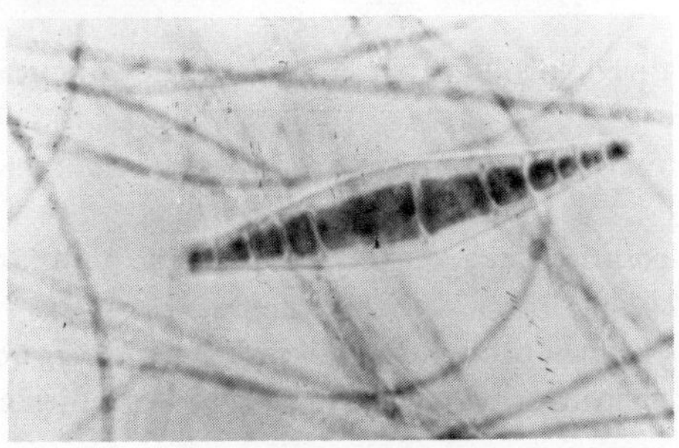	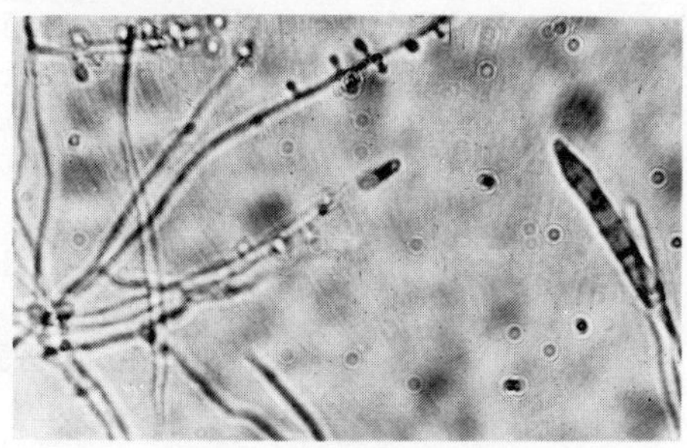

(2) Topical anesthetic, such as Skin Freeze
(3) Forceps
(4) Small, sharp scissors
(5) 10% formalin for preserving the specimen

c. The fungal elements can be easily demonstrated, as they have a high mucopolysaccharide content that is selectively stained a dark red color by such stains as periodic acid Schiff or modifications (Gridley's or Hotchkiss-McManus).

II. Subcutaneous mycoses

A. Candidiasis (moniliasis)
1. Predisposing factors
a. Moisture
b. Prolonged administration of antibiotics
c. Impaired or immature immunologic systems
d. Storing of sugar favors growth of the organism—diabetes, obesity
2. Predilection for:
a. Mucous membranes—white, thick, opaque plaques
b. Mucocutaneous junctions
c. Skin—rare
(1) Occurs where moist conditions macerate the skin producing red eroded areas; vesiculopustules covered with crusts
(a) Perineum
(b) External ear—doubtful if *Candida* is the initial pathogen
(c) Nail folds—paronychia
[1] Considerable pain
[2] Some nails fall out or are loosely attached.

B. Sporotrichosis
1. Two forms
a. Disseminated—reported only in the dog
b. Infection limited to the subcutaneous tissues and lymphatics.
(1) Firm spherical nodules form at the site of puncture wounds in the integumentary tissue.
(a) Later ulcerate and drain
(2) Nodules and, later, ulcers develop along lymph vessels in the ulcerative lymphangitis form.
(a) Reported in the horse and dog
2. The primary lesion of sporotrichosis is a granuloma.

C. Rhinosporidiosis
1. Chronic infection of the mucous membranes of the nasal cavity, characterized by polyps rarely larger than 2 to 3 cm in diameter
2. Rare infection in the United States, but has been reported in cattle and the horse, dog, and goat

D. Maduromycosis (mycetoma)
1. Maduromycosis denotes chronic, localized, proliferative lesions of the subcutaneous and submucosal tissues.
2. The lesions appear as nodular or ulcerative granulomas or fistulas of the feet or lower extremities in the dog and cat.
3. In cattle, mycetoma of the nasal mucosa is characterized by bilateral nodular growth without distortion of the turbinate cartilage.
4. In the horse, nodular granulomatous masses occur in the skin of the head, body, and feet.
5. The granules are usually brown or black in color, as they are microcolonies of the fungus.

E. Phycomycosis
1. Cutaneous or subcutaneous phycomycosis has been reported in the horse, cat, mink, deer, and mouse.
2. The best clinical descriptions have been reported for the horse, where two forms of subcutaneous phycomycosis can occur.
a. Hyphomycosis
(1) Chronic proliferative inflammation of the skin and mucous membranes of the legs, abdomen, mammary gland, neck, head, and lips; purulent exudate may drain from the openings.
(2) The majority of lesions develop slowly in areas believed to be injured previously by wire cuts.
b. Equine nasal granuloma

(1) Affects nasal skin and mucosa, as well as the lips
(2) Nodules are fibrous and contain numerous yellow foci that may range from 0.1 to 3 mm in diameter.

F. Aspergillosis
1. Cutaneous lesions have been reported in cattle.
a. Adult—mycotic granuloma in the skin
b. Aborted fetus—focal areas of necrosis with neutrophilic infiltration of the epidermis
2. The disease more commonly involves respiratory tissues.
a. Rhinitis and sinusitis—in the dog and cat
b. Guttural pouch infections—in the horse

III. Systemic or deep mycoses—although these organisms ordinarily involve internal organs such as lung, liver, spleen, and lymph nodes, they may cause fistulas and also involve the skin

A. Cryptococcosis
1. Infections of the skin and subcutaneous tissues have been reported in the cat.
2. Nasal and lip granulomas have been seen in the horse.
a. Myxomalike lesions are produced in these areas.

B. Coccidioidomycosis
1. Primary infection through the skin has never been reported in animals.
2. Cutaneous lesions rarely have been reported in the dog and cat, but have been associated with disseminated forms of the disease.

C. Blastomycosis
1. North American blastomycosis is often confined to the skin and subcutaneous tissues or to the lungs.
2. It produces a chronic granulomatous, suppurative infection.
3. A subcutaneous ulcerated nodule may be the first or the last clinical sign to appear.
a. Chronic localized cutaneous infections are the most common form seen in man, but they are quite uncommon in the dog.
4. Cutaneous and subcutaneous lesions in the dog usually indicate dissemination.

D. Histoplasmosis
1. Infections rarely affect the skin.

IV. Actinomycetosis

A. Dermatophilosis (cutaneous streptothricosis, mycotic dermatitis)
1. Clinical appearance is that of an exudative dermatitis.
a. In typical lesions there are small, elevated scabs that contain tufts of hair, epithelial cells, leukocytes, and coagulated serum.
b. Removal of crusts reveals a concave pus pocket beneath the scab.
c. Lesions are generally circumscribed, but can become confluent.
2. Affects several species of animal (cattle and the horse, sheep, goat, deer, monkey, and squirrel)
3. Predisposed by moist conditions

B. Nocardiosis
1. Localized and mycetoma-type infections may result from injury.
a. More common than the systemic form
2. Dog—nodules, ulcers, fistulas, and abscesses
a. Edematous feet release a reddish-brown, purulent exudate, and there is cutaneous hypertrophy.
3. Cat—subcutaneous nodules, ulcers, and cutaneous edema may accompany pyothorax
4. The characteristic tissue response is suppurative and granulomatous.

C. Actinomycosis

1. Characteristic bovine lesions involve the mandible, causing a suppurative or proliferative osteitis (called lumpy jaw), and in many of these cases there is marked production of connective tissue in the adjacent subcutaneous tissues.
   a. Typical cases will be followed by sinus tracts to the surface of the jaw, which discharge a thick, mucoid, yellow, purulent exudate that may contain "sulfur" granules.
2. Sheep, deer, elk, and antelope can develop lesions similar to those in cattle.
3. In the dog and cat subcutaneous abscesses can develop.

GLOSSARY

ACD—acid citrate dextrose
ACTH—adrenocorticotropic hormone
AD—acid dextrose
ADH—antidiuretic hormone (vasopressin)
ADP—adenosine diphosphate
A/G ratio—albumin:globulin ratio
AHF—antihemophilic factor
AIHA—autoimmune hemolytic anemia
ANA—antinuclear antibody
AP—alkaline phosphatase
ATP—adenosine triphosphate
ASCP—American Society of Clinical Pathologists

BMC—Boehringer Mannheim Company
Bod. unit—Bodansky unit
BSP—Bromsulphalein (trademark for a brand of sulfobromophthalein)
BVD—bovine virus diarrhea
BUN—blood urea nitrogen

CHPC—chloramphenicol
CNS—central nervous system
CMT—California mastitis test
CNP—circulating neutrophilic pool
CPB—competitive protein binding
CPK—creatine phosphokinase
CSF—cerebrospinal fluid

DIC—disseminated intravascular coagulation
DIT—diiodotyrosine
DLH—domestic long hair
DNA—deoxyribonucleic acid
DND—deoxyribonucleoprotein
DNP—sodium disophenol
DSH—domestic short hair

ECP—estradiol cyclopentylpropionate
EDTA—ethylenediamine-tetraacetate
ER—erythrocyte refractile
ESR—erythrocyte sedimentation rate

FDP—fibrinogen degradation product
FeLV—feline leukemia virus
FFA—free fatty acids
Fi—fibrinogen
FIP—feline infectious peritonitis
FPI—feline picornavirus infection
FSF—fibrin stabilizing factor
FVR—feline viral rhinotracheitis

GFR—glomerular filtration rate
GLDH—glutamic dehydrogenase
GOT—glutamic oxaloacetic transaminase; 1-aspartate:2-oxoglutarate aminotransferase
GPT—glutamic pyruvic transaminase; 2-oxoglutarate aminotransferase
G-6-Pase—glucose-6-phosphatase
G-6-PD—glucose-6-phosphate dehydrogenase
GSD—glycogen storage disease

HABA—2-(4′-hydroxyazobenzene)-benzoic acid
Hb—hemoglobin
HPF—high power field

IBR—infectious bovine rhinotracheitis
ICD—isocitric dehydrogenase
ICH—infectious canine hepatitis
IE—immunoelectrophoresis
Ig—immunoglobulin
IgG—immunoglobulin G
i.m.—intramuscular
IRI—immunoreactive insulin
ITP—idiopathic thrombocytopenia purpura
IU—international units
i.v.—intravenous

K-A-units—King-Armstrong units

LAP—leucine aminopeptidase
LE—lupus erythmatosus
LDH—lactic dehydrogenase
LPF—low power field

MCH—mean corpuscular hemoglobin
MCHC—mean corpuscular hemoglobin concentration
MCV—mean corpuscular volume
M:E ratio—myeloid:erythroid ratio
MIT—monoiodotyrosine
MNP—marginal neutrophilic pool

NAD—nicotinamide adenine dinucleotide (NADH = reduced form; NAD = oxidized form)
NF grade—National Formulary grade
N:L ratio—neutrophil:lymphocyte ratio
NMB stain—new methylene blue stain
NPN—nonprotein nitrogen

NZB—New Żealand black (mouse)

OCT—ornithine carbamyl transferase
OD—optical density

PAH—*p*-aminohippuric acid
PAS—periodic acid Schiff
PBI—protein-bound iodine
PCV—packed cell volume
PF-3—platelet factor 3
PHA—passive hemagglutination
PK—pyruvate kinase
PMN—polymorphonuclear
PP:F—plasma protein:fibrinogen ratio
PSP—phenolsulfonphthalein
PTA—plasma thromboplastin antecedent
PTC—plasma thromboplastin component
PTT—partial thromboplastin time

q.s.—*quantum sufficit;* as much as needed

RBC—red blood cell; erythrocyte
RCF—relative centrifugal force
RE—reticuloendothelial
RF units—Reitman-Frankel units
RIA—radioimmunoassay
RNA—ribonucleic acid
rpm—revolutions per minute

SAP—serum alkaline phosphatase
SDH—sorbitol dehydrogenase
SF units—Sigma Frankel units
SGOT—serum glutamic oxaloacetic transaminase
SGPT—serum glutamic pyruvic transaminase
SLE—systemic lupus erythmatosus
ST units—skin test units

TIBC—total iron-binding capacity
t.i.d.—*ter in die;* three times a day
TP—total protein
TRF—thyrotropin-releasing factor
TSH—thyroid-stimulating hormone
2, 3-DPG—2, 3-diphosphoglycerate

WBC—white blood cell; leukocyte

REFERENCES

Chapter 1

1. Abul-Fadl, M. A. M., and King, E. J. 1949. Properties of the acid phosphatases of erythrocytes and of the human prostate gland. Biochem. J. 45:51-60.
2. Altman, P. L., and Dittmer, D. S. 1964. Biology Data Book. Fed. Am. Soc. Exp. Biol., Washington, D.C.
3. Amador, Elias, and Wacker, Warren E. C. 1965. Enzymatic methods used for diagnosis. In: Methods of Biochemical Analysis, vol. 13, David Glick (ed.). Interstate, New York.
4. Ancill, R. J. 1956. The blood volume of the normal guinea pig. J. Physiol. 132:469-75.
5. Andersen, Allen C., and Schalm, Oscar W. 1970. Hematology. In: The Beagle as an Experimental Dog, Allen C. Andersen (ed.). Iowa State Univ. Press, Ames.
6. Archer, R. K. 1965. Haematological Technic for Use on Animals. Blackwell Scientific, Oxford.
7. Armin, J., Grant, R. T., Pels, H., and Reeve, E. B. 1952. The plasma, cell and blood volumes of albino rabbits as estimated by the dye (T-1824) and ^{32}P marked cell methods. J. Physiol. 116:59-73.
8. Baer, Daniel M., and Krause, Richard B. 1968. Spurious laboratory values resulting from simulated mailing conditions. A study of time and temperature variables. Am. J. Clin. Pathol. 50:111-19.
9. Behrendt, H. 1957. Chemistry of Erythrocytes. Charles C. Thomas, Springfield, Ill.
10. Bergmeyer, Hans-Ulrich (ed.). 1970. Methoden der Enzymatischen Analyse, vol. 1, 2nd ed. Verlag Chemie, Weinheim/Bergstr.
11. Cabaud, P. G., and Wróblewski, F. 1958. Colorimetric measurement of lactic dehydrogenase activity of body fluids. Am. J. Clin. Pathol. 30:234-36.
12. Caraway, Wendell T. 1962. Chemical and diagnostic specificity of laboratory tests. Effect of hemolysis, lipemia, anticoagulants, medications, contaminants, and other variables. Am. J. Clin. Pathol. 37:445-64.
13. Clark, Mary B. 1951. Studies based on errors observed in the use of anticoagulants in blood chemistry determinations. Am. J. Med. Technol. 17:190-97.
14. Conn, H. O. 1960. Effect of heparin on the blood ammonia determination, N. Eng. J. Med. 262:1103-7.
15. Courtice, F. C. 1943. The blood volume of normal animals. J. Physiol. 102:290-305.
16. Gambino, S. R. 1959. Heparinized vacuum tubes for determination of plasma pH, plasma CO_2 content, and blood oxygen saturation. Am. J. Clin. Pathol. 32:285-93.
17. Goodman, J. R., Vincent, J., and Rosen, I. 1954. Serum potassium changes in blood clots. Am. J. Clin. Pathol. 24:111-13.
18. Gregersen, Magnus I., Sear, H., Rawson, R. A., Chien, S., and Saiger, G. L. 1959. Cell volume, plasma volume, total blood volume and F cells factor in the rhesus monkey. Am. J. Physiol. 196:184-87.
19. Hansard, S. L., Sauberlich, H. E., and Comar, C. L. 1951. Blood volume of swine. Soc. Exp. Biol. Med. Proc. 78:544-45.
20. Hansard, S. L., Butler, W. O., Comar, C. L., and Hobbs, C. S. 1953. Blood volume of farm animals. J. Anim. Sci. 12:402-13.
21. Henry, R. J., Sobel, C., and Berkman, S. 1957. On the determination of "pancreatic lipase" in serum. Clin. Chem. 3:77-89.
22. Henry, R. J., and Berkman, S. 1957. Absorbance of various protein-free filtrates of serum. Clin. Chem. 3:711-15.
23. Henry, R. J. 1965. Clinical Chemistry, Principles and Technics. Harper and Row, New York.
24. Hodgetts, V. E. 1961. The dynamic red cell storage function of the spleen in sheep. III. Relationship to determination of blood volume, total red cell volume, and plasma volume. Aust. J. Exp. Biol. Med. Sci. 39:187-96.
25. Hoerlein, A. B., Hubbard, E. D., and Getty, R. 1951. The procurement and handling of swine blood samples on the farm. J. Am. Vet. Med. Assoc. 119:357-62.
26. Hovell, G. J. R. 1968. Jugular puncture in the dog. Vet. Rec. 83:289-90.

27. Julian, L. M., Lawrence, J. H., Berlin, N. I., and Hyde, G. M. 1956. Blood volume, body water, and body fat of the horse. J. Appl. Physiol. 8:651-53.
28. Lehnert, James P. 1967. New method for bleeding guinea pigs. Am. J. Clin. Pathol. 47:416-17.
29. McGann, C. J., and Carter, R. E. 1960. The effect of hemolysis on the van den Bergh reaction for serum bilirubin. J. Pediatr. 57:199-203.
30. McGeachin, R. L., Daugherty, H. K., Hargen, L. A., and Potter, B. A. 1957. The effect of blood anti-coagulants on serum and plasma activities. Clin. Chim. Acta 2:75-77.
31. McKelvie, D. H., Powers, Susan, and McKim, Frank. 1966. Microanalytical procedures for blood chemistry long-term study on Beagles. Am J. Vet. Res. 27:1405-12.
32. Marcilese, N. A., Valsecchi, R. M., Figueiras, H. D., Camberos, H. R., and Varela, J. E. 1964. Normal blood volumes in the horse. Am. J. Physiol. 207:223-27.
33. Martinek, Robert G. 1966. Specimens for clinical laboratory analysis. Collection and preservation. Postgrad. Med. 39:A-46, A-48, A-50, A-52, A-54, A-56.
34. Mather, A., and Mackie, N. R. 1960. Effects of hemolysis on serum electrolyte values. Clin. Chem. 6:223-27.
35. Moreland, Alvin F. 1965. Collection and withdrawal of body fluids and infusion techniqes. In: Methods of Animal Experimentation, vol. 1, William I. Gay (ed.). Academic Press, New York.
36. O'Hagan, J. E., Hamilton, T., Le Breton, E. G., and Shaw, A. E. 1957. Human serum bilirubin. An immediate method of determination and its application to the establishment of normal values. Clin. Chem. 3:609-23.
37. Overman, Richard R., and Feldman, Harry A. 1947. Circulatory and fluid compartment physiology in the normal monkey with especial reference to seasonal variations. Am. J. Physiol. 148:445-59.
38. Parkinson, J. E., and Dougherty, J. H. 1958. Effect of internal emitters on red cell and plasma volumes of Beagle dogs. Soc. Exp. Biol. Med. Proc. 97:722-25.
39. Quick, A. J., Georgatsos, J. G., and Hussey, C. V. 1954. The clotting activity of human erythrocytes: Theoretical and clinical implications. Am. Med. Sci. 228:207-13.
40. Reynolds, M. 1953. Plasma and blood volume in the cow using the T-1824 hematocrit method. Am. J. Physiol. 173:421-27.
41. Salenius, P. 1957. A study of the pH and buffer capacity of blood, plasma and red blood cells. J. Clin. Lab. Invest. 9:160-67.
42. Schermer, Siegmund. 1967. The Blood Morphology of Laboratory Animals, 3rd ed. F. A. Davis, Philadelphia.
43. Seligson, D., Marino, J., and Dodson, E. 1957. Determination of sulfobromophthalein in serum. Clin. Chem. 3:638-45.
44. Sherman, H. C., Caldwell, M. L., and Adams, M. 1928. A quantitative comparison of the influence of neutral salts on the activity of pancreatic amylase. J. Am. Chem. Soc. 50:2538-43.
45. Shinowara, G. Y. 1954. Spectrophotometric studies on blood serum and plasma. Am. J. Clin. Pathol. 24: 696-710.
46. Spink, Ronald R., Malvin, Richard L., and Cohen, Bennett J. 1966. Determination of erythrocyte half-life and blood volume in cats. Am. J. Vet Res. 27:1041-43.
47. Tollersrud, Sverre. 1969. Stability of some serum enzymes in sheep, cattle, and swine during storage at different temperatures. Acta Vet. Scand. 10:359-71.
48. Vincent, D., and Segonzac, G. 1960. Le dosage de l'arginase sérique en pratique clinique. Rev. Franç. Études Clin. Biol. 5:390-92.
49. Walford, Roy L., Sowa, Masako, and Daley, Donald. 1956. Stability of protein, enzyme and nonprotein constituents of stored frozen plasma. Am. J. Clin. Pathol. 26:376-80.
50. Wallach, J. D. 1970. A simple technique for the collection of blood from small zoo animals. J. Am. Vet. Med. Assoc. 157:694-95.
51. Wang, Louise. 1959. Plasma volume, cell volume, total blood volume and F cells factor in the normal and splenectomized Sherman rat. Am. J. Physiol. 196:188-92.
52. Webster, J., Schiaffino, S. S., and Richmond, A. M. 1952. Evaluation of serum potassium levels. Am. J. Clin. Pathol. 22:833-42.
53. Wirth, Wolfgang A., and Thompson, Richard L. 1965. The effect of various conditions and substances on the results of laboratory procedures. Am. J. Clin. Pathol. 43:579-90.
54. Wish, Leon, Furth, Jacob, and Storey, Robert H. 1950. Direct determinations of plasma, cell, and organ-blood volumes in normal and hypervolemic mice. Soc. Exp. Biol. Med. Proc. 74:644-48.
55. Woodward, Kent T., Berman, Ann R., Michaelson, Sol. M., and Odland, Lawrence T. 1968. Plasma, erythrocyte, and whole blood volume in the normal Beagle. Am. J. Vet. Res. 29:1935-44.

56. Yonan, V. L., and Reinhold, J. G. 1957. Effects of delayed examination on the results of certain hepatic tests. Clin. Chem. 3:685-90.
57. Zaroda, R. A. 1964. Effect of various anticoagulants on carbon dioxide combining power of blood. Am. J. Clin. Pathol. 41:377-80.
58. Zinkl, J. G., Bush, R. M., Cornelius, C. E., and Freedland, R. A. 1971. Comparative studies on plasma and tissue sorbitol, glutamic, lactic, and hydroxybutyric dehydrogenase and transaminase activities in the dog. Res. Vet. Sci. 12:211-14.
59. Zucker, M. B., and Borrelli, J. 1959. Platelets as a source of serum acid nitrophenylphosphatase. J. Clin. Invest. 38:148-54.

Chapter 2

1. Archer, R. K. 1954. Bone marrow biopsy in the horse. A study of the normal marrow cytology in cross-bred ponies. Vet. Rec. 66:261-63.
2. Archer, R. K. 1965. Haematological Techniques for Use on Animals. Blackwell Scientific, Oxford.
3. Backgren, A. W. Lymphatic leukosis in dogs. 1965. An epizoological, clinical and hematologic study. DVM thesis, Stockholm, Sweden.
4. Bloom, F., and Meyer, L. M. 1944. The morphology of bone marrow cells in normal dogs. Cornell Vet. 34:13-18.
5. Bohorfoush, Joseph G. 1964. Concentrating and staining bone marrow: An on-the-slide technique. Stain Technol. 39:339-43.
6. Calhoun, M. Lois. 1954. A cytological study of costal marrow. I. The adult horse. Am. J. Vet. Res. 15:181-96.
7. Calhoun, M. Lois. 1954. A cytological study of costal marrow. II. The adult cow. Am. J. Vet. Res. 15:395-404.
8. Conner, G. H., Gupta, B. N., and Krehbiel, J. D. 1971. A technique for bone marrow biopsy in the cat. J. Am. Vet. Med. Assoc. 158:1702-5.
9. Cornelius, C. E., Goodbary, R. F., and Kennedy, P. C. 1959. Plasma cell myelomatosis in a horse. Cornell Vet. 49:478-93.
10. Diggs, L. W., Sturm, Dorothy, and Bell, Ann. 1970. The Morphology of Human Blood Cells. Abbott Laboratories, North Chicago.
11. Doxey, D. L., Veterinary Clinical Pathology. 1971. Baillière Tindall, London.
12. Dungworth, D. L., Thielen, G. H., and Lengyel, J. 1964. Bovine lymphosarcoma in California. II. The thymic form. Pathol. Vet. 1:323-50.
13. Eyestone, W. H. 1951. Myelogenous leukemia in the cat. J. Natl. Cancer Inst. 12:599-613.
14. Gilmore, C. E., Gilmore, V. H., and Jones, T. C. 1965. Bone marrow and peripheral blood of cats: Technique and normal values. Pathol. Vet. 1:18-40.
15. Gilmore, C. E., Gilmore, V. H., and Jones, T. C. 1964. Reticuloendotheliosis. A myeloproliferative disorder of cats: A comparison with lymphocytic leukemia. Pathol. Vet. 1:161-83.
16. Gilmore, Charley E., and Holzworth, Jean. 1971. Naturally occurring feline leukemia: Clinical, pathologic, and differential diagnostic features. J. Am. Vet. Med. Assoc. 158:1013-25.
17. Greenberg, Michael L., Atkins, Harold L., and Schiffer, Lewis M. 1966. Erythropoietic and reticuloendothelial function in bone marrow in dogs. Science 152:526-28.
18. Grunsell, C. S. 1955. The marrow cells of normal sheep. J. Comp. Pathol. 65:8-16.
19. Hjärre, A. 1943. Om sternalpunktion och den normala benmargsbilden hos husdjuren. Skand. Vet.-tidskr. 33:457-72.
20. Holzworth, Jean. 1960. Leukemia and related neoplasms in the cat. I. Lymphoid malignancies. J. Am. Vet. Med. Assoc. 136:47-69.
21. Holzworth, Jean. 1960. Leukemia and related neoplasms in the cat. II. Malignancies other than lymphoid. J. Am. Vet. Med. Assoc. 136:107-21.
22. Hyde, J. L., King, J. M., and Bentinck-Smith, J. 1958. A case of bovine myelogenous leukemia. Cornell Vet. 48:269-76.
23. Lahey, M. E., Gubler, C. J., Chase, M. S., Cartwright, G. E., and Wintrobe, M. M. 1952. Studies on copper metabolism. II. Hematologic manifestations of copper deficiency in swine. Blood 7:1053-75.
24. Lawrence, J. S., Syverton, J. T., Shaw, J. S., and Smith, F. P. 1940. Infectious feline agranulocytosis. Am. J. Pathol. 16:333-54.

25. Medway, W., and Rapp, J. P. 1962. A case of chronic granulocytic leukemia with thrombocytopenic purpura in a dog. Cornell Vet. 52:247-60.
26. Medway, W., Weber, W. T., O'Brien, J., and Krawitz, L. 1967. Multiple myeloma in a dog. J. Am. Vet. Med. Assoc. 150:386-95.
27. Meier, H., and Patterson, D. F. 1956. Myelogenous leukemia in a cat. J. Am. Vet. Med. Assoc. 128:211-14.
28. Meier, H., and Gourley, G. 1957. Basophilic (myelocyte) or mast cell leukemia in the cat. J. Am. Vet Med. Assoc. 130:33-40.
29. Mulligan, R. M. 1941. Quantitative studies on the bone marrow of the dog. Anat. Rec. 79:101-8.
30. Penny, R. H. C., and Carlisle, Carol H. 1970. The bone marrow of the dog: A comparative study of biopsy material obtained from the iliac crest, rib and sternum. J. Small Anim. Pract. 11:727-34.
31. Reichel, K. 1962. Kinisch-haematologische Untersuchungen bei der Leukose des Schweines. Dtsch. Tieraerztl. Wochenschr. 69:297-303.
32. Roscher, A. A., Boatwright, R. S., Kupfer, H. G., and Egdhal, R. H. 1960. Acute myelogenous leukemia, with histopathologic studies, following total body irradiation of a dog. J. Am. Vet. Med. Assoc. 136:491-500.
33. Rywlin, Arkadi M., Marvan, Paul, and Robinson, Morton J. 1970. A simple technic for the preparation of bone marrow smears and sections. Am. J. Clin. Pathol. 53:389-93.
34. Saar, C., Hilliger, H. G., and Loppnow, H. 1963. Plasmazellulaere Retikulose mit kristallinen Paraporteinablagerungen bei einem Hund. Zentralbl. Veterinaermed. A 10:723-41.
35. Sawitsky, A., and Meyer, L. M. 1947. The bone marrow of normal cats. J. Lab. Clin. Med. 32:70-75.
36. Schalm, O. W., Jain, N. C., and Carroll, E. J. 1975. Veterinary Hematology, 3rd ed. Lea and Febiger, Philadelphia.
37. Schryver, H. F. 1963. The bone marrow of the cat. Am. J. Vet. Res. 24:1012-17.
38. Switzer, J. W., and Schalm, O. W. 1968. Bone marrow disorders in cats: Bone marrow sampling techniques. Calif. Vet. 22:20-24.
39. Theilen, G. H., and Dungworth, D. L. 1965. Bovine lymphosarcoma in California. III. The calf form. Am. J. Vet. Res. 26:696-709.
40. Valli, V. E., McSherry, B. J., and Hulland, T. J. 1969. A review of bone marrow handling techniques and description of a new method. Can. J. Comp. Med. 33:68-71.
41. Van Loon, E. J., and Clark, B. B. 1943. Hematology of the peripheral blood and bone marrow of the dog. J. Lab. Clin. Med. 28:1575-79.
42. Weber, W. T., and Marshak, R. R. 1963. A correlative study of bone marrow and peripheral blood in bovine lymphosarcoma. Am. J. Vet. Res. 24:515-24.
43. Weber, W. T. 1969. Evaluation of bone marrow. In: Textbook of Veterinary Clinical Pathology, W. Medway et al. (eds.). Saunders, Philadelphia.
44. Wilde, J. K. H. 1961. A technique for bone marrow biopsy in cattle. Res. Vet. Sci. 2:315-19.
45. Wilde, J. K. H. 1964. The cellular elements of the bovine bone marrow. Res. Vet. Sci. 5:213-27.
46. Winqvist, G. 1954. Morphology of the blood and the hemopoietic organs in cattle under normal and some experimental conditions. Acta Anat. Suppl. 21:1-159.
47. Winter, H. 1964. The myelogram of normal sheep. J. Comp. Pathol. Therap. 74:457-69.
48. Wintrobe, M. M. 1974. Clinical Hematology, 7th ed. Lea and Febiger, Philadelphia.
49. Zawidzka, Z. Z., Janzen, E., and Grice, H. C. 1964. Erythremic myelosis in a cat. Pathol. Vet. 1:530-41.

Chapter 3

1. Archer, R. K. 1965. Haematological Techniques for Use on Animals. Blackwell Scientific, Oxford.
2. Brecher, George. 1949. New methylene blue as a reticulocyte stain. Am. J. Clin. Pathol. 19:895-96.
3. Elton, Norman W., Fredenburgh, Edwin J., and Manning, David W. 1948. The Chanco technic in Wright's stain. Am. J. Clin. Pathol. 18:92-93.
4. Fowler, James L., Ruff, Michael D., and Hornof, William J. 1970. Modification of Field's stain for examination of growth forms of *Babesia gibsoni*. Am. J. Vet. Res. 31:1079-83.
5. Frankel, Sam, and Reitman, Stanley (eds.). 1963. Gradwohl's Clinical Laboratory Methods and Diagnosis, vol. 2, 6th ed. Mosby, St. Louis.
6. Granzien, Corinne K., and Newton, L. G. 1968. Siderocytes as a diagnostic aid in equine infectious anaemia. Aust. Vet. 44:406-9.
7. Humason, Gretchen L. 1966. Animal Tissue Techniques, 2nd ed. Freeman, San Francisco.

8. Oxer, D. T. 1962. equine infectious anaemia in two groups of horses. Aust. Vet. 38:190-200.
9. Rothenbacher, H. J., Ishida, K., and Barner, R. D. 1962. Equine infectious anemia. Part II. The sidero-leukocyte test as an aid in the clinical diagnosis. Vet. Med. 57:886-90.
10. Schalm, O. W., Jain, N. C., and Carroll, E. J. 1975. Veterinary Hematology, 3rd ed. Lea and Febiger, Philadelphia.
11. Schalm, O. W., Jain, N. C., and Carroll, E. J. 1961. A rapid method for staining blood films. Calif. Vet. 15:28-30.
12. Schalm, O. W., Jain, N. C., and Carroll, E. J. 1962. Absolute numbers for the differential leukocyte count. Calif. Vet. 16:39-40.
13. Thompson, Samuel W., and Hunt, Ronald D. 1966. Selected Histochemical and Histopathological Methods. Charles C. Thomas, Springfield, Ill.

Chapter 4

1. Committee for clarification of the nomenclature of cells and diseases of the blood and blood-forming organs. 1948. First report. Am. J. Clin. Pathol. 18:443-50.
2. Committee for clarification . . . . 1949. Second report. Am. J. Clin. Pathol. 18:56-60.
3. Committee for clarification . . . . 1950. Third, fourth, and fifth reports. Am. J. Clin. Pathol. 20:562-79.
4. Department of the Army. 1963. TM8-227-4: Laboratory procedures in clinical hematology. Supt. of Documents, USGPO, Washington, D.C.
5. Finch, Clement A. 1969. Red cell manual. Univ. Wash., Seattle.
6. Schalm, O. W., Jain, N. C., and Carroll, E. J. 1975. Veterinary Hematology, 3rd ed. Lea and Febiger, Philadelphia.

Chapter 5

1. Ackart, R. J., Shaw, J. S., Jr., and Lawrence, J. S. 1940. Blood cell picture of normal cats. Anat. Rec. 76:357-64.
2. Adler, A. E., Jr. 1940. Blood picture in normal dogs. North Am. Vet. 21:356-57.
3. Albritton, E. C. (ed.). 1952. Standard Values in Blood. Saunders, Philadelphia.
4. Allen, J. G., Sanderson, M., Milham, M., Kirschon, A., and Jacobson, L. O. 1948. Heparinemia (?). An anticoagulant in the blood of dogs with hemorrhagic tendency after total body exposure to roentgen rays. J. Exp. Med. 87:71-86.
5. Archer, R. K. 1959. The normal haemograms and coagulograms of the English Thoroughbred horse. J. Comp. Pathol. Therap. 69:390-99.
6. Becker, D. E., and Smith, S. E. 1950. A chemical and morphological study of normal sheep blood. Cornell Vet. 40:350-56.
7. Benjamin, M. M. 1953. Blood cytology of shipping fever in beef cattle. J. Am. Vet. Med. Assoc. 123:209-12.
8. Berrier, H. H. 1961. Diagnostic Aids in the Practice of Veterinary Medicine. Alban, St. Louis.
9. Brenon, H. C. 1958. Further erythrocyte and hemoglobin studies in Thoroughbred racing horses. J. Am. Vet. Med. Assoc. 133:102-4.
10. Britton, J. W. 1946. Changes of the blood constituents in diseases of ruminants. Cornell Vet. 36:25-30.
11. Bruner, H. D., and Wakerlin, G. E. 1937. The blood picture of the normal dog. Soc. Exp. Biol. Med. Proc. 36:667-70.
12. Calhoun, M. L., and Smith, E. M. 1975. Hematology and hematopoietic organs. In: Diseases of Swine, H. W. Dunne and A. D. Leman (eds.). Iowa State Univ. Press, Ames.
13. Coffin, D. L. 1953. Manual of Veterinary Clinical Pathology, 3rd ed. Comstock, Ithaca, N.Y.
14. Dukes, H. H. 1955. The Physiology of Domestic Animals, 7th ed. Comstock, Ithaca, N.Y.
15. Ederstrom, H. E., and DeBoer, B. 1946. Changes in the blood of the dog with age. Anat. Rec.94:663-70.
16. Ferguson, L. C., Irwin, M. R., and Beach, B. A. 1945. On variation in the blood cells of healthy cattle. J. Infect. Dis. 76:24-30.
17. Greatorex, J. C. 1954. Studies on the haematology of calves from birth to one year of age. Brit. Vet. J. 110: 120-38.
18. Grunsell, C. S. 1955. Seasonal variation in the blood and bone marrow of Scottish hill sheep. J. Comp. Pathol. Therap. 65:93-107.

19. Hammon, W. D., and Enders, J. F. 1939. A virus disease of cats, principally characterized by aleucocytosis, enteric lesions and the presence of intranuclear inclusion bodies. J. Exp. Med. 69:327-52.
20. Hansen, M. F., Todd, A. C., Kelley, G. W., and Hull, F. E. 1950. Studies on the hematology of the Thoroughbred horse. I. Mares in foal. Am. J. Vet. Res. 11:296-300.
21. Hansen, M. F., Todd, A. C., Kelley, G. W., Cawein, M., and McGee, W. R. 1950. Studies on the hematology of the Thoroughbred horse. II. Weanlings. Am. J. Vet. Res. 11:393-96.
22. Hansen, M. F., Todd, A. C., Cawein, M., and McGee, W. R. 1950. Studies on the hematology of the Thoroughbred horse. III. Stallions. Am. J. Vet. Res. 11:397-99.
23. Hansen, M. F., Todd, A. C., Kelley, G. W., and Cawein, M. 1951. Studies on the hematology of the Thoroughbred horse. IV. Barren mares. Am. J. Vet. Res. 12:31-34.
24. Holman, H. H. 1944. Studies on the haematology of sheep. I. The blood picture of healthy sheep. J. Comp. Pathol. Therap. 54:26-40.
25. Holman, H. H. 1956. Clinical haematology. In: Diagnostic Methods in Veterinary Medicine, G. F. Boddie, 4th ed. Lippincott, Philadelphia.
26. Hoorens, J. 1959. Blood studies in newborn pigs. Vlaams Diergeneeskd. Tijdschr. 26:37-53. (Abstr., Mod. Vet. Pract. 40:55, 1959.)
27. Jennings, A. R. 1947. Haematology of healthy kittens. Brit. Vet. 103:234-39.
28. Landsberg, J. W. 1939. The blood picture of young, normal dogs. J. Am. Vet. Med. Assoc. 94:595-600.
29. Landsberg, J. W. 1940. The blood picture of normal cats. Folia Haematol. 64:169.
30. Luke, D. 1953. The differential leucocyte count in the normal pig. J. Comp. Pathol. Therap. 63:346-54.
31. Miller, W. T. 1932-33. Erythrocyte, leukocyte and hemoglobin determinations on the blood of cattle, with a note on the blood in Johne's disease. N.Y. State Vet. Coll., Cornell Univ. Annual report.
32. Morris, M. L., Stelton, N. J., Allison, J. B., and Green, D. F. 1940. Blood cytology of the normal dog. J. Lab. Clin. Med. 25:353-60.
33. Mulligan, R. M. 1941. Studies on the blood of mongrel dogs at high altitude. Am. J. Physiol. 133:394.
34. Mundhenk, R. L. 1941. A study of the normal adult canine hemogram. North Am. Vet. 22:95-100, 167-70.
35. Riser, W. H. 1946. The normal blood count of the domestic cat. North Am. Vet. 27:93-98.
36. Scarborough, R. A. 1931. The blood picture of normal laboratory animals. Yale J. Biol. Med. 3:63, 168, 267, 359, 431, 547.
37. Schalm, O. W. 1956. The blood and blood-forming organs. In: Diseases of Cattle, M. G. Fincher (ed.). American Veterinary Publ., Evanston, Ill.
38. Schalm, O. W. 1958. The leukocytes. Calif. Vet. 12:18-19.
39. Schalm, O. W. 1959. The erythrocytes. Calif. Vet. 12:31-33.
40. Swenson, M. J., Goetsch, D. D., and Underbjerg, G. K. L. 1955. The effect of the sow's ration on the hematology of the newborn pig. Am. Vet. Med. Assoc. Proc., pp. 159-62.
41. Todd, A. C., McGee, W. R., Wyant, Z. N., and Hollingsworth, K. P. 1951. Studies on the hematology of the Thoroughbred horse. V. Sucklings. Am. J. Vet. Res. 12:364-67.
42. Vaulont, H. 1935. Untersuchungen des Katzen-und Pferdeblutes. Z. f. Biol. 96:241.
43. Wintrobe, M. M. 1974. Clinical Hematology, 7th ed. Lea and Febiger, Philadelphia.

Chapter 6

1. Arensburger, K. E. 1955. A modified direct method for enumeration and study of platelets. Am. J. Clin. Pathol. 25:1220-23.
2. Barkhan, P., Tomlin, S. C., and Archer, R. K. 1957. Comparative coagulation studies on horse and human blood. J. Comp. Pathol. 67:358-68.
3. Brecher, G., Schneiderman, M., and Cronkite, E. P. 1953. The reproducibility and constancy of the platelet count. Am. J. Clin. Pathol. 23:15-26.
4. Carper, H. A., and Schalm, O. W. 1962. A comparison of the direct and indirect methods for estimation of eosinophil numbers in blood. Calif. Vet. 16:16, 18.
5. Costello, Ronald T. 1970. A Unopette for eosinophil counts. Am. J. Clin. Pathol. 54:249-50.
6. Dodds, W. Jean, and Kaneko, J. J. 1971. Hemostasis and blood coagulation. In: Clinical Biochemistry of Domestic Animals, 2nd ed., vol. 2, J. J. Kaneko and C. E. Cornelius (eds.). Academic Press, New York.
7. Farrington, E. M., and Jetter, W. W. 1953. An improved staining solution for counting eosinophils in dogs. Am. J. Clin. Pathol. 23:836-37.

8. Finocchio, Ernest J., Coffman, James R., and Osbaldiston, George W. 1970. Platelet counts in horses. Cornell Vet. 60:518-27.
9. Gerarde, Horace W., and Anderson, Ellen. 1970. Hematology Manual. Unopette Disposable Diluting Pipette, 4th ed. Becton, Dickinson and Co., Rutherford, N.J.
10. Gerarde, Horace W. 1972. Personal communication.
11. Huntsman, Doris B., Doggett, Margaret C., and Holtkamp, Dorsey E. 1959. Hinkleman's solution as a diluent for counting eosinophils. Am. J. Clin. Pathol. 31:91-92.
12. Kaneko, J. J. 1960. Rapid tests for hemostatic defects. Calif. Vet. 13:22.
13. Miescher, P.A., and Gerarde, H. W. 1966. A one-step method for counting leukocytes and platelets. Am. J.Clin. Pathol. 46:576-81.
14. Pilot, M. L. 1950. Use of base in fluids for counting eosinophils. Am. J. Clin. Pathol. 20:870-71.
15. Schalm, O. W., and Murray, Ronald. 1964. Estimation of blood leukocyte numbers by means of a DNA viscosity test. J. Am. Vet. Med. Assoc. 145:1177-83.
16. Schalm, O. W., Jain, N. C., and Carroll, E. J. 1975. Veterinary Hematology, 3rd ed. Lea and Febiger, Philadelphia.
17. Schalm, O. W., Jain, N. C., and Carroll, E. J. 1969. Estimation of total leukocyte count in cat blood by DNA viscosity test. Calif. Vet. 23:8-11.
18. Weed, Robert I., Crump, S. Lee, and Swisher, Scott N. 1965. Evaluation of a technic for counting dog and human platelets. Blood 25:261-65.

Chapter 8

1. Andersen, A. C., and Gee, William. 1958. Normal blood values in the Beagle. Vet. Med. 53:135-38.
2. Baer, J. E., Peck, H. M., and McKinney, S. E. 1957. Some normal laboratory values in the dog. Soc. Exp. Biol. Med. Proc. 95:80-84.
3. Bild, C. E. 1956. Erythrocyte sedimentation rate and hematocrit. J. Am. Vet. Med. Assoc. 129:471-74.
4. Bloom, F. 1957. The laboratory diagnosis of canine distemper. North Am. Vet. 38:313-15.
5. Bottinger, L. E. 1967. Erythrocyte sedimentation rate and protein-bound carbohydrates in domestic animals. Acta Vet. Scand. 8:279.
6. Bunce, S. A. 1954. Observations on the blood sedimentation rate and the packed cell volume of some domestic farm animals. Brit. Vet. J. 110:322-28.
7. Coffin, D. L. 1953. Manual of Veterinary Clinical Pathology, 3rd ed. Comstock, Ithaca, New York.
8. Dalton, P. J. 1959. The erythrocyte sedimentation rate as a guide to the radio-sensitivity of neoplasms. Vet. Rec. 71:49-52.
9. Detweiler, D. K. 1959. The heart. In: Canine Medicine, 2nd ed., H. P. Hoskins (ed.). Am. Vet. Publ., Santa Barbara.
10. Eshenour, R. W., Newberne, J. W., and Burch, G. R. 1958. Accelerated (three-day) treatment with Filcide for canine heartworms. Allied Vet. 29:7-9, 22-23.
11. Ferguson, L. C. 1937. Studies on bovine blood. I. The sedimentation rate and percentage volume of erythrocytes in normal blood. J. Am. Vet. Med. Assoc. 91:163-75.
12. Gilman, A. R. 1952. The blood sedimentation rate in the horse. Am. J. Vet. Res. 13:77-82.
13. Greatorex, John C. 1957. Observations on the haematology of calves and various breeds of adult dairy cattle. Brit. Vet. J. 113:29-33.
14. Hammersland, H. L., Herrin, H. S., and Haynes, C. F. 1938. A study of the blood in horses infected with infectious anemia. J. Am. Vet. Med. Assoc. 93:320-24.
15. Holman, H. H. 1944. Studies on the haematology of sheep. I. The blood-picture of healthy sheep. J. Comp. Pathol. Therap. 54:26-40.
16. Knowles, R. P. 1955. Interpretation of white cell count, sedimentation rate and packed cell volume. Vet. Med. 50:127-30.
17. Low, Donald G., Hiatt, C. W., Gleiser, Chester A., and Bergman, E. N. 1956. Experimental canine leptospirosis. I. *Leptospira icterohemorrhagiae* infections in immature dogs. J. Inf. Dis. 98:249-59.
18. Miale, J. B. 1972. Laboratory Medicine—Hematology, 4th ed. C. V. Mosby, St. Louis.
19. Miller, S. E., and Weller, J. M. (eds.). 1971. A Textbook of Clinical Pathology, 8th ed. Williams and Wilkins, Baltimore.
20. Monlux, W. S. 1948. Leptospirosis. III. The clinical pathology of canine leptospirosis. Cornell Vet. 38:109-21.

21. Olsen, R. E. 1966. Determining the erythrocyte sedimentation rate of cattle. J. Am. Vet. Med. Assoc. 148:801-3.
22. Osbaldiston, G. W. 1971. Erythrocyte sedimentation rate studies in sheep, dog, and horse. Cornell Vet. 61:386-99.
23. Sacher, G. A. 1956. A sign of severe radiation injury observed in the erythrocyte sedimentation of dogs. Blood 11:174-83.
24. Schalm, O. W., and Wood, M. 1954. Observations on the use of certain hematological techniques in canine medicine. Am. Vet. Med. Assoc. Proc., pp. 286-94.
25. Schalm, O. W., Jain, J. C., and Carroll, E. J. 1975. Veterinary Hematology, 3rd ed. Lea and Febiger, Philadelphia.
26. Schnitzlein, W. 1968. Evaluation of the erythrocyte sedimentation reaction in laboratory cats. Z. Versuchstierkd. 10:91-106.
27. Sesaki, Kizo. 1960. Studies on the erythrocyte sedimentation rate in domestic animals. Utsunomiya Univ. Coll. Agr. Spec. Bull.
28. Simms, B. T. 1940. Erythrocyte sedimentation studies in dogs. J. Am. Vet. Med. Assoc. 96:77-80.
29. Simov, I. 1965. I. Sedimentation rate of bovine blood in tubes held at different angles. II. Effect of anti-coagulants on sedimentation rate. Nauchni. Tr. Vissh. Vet.-Med. Inst. Prof. G. Pavlov 15:47-57, 59-66.
30. Sippel, W. L. 1958. Sedimentation rate. Vet. Med. 53:339-40.
31. Tietz, W. J., Jr., Benjamin, Maxine M., and Angleton, G. M. 1967. Anemia and cholesterolemia during estrus and pregnancy in the Beagle. Am. J. Physiol. 212:693-97.
32. Torten, Michael, and Schalm, O. W. 1962. The relation of sedimentation rate of erythrocytes to packed cell volume in the horse. Calif. Vet. 16:34-36.
33. Wintrobe, M. M. 1974. Clinical Hematology, 7th ed. Lea and Febiger, Philadelphia.

Chapter 9

1. Allen, B. V., and Archer, R. K. 1973. Studies with normal erythrocytes of the English Thoroughbred horse. Equine Vet. J. 5:135-36.
2. Archer, R. K. 1955. Haematological Techniques for Use on Animals. Blackwell Scientific, Oxford.
3. Bulgin, Marie S., Munn, Susan L., and Gee, William. 1970. Hematologic changes to 4½ years of age in clinically normal Beagles. J. Am. Vet. Med. Assoc. 157:1064-70.
4. Clarkson, G. T. 1968. Haematology and serum iron in the racehorse. Thesis, Univ. of Melbourne, Australia.
5. Holman, H. H. 1956. Changes associated with age in the blood picture of calves and heifers. Brit. Vet. J. 112:91-104.
6. Johnson, Kenneth H., and Perman, Victor. 1968. Normal values for jugular blood in the cat. Vet. Med./Small Anim. Clin. 63:851-54.
7. Miller, E. R., Ullrey, D. E., Ackermann, I., Schmidt, D. A., Luecke, R. W., and Hoefer, J. A. 1961. Swine hematology from birth to maturity. II. Erythrocyte population, size and hemoglobin concentration. J. Anim. Sci. 20:890-97.
8. Schalm, O. W. 1957. The hematocrit. Calif. Vet. 10:27-28.
9. Schalm, O. W. 1975. Veterinary Hematology, 3rd ed. Lea and Febiger, Philadelphia.
10. Stewart, G. A., Clarkson, G. T., and Steel, J. D. 1970. Hematology of the racehorse and factors affecting interpretation of the blood count. Am. Assoc. Equine Pract. Proc. 16:17.
11. Sréter, F. A. 1959. The effect of systematic training on plasma electrolytes, haematocrit values, and blood sugar in Thoroughbred racehorses. Can. J. Biochem. Physiol. 37:273-83.
12. Ullrey, D. E., Miller, E. R., Long, C. H., and Vincent, B. H. 1965. Sheep hematology from birth to maturity. I. Erythrocyte population, size and hemoglobin concentration. J. Anim. Sci. 24:135-40.
13. Wintrobe, M. M. 1974. Clinical Hematology, 7th ed. Lea and Febiger, Philadelphia.

Chapter 10

1. Aanes, W. A. 1961. Pingue (*Hymenoxys richardsonii*) poisoning in sheep. Am J. Vet. Res. 22:47-52.
2. Adams, H. Richard, Dixit, Balwant N., Smookler, Harold H., and Buckley, Joseph P. 1972. Clinical and biochemical effects of chronic reserpine administration in mongrel dogs. Am. J. Vet. Res. 33:699-708.

3. Alexander, F., and Ash, R. W. 1955. The effect of emotion and hormones on the concentration of glucose and eosinophils in horse blood. J. Physiol. 130:703-10.
4. Alexander, F. 1958. The effect of adrenaline, ACTH and insulin on the circulating eosinophils of the cow. J. Comp. Pathol. Therap. 68:64-70.
5. Allen, W. M., Berrett, Sylvia, and Patterson, D. S. P. 1967. A haematological study of clinical cases of Johne's disease and the assessment of an intravenous Johnin diagnostic test. J. Comp. Pathol. 77:71-79.
6. Archer, R. K. 1957. The mechanism of eosinopenia produced by ACTH and corticoids in the horse. J. Pathol. Bact. 74:387-95.
7. Archer, R. K., and Poynter, D. 1957. Anaemia and eosinophilia associated with helminthiasis in young horses. J. Comp. Pathol. Therap. 67:196-207.
8. Archer, R. K., and Clabby, J. 1965. The effect of excitation and exertion on the circulating blood of horses. Vet. Rec. 77:689-90.
9. Arlein, M. S. 1940. So-called infectious feline enteritis or panleukopenia. North Am. Vet. 21:733-37.
10. Arthur, G. H. 1947. The diagnosis of traumatic reticulitis and pericarditis of bovines. Vet. Rec. 59:69-72.
11. Athens, J. W., Cartwright, G. E., and Wintrobe, M. M. 1958. Hematologic manifestations of lysine deficiency in swine. Soc. Exp. Biol. Med. Proc. 97:909-12.
12. Baker, J. A., Richards, M. G., Brown, A. L., and Rickard, C. G. 1950. Infectious hepatitis in dogs. Am. Vet. Med. Assoc. Proc., pp. 242-48.
13. Baker, J. A., and Gillespie, J. H. 1958. Viral diseases. II. Mod. Vet. Pract. 39:34-39.
14. Baker, W. L. 1960. Septicemia in swine. Vet. Med. 55:32-33.
15. Bell, F. N., and Irwin, M. R. 1938. Studies on the variation of the blood cells of cattle in health and during *Brucella* infections. J. Inf. Dis. 63:251-62.
16. Benjamin, M. M. 1953. Blood cytology of shipping fever in beef cattle. J. Am. Vet. Med. Assoc. 123:209-12.
17. Benjamin, M. M., and Lumb, W. V. 1959. *Haemobartonella canis* infection in a dog. J. Am. Vet. Med. Assoc. 135:388-90.
18. Bentinck-Smith, John. 1949. Feline panleukopenia (feline infectious enteritis). North Am. Vet. 30:379-84.
19. Bentinck-Smith, J., Kennedy, P. C., and Saunders, L. Z. 1952. Histoplasmosis in a dog. Cornell Vet. 42:61-66.
20. Blake, Joseph T. 1965. Certain hematopathologic conditions associated with brisket disease. Am. J. Vet. Res. 26:68-75.
21. Bloom, Frank. 1944. The blood and bone marrow in pyometra. North Am. Vet. 25:483-84, 486, 488.
22. Bloom, Frank. 1957. The laboratory diagnois of canine leptospirosis. North Am. Vet. 38:273-76, 284.
23. Bloom, Frank. 1957. The laboratory diagnosis of canine distemper. North Am. Vet. 38:313-15.
24. Bohn, H. E. 1962. The effects of *Ancylostoma caninum* on the hemogram of the dog. Southeastern Vet. 13: 58-60, 64, 67.
25. Bohning, Richard H., Suter, Peter F., Hohn, R. Bruce, and Marshall, John. 1970. Clinical and radiologic survey of canine panosteitis. J. Am. Vet. Med. Assoc. 156:870-83.
26. Bond, E., and Kubin, R. 1949. Lead poisoning in dogs. Vet. Med. 44:118-23.
27. Borson, H. J., and Mettier, S. R. 1940. Relief of hypochromic anemia in dogs with synthetic vitamin B_6: Influence of "filtrate factors." Soc. Exp. Biol. Med. Proc. 43:429-32.
28. Britton, J. W. 1946. Changes of the blood constituents in diseases of ruminants. Cornell Vet. 36:25-30.
29. Brown, J. M., Kingrey, B. W., and Rosenquist, B. D. 1959. The hematology of chronic reticuloperitonitis. Am. J. Vet. Res. 20:255-64.
30. Bunce, D. F. M. II. 1956. Urinary problems in small animals. I. Cystitis and its treatment. North Am. Vet. 37:765-69.
31. Burnett, S. H. 1917. The Clinical Pathology of the Blood of Domesticated Animals. Macmillan, N.Y.
32. Burnside, J. E., and Sippel, W. L. 1956. Trichloroethylene-extracted soybean oil meal poisoning. In: Diseases of Cattle, M. G. Fincher (ed.). Am. Vet. Publ., Evanston, Ill.
33. Burrows, George E., and Cannon, Joseph. 1970. Endotoxemia induced by rapid intravenous injection of *Escherichia coli* in anesthetized ponies. Am. J. Vet. Res. 31:1967-73.
34. Burrows, George E. 1971. *Escherichia coli* endotoxemia in the conscious pony. Am. J. Vet. Res. 32:243-48.
35. Carll, W. T., Forgacs, J., Herring, A. S., and Mahlandt, B. G. 1955. Toxicity of *Aspergillus fumigatus* substrates to animals. Vet. Med. 50:210-12.
36. Carroll, E. J., Schalm, O. W., and Wheat, J. D. 1965. Endotoxemia in a horse. J. Am. Vet. Med. Assoc. 146: 1300-1303.

37. Christian, R. G., and Tryphonas, L. 1971. Lead poisoning in cattle: Brain lesions and hematologic changes. Am. J. Vet. Res. 32:203-16.

38. Christensen, J. F. 1963. Protozoal diseases: Anaplasmosis. In: Diseases of Cattle, 2nd ed., W. J. Gibbons (ed). Am. Vet. Publ., Santa Barbara, Calif.

39. Churchill, E. A. 1950. Diagnosis and surgical treatment of traumatic gastritis. J. Am. Vet. Med. Assoc. 116: 196-98.

40. Coffin, D. L., and Cabasso, V. J. 1953. The blood and urine findings in infectious canine hepatitis. Am. J. Vet. Res. 14:254-59.

41. Cole, C. G. 1932. Leucocyte counts on the blood of normal, cholera-infected and recently immunized pigs. J. Am. Vet. Med. Assoc. 81:392-400.

42. Collette, W. L., and Meriwether, W. F. 1965. Some changes in the peripheral blood of dogs after administration of certain tranquilizers and narcotics. Vet. Med./Small Anim. Clin. 60:1223-26.

43. Conner, G. H. 1945. Prognostic value of blood determinations in certain surgical conditions of the horse. Am. J. Vet. Res. 6:45-53.

44. Cordy, D. R., and Gorham, J. R. 1950. The pathology and etiology of salmon disease in the dog and fox. Am. J. Pathol. 26:617-37.

45. Cox, D. H., and Pitts, J. C. 1957. The clinical picture of salt poisoning of swine. J. Am. Vet. Med. Assoc. 130:176-77.

46. Crafts, R. C. 1948. The effects of estrogens on the bone marrow of adult female dogs. Blood 3:276-85.

47. Curtin, T. M., Goetsch, G. D., and Hollandbeck, R. 1963. Clinical and pathologic characterization of esophago-gastric ulcers in swine. J. Am. Vet. Med. Assoc. 143:854-60.

48. Dalton, R. G., Fisher, E. W., and McIntyre, W. I. M. 1965. Changes in blood chemistry, body weight and haematocrit of calves affected with neonatal diarrhoea. Brit. Vet. J. 121:34-41.

49. Davis, J. W., and Libke, K. G. 1968. Hematologic studies in pigs fed clay pigeon targets. J. Am. Vet. Med. Assoc. 152:382-84.

50. Davis, J. W., and Smibert, R. M. 1963. Studies on hemolytic *Escherichia coli* associated with edema disease of swine. III. The effect of hemolytic and nonhemolytic *Escherichia coli* endotoxin on the blood of swine. Am. J. Vet. Res. 24:324-28.

51. Delaune, Elaine. 1939. Observations on the bovine blood picture in health and under parasitism. Soc. Exp. Biol. Med. Proc. 41:482-83.

52. De Tray, D., and Scott, G. 1957. Blood changes in swine with African swine fever. Am. J. Vet. Res. 18: 484-90.

53. Donovan, E. F., and Loeb, W. F. 1959. Polycythemia rubra vera in the dog. J. Am. Vet. Med. Assoc. 134:36-37.

54. Dreguss, M. N., and Lombard, L. S. 1954. Experimental Studies in Equine Infectious Anemia. Univ. Pa. Press, Philadelphia.

55. Drudge, J. H., Lyons, E. T., and Szanto, Joseph. 1966. Pathogenesis of migrating stages of helminths, with special reference to *Strongylus vulgaris*. In: Biology of Parasites. Academic Press, New York.

56. Dunne, H. W. 1975. Hog cholera. In: Diseases of Swine, 4rd ed., H. W. Dunne and A. D. Leman (eds.). Iowa State Univ. Press, Ames.

57. Easterday, B. C., Murphy, L. C., and Bennett, D. G. 1962. Experimental Rift Valley fever in calves, goats, and pigs. Am. J. Vet. Res. 23:1224-30.

58. Easterday, B. C.; Murphy, L. C., and Bennett, D. G. 1962. Experimental Rift Valley fever in lambs and sheep. Am. J. Vet. Res. 23:1231-39.

59. El Hindawy, M. R. 1950. Studies on the blood of dogs. IV. Haematological findings in the dogs suffering from some common diseases. (a) Pneumonia; (b) Distemper. Brit. Vet. J. 106:119-27.

60. Eshenour, R. W., Newberne, J. W., and Burch, G. R. 1958. Accelerated (three-day) treatment with Filcide for canine heartworms. Allied Vet. 29:7-9, 22-23.

61. Evans, J. V., Blunt, M. H., and Southcott, W. H. 1963. The effects of infection with *Haemonchus contortus* on the sodium and potassium concentrations in the erythrocyte and plasma in sheep of different haemoglobin types. Aust. J. Agric. Res. 14:549-58.

62. Ferguson, L. C., Irwin, M. R., and Beach, B. A. 1941. The effect of parturition on the blood picture of cows in health and during infection with *Brucella abortus*. Am. J. Vet. Res. 2:394-99.

63. Ferguson, L. C., Irwin, M. R., and Beach, B. A. 1945. Variations in the blood picture of cattle following an induced infection with *Brucella abortus*. J. Inf. Dis. 76:31-39.

64. Ferguson, L. C. 1970. Leptospirosis. In: Diseases of Swine, 3rd ed., H. W. Dunne (ed.). Iowa State Univ. Press, Ames.
65. Fitzgerald, Paul R., and Mansfield, M. E. 1972. Effects of bovine coccidiosis on certain blood components, feed consumption, and body weight changes of calves. Am. J. Vet. Res. 33:1391-97.
66. Flint, J. C., Roepke, M. H., and Jensen, R. 1958. Feline infectious anemia. I. Clinical aspects. Am. J. Vet. Res. 19:164-68.
67. Follis, R. H., Jr. 1958. Deficiency Disease. Charles C. Thomas, Springfield, Ill.
68. Fowler, Murray E. 1965. Clinical manifestations of primary hepatic insufficiency in the horse. J. Am. Vet. Med. Assoc. 147:55-64.
69. George, L. A., Hackett, P. L., and Bustad, L. K. 1957. Leukocytic response in lambs exposed to whole-body X irradiation. J. Am. Vet. Res. 18:631-33.
70. Gerber, H. 1969. Clinical features, sequelae and epidemiology of equine influenza. Equine Inf. Dis. 2nd Int. Conf. Proc., Paris.
71. Gibbons, W. J., and Wiggins, A. M. 1970. Bracken poisoning. In: Bovine Medicine and Surgery, W. J. Gibbons, E. J. Catcott, and J. F. Smithcors (eds.). Am. Vet. Publ., Wheaton, Ill.
72. Gillespie, J. H. 1952. Clinical features of infectious canine hepatitis. Am. Vet. Med. Assoc. Proc., pp. 224-25.
73. Gillespie, J. H., Lee, K. M., and Baker, J. A. 1957. Infectious bovine rhinotracheitis. Am. J. Vet. Res. 18:530-35.
74. Goetsch, D. D., McDonald, L. E., and Odell, G. 1959. The effects of four synthetic corticosteroids on leukocytes, blood glucose, and plasma sodium and potassium in the cow. Am. J. Vet. Res. 20:697-701.
75. Graca, J. G., and Garst, E. L. 1957. Early blood changes in dogs following intravenous pentobarbital anesthesia. Anesthesiology 18:461-65.
76. Greatorex, J. C. 1958. Changes in the blood picture of calves following vaccination with *Brucella abortus* (strain 19) vaccine. J. Comp. Pathol. Therap. 68:36-44.
77. Greenway, J. A., and McCraw, B. M. 1970. *Ascaris suum* infection in calves. II. Circulating and marrow eosinophil responses. Can. J. Comp. Med. 34:238-46.
78. Gwatkin, R., and L'Ecuyer, C. 1960. Rhinitis of swine. XIV. Haematology of infected and normal pigs. Can. J. Comp. Med. Vet. Sci. 24:6-9.
79. Haigler, S. W., and Hawkins, H. P. 1940. Pyometra in dogs. North Am. Vet. 21:743-44.
80. Hall, C. E., and Bryans, J. T. 1954. A case of leptospirosis in a horse. Cornell Vet. 44:345-48.
81. Heuschele, W. P., and Barber, T. L. 1963. Hematologic studies of rinderpest-infected swine. Can. J. Comp. Med. Vet. Sci. 27:56-60.
82. Hillman, Robert S. 1969. Hematology Laboratory Manual. Univ. Wash. Med. School.
83. Hirsch, J. G., and Church, A. B. 1961. Adrenal steroids and infection: The effect of cortisone administration on polymorphonuclear leukocytic functions and on serum opsonins and bactericidins. J. Clin. Invest. 40:794-802.
84. Hjerpe, C. A. 1961. Studies on acute bovine traumatic reticulo-peritonitis. III. Hematology. J. Am. Vet. Med. Assoc. 139:233-35.
85. Hjerpe, C. A. 1963. Clinical and hematologic observations on acute indigestion in dairy cattle. J. Am. Vet. Med. Assoc. 143:1322-25.
86. Hoe, C. M., and Wilkinson, J. S. 1957. A diluting effect of chlorpromazine hydrochloride on the circulating blood of dogs. Vet. Rec. 69:734-35.
87. Hoerlein, A. B., and Marsh, C. L. 1957. Studies on the epizootiology of shipping fever in calves. J. Am. Vet. Med. Assoc. 131:123-27.
88. Holman, H. H. 1945. Studies on the haematology of sheep. IV. Erythrocytic and thrombocytic pictures, and variations in physical attributes. J. Comp. Pathol. Therap. 55:146-57.
89. Holzworth, Jean. 1958. Disease conditions prominent in cats. Univ. Pa. Bull., Vet. Ext. Quart. 151:101-15.
90. James, Lynn F., and Binns, Wayne. 1967. Blood changes associated with locoweed poisoning. Am. J. Vet. Res. 28:1107-10.
91. Jennings, A. R. 1952. The peripheral blood picture in some diseases of animals. J. Comp. Pathol. Therap. 62:161-77.
92. Jennings, P. B., Simmons, R. L., Sleeman, H. K., and Hardaway, R. M. 1968. III. Hemodynamic, biochemical and coagulation alterations in endotoxin shock: Modification by induced tolerance in the dog. Ann. Surg. 167: 204-14.
93. Johnston, R. J. 1957. Feline pneumonitis and panleucopenia. Vet. Med. 52:499.
94. Jones, E. W. 1959. Gastric obstruction in cattle. Mod. Vet. Pract. 40:35-39.

95. Jones, T. C. 1969. Clinical and pathologic features of equine viral arteritis. II. J. Am. Vet. Med. Assoc. 155: 315-17.
96. Kernkamp, H. C. H. 1964. Pasteurellosis. In: Diseases of Swine, 2nd ed., H. W. Dunne (ed.). Iowa State Univ. Press, Ames.
97. Kernkamp, H. C. H. 1964. Coal-tar poisoning and mercury poisoning. In: Diseases of Swine, 2nd ed., H. W. Dunne (ed.). Iowa State Univ. Press, Ames.
98. Khuen, E. C., Park, S. E., and Adler, A. E., Jr. 1940. The hemogram in the differential diagnosis of metritis and pyometra. North Am. Vet. 21:666-70.
99. Kingrey, B. W. 1955. Experimental bovine traumatic gastritis. J. Am. Med. Assoc. 127:477-82.
100. Kirkham, Wayne W., Guttridge, Harold, Bowden, John, and Edds, George T. 1971. Hematopoietic response to hematinics in horses. J. Am. Vet. Med. Assoc. 159:1316-18.
101. Kirkpatrick, W. C., Roller, M. H., and Swanson, R. N. 1972. Hemogram of sheep acutely intoxicated with ammonia. Am. J. Vet. Res. 34:587-89.
102. Kleine, Lawrence J., Zook, Bernard C., and Munson, Todd O. 1970. Primary cardiac hemangiosarcomas in dogs. J. Am. Vet. Med. Assoc. 157:326-37.
103. Kral, Frank. 1958. Allergic dermatosis in small animals. Mod. Vet. Pract. 39:22-23.
104. Lawrence, J. S., Syverton, J. T., Shaw, J. S., and Smith, F. P. 1940. Infectious feline agranulocytosis. Am. J. Pathol. 16:333-54.
105. Lee, K. M., Moro, M., and Baker, J. A. 1954. Transmissible gastroenteritis in pigs. Am. J. Vet. Res. 15:364-72.
106. Lewis, P. A., and Shope, R. E. 1929. The blood in hog cholera. J. Exp. Med. 50:719.
107. Link, R. P., and Pensinger, Robert R. 1966. Lead toxicosis in swine. Am. J. Vet. Res. 27:759-63.
108. Link, R. P. 1975. Toxic plants, rodenticides, herbicides, and yellow fat disease. In: Diseases of Swine, 4th ed., H. W. Dunne and A. D. Leman (eds.). Iowa State Univ. Press, Ames.
109. Low, D. C. 1954. Pyometra in the bitch. Vet. Med. 49:527-30.
110. Luedke, A. J., Bowne, J. G., Jochim, M. M., and Doyle, C. 1964. Clinical and pathologic features of bluetongue in sheep. Am. J. Vet. Res. 25:963-70.
111. Luke, D. 1953. The reaction of the white blood cells at parturition in the sow. Brit. Vet. J. 109:241-44.
112. Luke, D. 1953. The effect of adrenocorticotrophic hormone and adrenal cortical extract on the differential white blood cell count in the pig. Brit. Vet. J. 109:434-36.
113. McChesney, A. E., England, J. J., Adcock, J. L., Stackhouse, L. L., and Chow, T. L. 1970. Adenoviral infection in suckling Arabian foals. Vet. Pathol. 7:547-65.
114. McChesney, A. E., England, J. J., and Rich, L. J. 1973. Adenoviral infection in foals. J. Am. Vet. Med. Assoc. 162:545-49.
115. McKercher, D. G., and Saito, J. K. 1951. Feline pneumonitis in California. Calif. Vet. 5:15-16.
116. McSherry, B. J., and Smith, D. L. T. 1953. Hematological changes noted in three dogs experimentally infected with the virus of infectious canine hepatitis. Cornell Vet. 43:104-9.
117. Mahrt, J. L., Hammond, D. M., and Miner, M. L. 1964. Changes in serum proteins and other blood values associated with experimental *Ostertagia ostertagi* infections in calves. Cornell Vet. 54:453-74.
118. Marshak, R. R., Webster, G. D., and Skelley, J. F. 1960. Observations on a case of primary adrenocortical insufficiency in a dog. J. Am. Vet. Med. Assoc. 136:274-80.
119. Martin, J. E., Skillen, R. G., and Deubler, M. J. 1954. The action of adrenocorticotropic hormone on circulating eosinophils in dogs—A proposed screening method for evaluating adrenal cortical function. Am. J. Vet. Res. 15:489-94.
120. Matteson, A. M., Ebert, E. F., and Case, A. A. 1953. The value of blood counts in traumatic gastritis. Vet. Med. 48:345-48.
121. Maurer, F. D. 1970. Rinderpest. In: Bovine Medicine and Surgery, W. J. Gibbons, E. J. Catcott, and J. F. Smithcors (eds.). Am. Vet. Publ., Wheaton, Ill.
122. Meier, H., Clark, S. T., Schnelle, G. B., and Will, D. H. 1957. Hypertrophic osteodystrophy associated with disturbance of vitamin C synthesis in dogs. J. Am. Vet. Med. Assoc. 130:483-91.
123. Mercer, H. D., Neal, F. C., Himes, J. A., and Edds, G. T. 1967. *Cassia occidentalis* toxicosis in cattle. J. Am. Vet. Med. Assoc. 151:735-41.
124. Miller, W. T. 1932-1933. Erythrocyte, leukocyte and hemoglobin determinations on the blood of cattle, with a note on the blood in Johne's disease. New York State Vet. Coll. Ann. Rept.
125. Moberg, Ralph. 1955. The White Blood Picture in Sexually Mature Female Cattle with Special Reference to Sexual Conditions. A Clinical and Experimental Study. Almqvist & Wiksells, Uppsala.

126. Monlux, W. S. 1948. Leptospirosis. III. The clinical pathology of canine leptospirosis. Cornell Vet. 38:109-21.
127. Moore, G. R. 1946. The blood picture in cases of retained fetal membranes in cattle. J. Am. Vet. Med. Assoc. 109:39-45.
128. Morris, M. L., Allison, J. B., and White, J. I. 1942. The effects of hyperplastic endometritis on the blood cytology of the dog. Am. J. Vet. Res. 3:100-105.
129. Morris, P. G. D. 1944. Blood picture of a cow during a normal pregnancy and parturition. Brit. Vet. J. 100:225-33.
130. Morter, R. J., Williams, R. D., Bolte, H., and Freeman, M. J. 1969. Equine leptospirosis. J. Am. Vet. Med. Assoc. 155:436-42.
131. Mosier, J. E., and Coles, E. H. 1958. Urinary tract infection of small animals. Vet. Med. 53:649-54.
132. Moulton, J. E., Cornelius, C. E., and Osburn, B. I. 1963. Acute pulmonary emphysema in cattle. J. Am. Vet. Med. Assoc. 142:133-37.
133. Munson, T. O., Holzworth, J., Small, E., Witzel, S., Jones, T. C., and Luginbühl, H. 1958. Steatitis ("yellow fat") in cats fed canned red tuna. J. Am. Vet. Med. Assoc. 133:563-68.
134. Muylle, E., and Oyaert, W. 1966. Effect of coli endotoxin on some blood constituents of the pig. Zentralbl. Veterinaermed [A] 13:405-9.
135. Nachreiner, R. F., Ginther, O. J., Ribelin, W. E., and Carlson, I. H. 1971. Pathologic and endocrinologic changes associated with porcine agalactia. Am. J. Vet. Res. 32:1065-75.
136. Nachreiner, R. F., and Ginther, O. J. 1972. Porcine agalactia: Hematologic, serum chemical, and clinical changes during the preceding gestation. Am. J. Vet. Res. 33:799-809.
137. Nafstad, Inger. 1965. Studies of hematology and bone marrow morphology in vitamin-E deficit pigs. Pathol. Vet. 2:277-87.
138. Nelson, A. W., Collier, J. R., and Griner, L. A. 1968. Acute surgical colonic infarction in the horse. Am. J. Vet. Res. 29:315-27.
139. Newberne, J. W., Neal, J. E., and Heath, M. K. 1955. Some clinical and microbiological observations on four cases of canine blastomycosis. J. Am. Vet. Med. Assoc. 127:220-23.
140. Newberne, J. W., Bittle, J. L., and Mayer, K. 1959. Clinical differentiation of feline viral diseases. Allied Vet. 30:50-53.
141. Nisbet, D. I., Butler, E. J., and MacIntyre, I. J. 1959. Muscular dystrophy in experimental lambs. J. Comp. Pathol. Therap. 69:339-52.
142. Nunamaker, D. M., Medway, W., and Berg, P. 1971. Treatment of ethylene glycol poisoning in the dog. J. Am. Vet. Med. Assoc. 159:310-14.
143. Olson, C., Jr., Cook, R. H., and Blore, I. C. 1950. The reaction of blood cells in experimental listeriosis of sheep. Am. J. Vet. Res. 11:29-40.
144. Osborne, Carl A., Low, Donald G., and Finco, Delmar R. 1972. Canine and Feline Urology. Saunders, Philadelphia.
145. Osweiler, Gary D., and Eness, P. G. 1972. Ethylene glycol poisoning in swine. J. Am. Vet. Med. Assoc. 160: 746-49.
146. Perman, V., and Stevens, J. B. 1971. Leukocyte responses in health and disease. Am. Anim. Hosp. Assoc. Proc.
147. Pierson, R. E., and Aanes, W. A. 1958. Treatment of chronic copper poisoning in sheep. J. Am. Vet. Med. Assoc. 133:307-11.
148. Plowright, W. 1953. The blood leucocytes in infectious malignant catarrh of the ox and rabbit. J. Comp. Pathol. Therap. 63:318-34.
149. Pollack, S. 1956. Prostatic abscess in the dog. J. Am. Vet. Med. Assoc. 129:274-75.
150. Powers, K. G., Todd, A. C., and McNutt, S. H. 1960. Experimental infections of swine with *Trichuris suis*. Am. J. Vet. Res. 21:262-68.
151. Pritchard, W. R., and Carlson, R. G. 1957. Symposium on the mucosal disease complex. III. Virus diarrhea in cattle. J. Am. Vet. Med. Assoc. 130:383-85.
152. Raker, C. W., and English, Blair. 1959. Promazine—Its pharmacological and clinical effects in horses. J. Am. Vet. Med. Assoc. 134:19-24.
153. Ramsey, F. K., and Chivers, W. H. 1957. Symposium on the mucosal disease complex. II. Pathology of a mucosal disease of cattle. J. Am. Vet. Med. Assoc. 130:381-83.
154. Records, E., and Vawter, L. R. 1945. Bacillary hemoglobinuria of cattle and sheep. Univ. Neb. Agr. Exp. Bull. 173:1-48.

155. Reda, H., and Hathout, A. F. 1951. The hematologic examination of the blood of sheep under physiologic and pathologic conditions. J. Am. Vet. Med. Assoc. 118:253-55.
156. Report of the panel for the symposium on immunity to bovine respiratory disease complex. 1968. J. Am. Vet. Med. Assoc. 152:713-19.
157. Rice, C. E., Konst, H., and Carrière, J. 1964. Studies of Johne's disease in Canada. XI. Complement-fixation titres and blood cell picture. Can. J. Comp. Med. Vet. Sci. 28:248-52.
158. Roberts, S. J. 1957. Winter dysentery in dairy cattle. Cornell Vet. 47:372-88.
159. Robertson, J. M. 1965. Diagnosis of left displacement of the bovine abomasum. J. Am. Vet. Med. Assoc. 146: 820-27.
160. Rodgers, S. E. 1965. Observations on the eosinophil leukocyte response and its specificity after vaccination and infection of cattle with *Dictyocaulus viviparus*. Vet. Rec. 77:92.
161. Roenigk, W. J. 1955. Observations on kennel cough. Speculum 8:16, 58.
162. Rooney, J. R., Bryans, J. T., and Doll, E. R. 1963. Colitis "X" of horses. J. Am. Vet. Med. Assoc. 142:510-11.
163. Rosner, Stephen F. 1968. Infectious bovine rhinotracheitis: Clinical review, immunity, and control. J. Am. Vet. Med. Assoc. 153:1631-38.
164. Rubin, R., and Lucker, J. T. 1956. The course and pathogenicity of initial infections with *Dictyocaulus viviparus*, the lungworm of cattle. Am. J. Vet. Res. 17:217-26.
165. Ryff, J. F. 1957. Brisket disease syndrome. J. Am. Vet. Med. Assoc. 131:425-30.
166. Sarles, M. P. 1929. Studies on the blood changes occurring in young and old dogs during cutaneous and oral infection with the dog hookworm, *Ancylostoma caninum*. Am. J. Hyg. 10:693-704.
167. Schalm, O. W. 1958. The leukocytes. Calif. Vet. 12:18-19.
168. Schalm, O. W. 1962. Equine clinical hematology. Am. Assoc. Equine Pract. Proc. 8:107-22.
169. Schalm, O. W. 1963. Interpretation of leukocyte responses in the dog. J. Am. Vet. Med. Assoc. 142:147-53.
170. Schalm, O. W., and Hughes, J. P. 1964. Some observations on physiologic leukocytosis in the cat and horse. Calif. Vet. 18:23-25.
171. Schalm, O. W., Jain, N. C., and Carroll, E. J. 1975. Veterinary Hematology, 3rd ed. Lea and Febiger, Philadelphia.
172. Schalm, O. W., Lasmanis, J., and Carroll, E. J. 1965. The use of a synthetic corticoid on experimental coliform (*Aerobacter aerogenes*) mastitis in cattle: The response of leukocytes and the effect of hormone-induced neutrophilia. Am. J. Vet. Res. 26:851-64.
173. Schalm, O. W., Hughes, John, and Hardy, Dennis. 1967. Dynamics of the neutrophil leukocyte and a unique response in acute indigestion in the cow. Calif. Vet. 21:20-23.
174. Schalm, O. W. 1970. The blood and blood-forming organs. In: Bovine Medicine and Surgery, W. J. Gibbons, E. J. Catcott, and J. F. Smithcors (eds.). Am. Vet. Publ., Wheaton, Ill.
175. Schwarte, L. H. 1964. Listeriosis. In: Diseases of Swine, 2nd ed., H. W. Dunne (ed.). Iowa State Univ. Press, Ames.
176. Shouse, C. L., and Meier, H. 1956. Acute vegetative endocarditis in the dog and cat. J. Am. Vet. Med. Assoc. 129:278-89.
177. Shuman, R. D., and Wood, R. L. 1970. Swine erysipelas. In: Diseases of Swine, 3rd ed., H. W. Dunne (ed.). Iowa State Univ. Press, Ames.
178. Siebold, H. R., and Bailey, W. S. 1957. Babesiasis (piroplasmosis) in dogs. J. Am. Vet. Med. Assoc. 130:46-48.
179. Sippel, W. L. 1952. White blood cell count in hog cholera. Vet. Med. 47:497-501.
180. Sippel, W. L. 1975. Moldy corn poisoning, vulvovaginitis, and ergotism. In: Diseases of Swine, 4th ed., H. W. Dunne and A. D. Leman (eds.). Iowa State Univ. Press, Ames.
181. Soliman, M. K., Amrousi, S. El, Khamis, M. Y. 1965. The influence of tranquillisers and barbiturate anaesthesia on the blood picture and electrolytes of dogs. Vet. Rec. 77:1256-58.
182. Storz, J., Kaneko, J. J., and Wada, E. M. 1962. The leukocytic response of cows and calves to acute infection with an agent of the psittacosis-lymphogranuloma group. Am. J. Vet. Res. 23:1200-1204.
183. Straub, O. C., Schalm, O. W., Hughes, J. P., and Theilen, G. H. 1959. Bovine hematology. II. Effect of parturition and retention of fetal membranes on blood morphology. J. Am. Vet. Med. Assoc. 135:618-22.
184. Stünzi, Von H., and Poppensiek, G. C. 1952. Zur Pathogenese der Hepatitis contagiosa canis. I. Teil: Perakute und akute Krankheitsstadien. Schweiz. Z. Allg. Path. Bakt. 15:722-34.
185. Theilen, G. H., Schalm, O. W., Straub, O. C., and Hughes, J. P. 1959. Bovine hematology. I. Leukocyte response to acute bovine mastitis. J. Am. Vet. Med. Assoc. 135:481-85.

186. Thordal-Christensen, A. 1957. Infectious canine hepatitis (Rubarth). Univ. Pa. Bull., Vet. Ext. Quart. 145: 36-88.
187. Torten, M., and Schalm, O. W. 1964. Influence of the equine spleen on rapid changes in the concentration of erythrocytes in peripheral blood. Am. J. Vet. Res. 25:500-504.
188. Trautman, A., and Fiebiger, J. 1952. Fundamentals of the Histology of Domestic Animals. Comstock, Ithaca, New York.
189. Tumbleson, M. E., Burks, M. F., Spate, M. P., Hutcheson, D. P., and Middleton, C. C. 1970. Serum biochemical and hematological parameters of Sinclair (S-1) miniature sows during gestation and lactation. Can. J. Comp. Med. 34:312-19.
190. Ullrey, D. E., Miller, E. R., Long, C. H., and Vincent, B. H. 1965. Sheep hematology from birth to maturity. II. Leukocyte concentration and differential distribution. J. Anim. Sci. 24:141-44.
191. Van Kruiningen, H. J., and Bartholomew, R. C. 1964. Infectious bovine rhinotracheitis diagnosed by lesions in a calf. J. Am. Vet. Med. Assoc. 244:1008-12.
192. Van Kruiningen, H. J. 1966. Granulomatous colitis of dogs. In: Newer Knowledge about Dogs. Sixteenth Gaines Vet. Symp., Gaines Res. Center, Philadelphia, pp. 19-24.
193. Van Pelt, R. W., and Riley, W. F., Jr. 1969. Clinicopathologic findings and therapy in septic arthritis in foals. J. Am. Vet. Med. Assoc. 155:1467-80.
194. Van Wyk, J. J., Baxter, J. H., Akeroyd, J. H., and Motulsky, A. G. 1953. The anemia of copper deficiency in dogs compared with that produced by iron deficiency. Johns Hopkins Hosp. Bull. 93:41-49.
195. Villalobos, T. J., Adelson, E., and Barila, T. G. 1955. Hematologic changes in hypothermic dogs. Soc. Exp. Biol. Med. Proc. 89:192-96.
196. Wass, Wallace M., and Hoyt, Harvey H. 1965. Bovine congenital porphyria: Hematologic studies, including porphyrin analyses. Am. J. Vet. Res. 26:659-67.
197. Weber, T. B., and Rubin, Robert. 1958. The eosinophilic response to infection with the cattle lungworm, *Dictyocaulus viviparus*. J. Inf. Dis. 102:214-18.
198. Weide, K. D., and Twiehaus, M. J. 1959. Hematological studies of normal, ascarid-infected, and hog cholera vaccinated swine. Am. J. Vet. Res. 20:562-67.
199. Westermarck, H. 1952. Studies on the condition and the blood composition of emaciated horses treated with certain nutritional supplements during recovery and during contagious bronchopneumonia. Diss., Vet. Coll., Helsinki, Finland.
200. Whitehair, C. K., and Miller, E. R. 1975. Nutritional deficiencies. In: Diseases of Swine, 4th ed., H. W. Dunne and A. D. Leman (eds.). Iowa State Univ. Press, Ames.
201. Whitlock, J. H. 1950. The anemias in the trichostongylidoses. Cornell Vet. 40:288-89.
202. Whitney, J. C. 1957. Atrophic myositis in a dog: The differentiation of this disease from eosinophilic myositis. Vet. Rec. 69:130-31.
203. Will, D. H., Alexander, A. F., Reeves, J. T., and Grover, R. F. 1962. High altitude-induced pulmonary hypertension in normal cattle. Circ. Res. 10:172-77.
204. Winter, A. J., and Hokanson, J. F. 1964. Effects of long-term feeding of nitrate, nitrite, or hydroxylamine on pregnant dairy heifers. Am. J. Vet. Res. 25:353-61.
205. Winter, H., and Stephenson, H. C. 1952. A case of eosinophilic myositis in a dog. Cornell Vet. 42:531-37.
206. Wintrobe, M. M. 1974. Clinical Hematology, 7th ed. Lea and Febiger, Philadelphia.
207. York, C. J. 1956. Miscellaneous and unclassified diseases. In: Diseases of Cattle, M. G. Fincher (ed.). Am. Vet. Publ., Evanston, Ill.
208. Younger, R. L., and Young, J. E. 1963. Toxicologic studies and associated clinical and hematologic effects of apholate (an alkylating agent) in sheep. A preliminary report. Am. J. Vet. Res. 24:659-69.
209. Zarrow, M. X., Denison, M. E., Rosenberg, B., Mann, D. E., Jr., and Neher, G. M. 1952. Effect of insulin and epinephrine on the eosinophil and blood glucose levels in sheep; lack of diurnal rhythm. Am. J. Physiol. 171: 636-40.
210. Zook, B. C., and Gilmore, C. E. 1967. Thallium poisoning in dogs. J. Am. Vet. Med. Assoc. 151:206-17.
211. Zook, B. C., Carpenter, J. L., and Leeds, E. B. 1969. Lead poisoning in dogs. J. Am. Vet. Med. Assoc. 155: 1329-42.

Chapter 11

1. Archer, R. K. 1965. Haematological Techniques for Use on Animals. Blackwell Scientific, Oxford.
2. Bennington, James L., Fouty, Robert A., and Hougie, Cecil. 1970. Laboratory Diagnosis. Macmillan, Toronto.
3. Bjørneboe, M. 1943. Serum proteins during immunization. Acta Pathol. Microbiol. Scand. 20:221-39.
4. Boguth, W. 1954. Papierelektrophoretische Serumuntersuchungen bei Haussäugetierem. (Paper electrophoretic serum examination of domestic animals.) I. Zentralbl. Veterinaermed. Band I:168-87.
5. Boguth, W. 1954. Papierelektrophoretische Serumuntersuchungen bei Haussäugetierem. II. Zentralbl. Veterinaermed. Band I:311-29.
6. Bradish, C. J., Henderson, W. M., and Brooksby, J. B. 1954. Electrophoretic studies of ox serum. I. The sera of normal cattle. Biochem. J. 56:329-35.
7. Bradish, C. J., Henderson, W. M., and Brooksby, J. B. 1954. Electrophoretic studies of ox serum. II. The sera of cattle injected with the virus of foot-and-mouth disease. Biochem. J. 56:335-41.
8. Contreras, A. G. 1967. Electrophoretic and immuno-electrophoretic research on blood serum of domestic ruminants. Arch. Zootec. 16:257-86.
9. Cornelius, C. E. 1957. New concepts and methods in the laboratory diagnosis of canine liver disease. Seventh Gaines Vet. Symp.
10. Dalton, R. G. 1967. Variations in calf plasma composition with age. Brit. Vet. J. 123:48-52.
11. Dalton, R. G. 1972. The significance of variations with activity and sedation in the haematocrit, plasma protein concentration and erythrocyte sedimentation rate of horses. Brit. Vet. J. 128:439-45.
12. Deavers, S., Huggins, R. A., and Smith, E. L. 1971. Extravascular-vascular distribution of I-131-tagged albumin in the growing Beagle. Am. J. Vet. Res. 32:1169-77.
13. Dimopoullos, George T. 1970. Plasma proteins. In: Clinical Biochemistry of Domestic Animals, vol. 1, 2nd ed., J. J. Kaneko and C. E. Cornelius (eds.). Academic Press, New York.
14. Forstner, M. J. 1967. Electrophoretic examination of serum from helminth-infected slaughter pigs. Dtsch. Tieraerztl. Wochenschr. 94:392-94.
15. Gleason, Thomas L., and Friedberg, Felix. 1953. Filter-paper electrophoresis of serum proteins. Physiol. Zool. 26:95-100.
16. Gorczyca, L. R., McCarty, R. T., and Lazaroni, J. A., Jr. 1960. Further study of goat serum proteins by paper electrophoresis. Am. J. Vet. Res. 21:851-55.
17. Greenberg, L. D., Hoessly, U. J. P., Brooks, R., and Rinehart, J. F. 1952. Electrophoretic studies on serum and plasma of control and vitamin-deficient monkeys. Soc. Exp. Biol. Med. Proc. 79:425-30.
18. Hort, I. 1968. Paper electrophoretic fractionation and chemical determination of horse serum proteins and lipoproteins. Am. J. Vet. Res. 29:813-15.
19. Howarth, William A., Luck, David R., Sinton, Eleanor, and Taylor, Tim. 1972. I. The use of a Technicon SMA autoanalyzer in small animal practice. II. The use of 2-(4-hydroxyazobenzene)-benzoic acid (HABA) in determining canine albumin. J. Am. Anim. Hosp. Assoc. 8:128-32.
20. Hudgins, Paul C., Cummings, Martin M., and Patnode, Robert A. 1956. Electrophoretic distribution of serum proteins in rabbit, guinea pig and rat following BCG administration. Soc. Exp. Biol. Med. Proc. 92:75-77.
21. Irfan, M. 1967. The electrophoretic pattern of serum proteins in normal animals. Res. Vet. Sci. 8:137-42.
22. Jennings, F. W., and Mulligan, W. 1953. Levels of some chemical constituents in normal horse sera. J. Comp. Pathol. Therap. 63:286-93.
23. Kaneko, J. J., and Carroll, E. J. 1967. The clinical significance of serum protein fractionation by electrophoresis: Interpretations in clinical veterinary medicine. Calif. Vet. 21:22, 28.
24. Kaneko, J. J., and Mills, R. 1970. Hematological and blood chemical observations in calves. Cornell Vet. 60:52-60.
25. Knill, L. M., Podleski, T. R., and Childs, W. A. 1958. Normal values of swine serum proteins. Soc. Exp. Biol. Med. Proc. 97:224-26.
26. Kuttler, K. L., and Marble, D. W. 1960. Serum protein changes in lambs with naturally acquired nematode infections. Am. J. Vet. Res. 21:445-48.
27. Lane, D. R., and Robinson, R. 1970. The utility of biochemical screening in dogs. Brit. Vet. J. 126:230-37.
28. Larson, B. L., and Touchberry, R. W. 1959. Blood serum protein level as a function of age. J. Anim. Sci. 18:983-90.

29. Lynch, J. E., and Stafseth, H. J. 1953. Electrophoretic studies on the serum proteins of turkeys. Poult. Sci. 32:1068-73.
30. McEwan, A. D., Fisher, E. W., Selman, I. E., and Penhale, W. J. 1970. A turbidity test for the estimation of immune globulin levels in neonatal calf serum. Clin. Chim. Acta 27:155-63.
31. Miller, E. R., Ullrey, D. E., Ackerman, Inge, Schmidt, D. A., Hoefer, J. A., and Luecke, R. W. 1961. Swine hematology from birth to maturity. I. Serum proteins. J. Anim. Sci. 20:31-35.
32. Németh, I., and Juhász, S. 1968. Effect of aflatoxin on serum protein fractions of day-old ducklings. Acta Vet. Acad. Sci. Hung. 18:95-105.
33. Osbaldiston, G. W. 1972. Serum protein fractions in domestic animals. Brit. Vet. J. 128:386-93.
34. Osborne, Carl A., Low, Donald G., and Finco, Delmar R. 1972. Canine and Feline Urology. Saunders, Philadelphia.
35. Patterson, D. S. P., Allen, W. M., Berrett, S., Ivins, L. N., and Sweasey, D. 1968. Some biochemical aspects of clinical Johne's disease in cattle. Res. Vet. Sci. 9:117-29.
36. Payne, J. M., Dew, S. R., Manston, R., and Faulks, M. 1970. The use of a metabolic profile test in dairy herds. Vet. Rec. 87:150-58.
37. Perk, K., and Lobl, K. 1961. Chemical and electrophoretic studies of the serums of cattle infected naturally with Asia-1 type foot-and-mouth disease virus. Am. J. Vet. Res. 22:217-23.
38. Rüsse, I. 1971. Veränderungen der Blutzusammensetzung bei neugeborenen Hundewelpen. (Changes in the blood composition of new-born puppies.) Berl. Muench. Tieraerztl. Wochenschr. 84:249-52.
39. Schalm, O. W., Jain, N. C., and Carroll, E. J. 1975. Veterinary Hematology, 3rd ed. Lea and Febiger, Philadelphia.
40. Schalm, O. W. 1965. The Goldberg refractometer or TS meter. Calif. Vet. 19:28-30.
41. Schalm, O. W. 1965. Plasma protein concentration, PCV and erythrocyte sedimentation rate in interpretation of disease in the dog. Calif. Vet. 19:28-30, 35.
42. Schalm, O. W. 1965. The Goldberg refractometer in acute blood loss in the horse. Calif. Vet. 19:27-29.
43. Schalm, O. W. 1970. Clinical significance of plasma protein concentration. J. Am. Vet. Med. Assoc. 157:1672-75.
44. Stone, S. S., and Gitter, M. 1969. The validity of the sodium sulfite test for detecting immuno-globulins in calf sera. Brit. Vet. J. 125:68-73.
45. Tennant, B. C., and Ewing, G. O. 1970. Gastrointestinal function. In: Clinical Biochemistry of Domestic Animals, vol. 2, 2nd ed., J. J. Kaneko and C. E. Cornelius (eds.). Academic Press, New York.
46. Tumbleson, M. E., and Kalish, P. R. 1972. Serum biochemical and hematological parameters in crossbred swine from birth through eight weeks of age. Can. J. Comp. Med. 36:202-9.
47. Weber, T. B. 1964. Electrophoretic analysis of bovine serum by vertical and horizontal types of apparatus. Am. J. Vet. Res. 25:386-90.

Chapter 12

1. Anderson, G. F., and Barnhart, M. I. 1964. Prothrombin synthesis in the dog. Am. J. Physiol. 206:929-38.
2. Barnhart, M. I., and Anderson, G. F. 1962. Intracellular localization of fibrinogen. Soc. Exp. Biol. Med. Proc. 110:734-37.
3. Bennington, James L., Fouty, Robert A., and Hougie, Cecil. 1970. Laboratory Diagnosis. Macmillan, Toronto.
4. Bentinck-Smith J., Roberts, J. S., and Katz, E. M. 1960. A bleeding disease of new-born calves. Cornell Vet. 50:15-25.
5. Blaisdell, F. S., and Dodds, W. J. 1977. Evaluation of two microhematocrit methods for quantitating plasma fibrinogen. J. Am. Vet. Med. Assoc. 171:340-42.
6. Finco, D. R., and Low, D. G. 1968. Fibrinogen content and fibrinolytic activity of plasma from dogs infected with *Leptospira canicola*. Am. J. Vet. Res. 29:2037-40.
7. Forman, W. B., and Barnhart, M. I. 1964. Cellular site for fibrinogen synthesis. J. Am. Med. Assoc. 187:128-32.
8. Foster, J. B. T., De Natale, A., and Dott, L. B. 1959. Determination of plasma fibrinogen by means of centrifugation after heating. Am. J. Clin. Pathol. 31:42-45.
9. Hall, D. E. 1972. Blood Coagulation and Its Disorders in the Dog. Baillière, Tindall, London.

10. Hardaway, R. M., McKay, D. G., Wahe, G. H., Tartock, D. E., and Edelstein, R. 1956. Pathologic study of intravascular coagulation following incompatible blood transfusion in dogs. Am. J. Surg. 91:24.
11. Kaneko, J. J., and Smith, R. 1967. The estimation of plasma fibrinogen and its clinical significance in the dog. Calif. Vet. 21:21-24.
12. Low, Edmund M. Y., Hill, H. Bradley, and Searcy, Ronald L. 1967. Simple method for detection of abnormal plasma fibrinogen levels. Am. J. Clin. Pathol. 47:538-40.
13. McSherry, B. J., Horney, F. D., and de Groot, J. J. 1970. Plasma fibrinogen levels in normal and sick cows. Can. J. Comp. Med. 34:191-97.
14. Millar, H. R., Simpson, J. G., and Stalker, A. L. 1971. An evaluation of the heat precipitation method for plasma fibrinogen estimation. J. Clin. Pathol. 24:827-30.
15. Schalm, O. W., Smith, R., and Kaneko, J. J. 1970. Plasma protein: Fibrinogen ratios in dogs, cattle and horses. I. Influence of age on normal values and explanation of use in disease. Calif. Vet. 24:9-11.
16. Schalm, O. W., Smith, R., and Kaneko, J. J. 1970. Plasma protein: Fibrinogen ratios in disease in the dog and horse. II. Calif. Vet. 24:19-22.
17. Schalm, O. W., Smith, R., and Kaneko, J. J. 1970. Plasma protein: Fibrinogen ratios in routine clinical material from cats, dogs, horses, and cattle. III. Calif. Vet. 24:6-7, 9-10.

Chapter 16

1. Biggers, J. D., Ingram, P. L., and Murray, C. B. 1949. Studies on equine purpura haemorrhagica. Brit. Vet. J. 105:191-200.
2. Bowie, E. J. W., Owen, C. A., Jr., Zollman, P. E., Thompson, J. H., and Fass, D. N. 1973. Tests of hemostasis in swine: Normal values and values in pigs affected with von Willebrand's disease. Am. J. Vet Res. 34:1405-7.
3. Dodds, W. J. 1968. Current concepts of hereditary coagulation disorders in dogs. Exp. Anim. 1:243.
4. Dodds, W. J., and Kaneko, J. J. 1970. Hemostasis and blood coagulation. In: Clinical Biochemistry of Domestic Animals, vol. 2, J. J. Kaneko and C. E. Cornelius (eds.). Academic Press, New York.
5. Dodds, W. J. 1971. Hemorrhagic disorders. In: Current Veterinary Therapy, vol. 4, R. W. Kirk (ed.). Saunders, Philadelphia.
6. Dodds, W. J. 1972. Hereditary and acquired hemorrhagic disorders in animals. In: Progress in Hemostasis and Thrombosis, vol. 2, T. H. Spaet (ed.). Grune and Stratton, New York.
7. Dodds, W. J. 1974. Diagnosis of bleeding diseases. Presented at Am. Vet. Med. Assoc., annual meeting, Denver, Colo.
8. Dodds, W. J. 1975. Bleeding disorders. In: Textbook of Veterinary Internal Medicine, vol. 1, S. J. Ettinger (ed.). Saunders, Philadelphia.
9. Dodds, W. J. 1977. Inherited hemostatic defects. In: Current Veterinary Therapy, vol. 4, R. W. Kirk (ed.). Saunders, Philadelphia.
10. Dodds, W. J. 1977. The diagnosis, management and treatment of bleeding disorders. I. Mod. Vet. Pract. 58:680-84.
11. Dodds, W. J. 1977. The diagnosis, management and treatment of bleeding disorders. II. Mod. Vet. Pract. 58:756-62.
12. Dodds, W. J. 1977. Autoimmune hemolytic disease and other causes of immune-mediated anemia; An overview. J. Am. Anim. Hosp. Assoc. 13:437-41.
13. Hall, D. E. 1972. Blood Coagulation and Its Disorders in the Dog. Baillière Tindall, London.
14. Harker, L. A. 1970. Hemostasis Manual. Univ. Washington, Seattle.
15. Hathaway, J. E., and Kitchen. 1973. Management of the bleeding disorders and hemoglobinopathies. Am. Anim. Hosp. Assoc. Proc.
16. Hovig, T., Rowsell, H. C., Dodds, W. J., Jorgensen, L., and Mustard, J. F. 1967. Experimental hemostasis in normal dogs and dogs with congenital disorders of blood coagulation. Blood 30:636-68.
17. Irfan, M. 1967. Studies on factor V in animals. J. Comp. Pathol. 77:13-20.
18. Kociba, G. J. 1974. Hemostatic defects. In : Current Veterinary Therapy, vol. 5, R. W. Kirk (ed.). Saunders, Philadelphia.
19. Mustard, J. F. 1972. Platelets and thrombosis in acute myocardial infarction. Hosp. Pract. 7:115-28.
20. Perman, V. 1971. Laboratory evaluation of blood coagulation. Am. Anim. Hosp. Assoc. Proc., annual meeting, Bal Harbour, Fla.

21. Schalm, O. W., Jain, N. C., and Carroll, E. J. 1975. Veterinary Hematology, 3rd ed. Lea and Febiger, Philadelphia.
22. Soloway, H. B. 1974. Drug-induced bleeding. Am. J. Clin. Pathol. 61:622-27.
23. Wilkins, R. J., Hurvitz, A. I., and Dodds-Laffin, W. J. 1973. Immunologically mediated thrombocytopenia in the dog. J. Am. Vet. Med. Assoc. 163:277-82.
24. Wilkins, R. J., and Dodds, W. J. 1974. Idiopathic (immunologic) thrombocytopenic purpura. In: Current Veterinary Therapy, vol. 5, R. W. Kirk (ed.). Saunders, Philadelphia.

Chapter 18

1. Coffin, D. L. 1949. Diagnosis of diseases of the urinary tract of the dog. J. Am. Vet. Med. Assoc. 114:318-21.
2. Cornelius, C. E. 1957. Urinalysis—The microscopic sediment. Calif. Vet. 10:30-31.
3. Dreifus, L. S., Stamler, J., and Lichton, I. J. 1959. Production of hypernatremia and hyperosmolarity in the diabetes insipidus dog infused with Ringer's solution. Circ. Res. 7:314-17.
4. Lippman, R. W. 1957. Urine and the Urinary Sediment, 2nd ed. Charles C. Thomas, Springfield, Ill.
5. Pollock, S. 1955. Cystinuria in the dog. J. Am. Vet. Med. Assoc. 126:188-91.
6. Roberts, S. J., Rickard, C. G., and Bentinck-Smith, J. 1951. A clinical and laboratory evaluation of the Sulkowitch test as a diagnostic aid in bovine hypocalcemia. J. Am. Vet. Med. Assoc. 119:380-82.
7. Spector, W. S. (ed.). 1956. Handbook of Biological Data. Saunders, Philadelphia.
8. Worden, A. N., Waterhouse, C. E., and Sellwood, E. H. B. 1960. Studies on the composition of normal cat urine. J. Small Anim. Pract. 1:11-23.

Chapter 19

1. Abbott Laboratories. 1974. Fluid and Electrolytes. Abbott Laboratories, Chicago.
2. Albritton, E. C. (ed.). 1952. Standard Values in Blood. Saunders, Philadelphia.
3. Dukes, H. H. 1970. Dukes' Physiology of Domestic Animals, 8th ed., M. J. Swenson (ed.). Comstock, Ithaca, N.Y.
4. Gamble, J. L. 1951. Chemical Anatomy, Physiology and Pathology of Extracellular Fluid, 5th ed. Harvard Univ. Press, Cambridge, Mass.
5. Helmer, O. M. 1955. Symposium on parenteral fluids, nutrition and electrolytes. The milliequivalent as a unit of measure in the interpretation and correction of electrolyte disturbances. Minnesota Med. (supp.) 38:1-3.
6. Jones, L. M. 1965. Veterinary Pharmacology and Therapeutics, 3rd ed. Iowa State Univ. Press, Ames.
7. McSherry, B. J., and Grinyer, I. 1954. The pH values, carbon dioxide content, and the levels of sodium, potassium, calcium, chloride, and inorganic phosphorus in the blood serum of normal cattle. Am. J. Vet. Res. 15:509-10.
8. McSherry, B. J., and Grinyer, I. 1954. Disturbances in acid-base balance and electrolyte in calf diarrhea and their treatment. A report of 18 cases. Am. J. Vet. Res. 15:535-41.
9. Miller, S. E. 1966. A Textbook of Clinical Pathology, 7th ed. Williams and Wilkins, Baltimore.
10. Nadeau, G. 1953. Simple method for combined determination of plasma bicarbonate, pH and chloride. Am. J. Clin. Pathol. 23:710-12.
11. Scribner, B. H., and Caillouette, J. C. 1954. Improved method for the bedside determination of bicarbonate in serum. J. Am. Med. Assoc. 155:644-48.
12. Scribner, B. H. 1950. Bedside determination of chloride: Method for plasma, urine and other fluids and its application to fluid balance problems. Mayo Clinic Staff Meeting Proc. 25:209-18.
13. Snively, W. D., and Sweeney, M. J. 1956. Fluid Balance Handbook for Practitioners, Charles C. Thomas, Springfield, Ill.
14. Spector, W. S. (ed.). 1956. Handbook of Biological Data. Saunders, Philadelphia.
15. Stewart, B. D., Swan, H., and Kortz, A. B. 1954. The bedside clinic and laboratory of the management of acute dehydration . Am. Surg. 20:93-111.
16. Talbot, N. B., Kerrigan, G. A., Crawford, J. D., Cochran, W., and Terry M. 1955. Medical progress: Application of homeostatic principles to the practice of parenteral fluid therapy. New Eng. J. Med. 252:856-62, 898-906.

Chapter 21

1. Allcroft, W. M., and Folley, S. J. 1941. Observations on the serum phosphatase of cattle and sheep. Biochem. J. 35:254-66.
2. Benjamin, M. M. 1978. Outline of Veterinary Clinical Pathology. Iowa State Univ. Press, Ames.
3. Cornelius, C. E., Bishop, J., Switzer, J., and Rhode, E. A. 1959. Serum and tissue transaminase activities in domestic animals. Cornell Vet. 49:116-26.
4. Cornelius, C. E. 1961. Serum isocitric dehydrogenase (SIC-D) activities in domestic animals with experimental hepatic necrosis and in equine hepatopathy. Cornell Vet. 51:559-68.
5. Cornelius, C. E., Douglas, G. M., Gronwall, R. R., and Freedland, R. A. 1963. Comparative studies on plasma arginase and transaminases in hepatic necrosis. Cornell Vet. 53:181-91.
6. Dunavant, Michael L., and Rich, L. J. 1974. Clinical applications of serum enzyme determinations. Am. Soc. Vet. Clin. Pathol. 3:3-26.
7. Ford, E. J. H., and Lawrence, J. A. 1965. Hepatic and serum changes following repeated administration of small smounts of carbon tetrachloride to sheep. J. Comp. Pathol. Therap. 75:185-200.
8. Gerber, Heinz. 1969. Serum enzyme determination in equine medicine. Equine Vet. J. 1:129-139.
9. Hamar, Dwayne. 1978. Personal communication.
10. Healy, P. J. 1968. Serum ornithine carbamyl transferase activity in sheep and cattle. Clin. Chim. Acta 22:603-9.
11. Hoe, C. M., and Harvey, D. G. 1961. An investigation into liver function tests in dogs. II. Tests other than transaminase estimations. J. Small Anim. Pract. 2:109-27.
12. Holtenius, P., and Jacobsson, S-O. 1966. Ornithine carbamyl transferase (OCT) activity in ruminants. Cornell Vet. 56:187-95.
13. Jennings, F. W., and Mulligan, W. 1953. Levels of some chemical constituents in normal horse sera. J. Comp. Pathol. 63:286-93.
14. Kaneko, J. J. 1974. Standard values in domestic animals. Univ. Calif., Davis.
15. Kramer, J., and Sleight, S. D. 1968. Isoenzymes of serum alkaline phosphatase in cats. Am. J. Vet. Clin. Pathol. 2:87-91.
16. Kronfeld, D. S., and Medway, W. 1969. Blood chemistry. In: Textbook of Veterinary Clinical Pathology, W. Medway, J. F. Prier, and J. S. Wilkinson (eds.). Williams and Wilkins, Baltimore.
17. Lagáce, A., Bell, D. S., Moxon, A. L., and Pounden, W. D. 1961. Serum transaminase in the blood of lambs given preventive treatments for white muscle disease. Am. J. Vet. Res. 22:686-88.
18. Laird, C. W. 1972. Representative Values for Animal and Veterinary Populations and Their Clinical Significances. Hycel, Houston.
19. Roussel, J. D., and Stallcup, O. T. 1967. Blood serum enzymes within the estrous cycle. J. Dairy Sci. 50:1341-42.
20. Schalm, O. W., Jain, N. C., and Carroll, E. J. 1975. Veterinary Hematology, 3rd ed. Lea and Febiger, Philadelphia.
21. Sinton, Eleanor. 1972. Personal communication.
22. Sinton, Eleanor, and Taylor, Tim. 1972. II. The use of 2-(4-hydroxyazobenzene)-benzoic acid (HABA) in determining canine albumin. J. Am. Anim. Hosp. Assoc. 8:130-32.
23. Svirbely, J. L. 1946. The comparative efficiency of various liver function tests in detecting hepatic damage produced in dogs by xylidine. J. Lab. Clin. Med. 31:1133.
24. Swenson, M. J. 1970. Composition of body fluids. In: Diseases of Swine, 3rd ed., H. W. Dunne (ed.). Iowa State Univ. Press, Ames.
25. University of Pennsylvania. 1975. Standard values.
26. Van Vleet, J. F., and Alberts, J. O. 1968. Evaluation of liver function tests and liver biopsy in experimental carbon tetrachloride intoxication and extrahepatic bile duct obstruction in the dog. Am. J. Vet. Res. 29:2119-31.
27. Van Kampen, Kent. 1972. Data presented at the 33rd annual conference for veterinarians, Colorado State Univ., Fort Collins.
28. Veterinary Reference Laboratory. 1977. Report form. Vet. Ref. Lab., Fullerton, Calif.
29. Wolff, W. A., Tumbleson, M. E., and Littleton, C. A. 1970. Serum chemistry in normal and diseased horses. In: Advances in Automated Analysis. Technicon, Tarrytown, N.Y.

Chapter 22

1. Alsever, R. N. 1975. Clinical problems in carbohydrate testing. Lab. Med. 6:31-45.
2. Anderson, N. V., and Low, D. G. 1965. Juvenile atrophy of the canine pancreas. Anim. Hosp. 1:101-9.
3. Anderson, N. V., and Low, D. G. 1965. Diseases of the canine pancreas: A comparative summary of 103 cases. Anim. Hosp. 1:189-94.
4. Anderson, N. V., and Strafuss, A. C. 1971. Pancreatic disease in dogs and cats. J. Am. Vet. Med. Assoc. 159:885-91.
5. Anderson, N. V. 1972. Pancreatitis in dogs. Vet. Clin. North Am. 2:79-97.
6. Anderson, N. V. 1973. The pancreas. J. Am. Anim. Hosp. Assoc. 9:89-100.
7. Archibald, J. 1953. Canine atrophic pancreatitis. Am. Vet. Med. Assoc. Proc., pp. 264-66.
8. Archibald, J. 1955. Canine pancreatitis. Calif. Vet. 9:28-32.
9. Bardens, J. W. 1966. Glycogen storage disease in puppies. Vet. Med./Small Anim. Clin. 61:1174-76.
10. Bennington, J. L., Fouty, R. A., and Hougie, C. 1970. Laboratory Diagnosis. Macmillan, London.
11. Berk, J. E., Searcy, R. L., Hayashi, S., and Ujihira, I. 1965. Distribution of serum amylase in man and animals. Electrophoretic and chromatographic studies. J. Am. Med. Assoc. 192:389-93.
12. Brobst, D., and Brester, J. E. 1967. Serum lipase determination in the dog using a one-hour test. J. Am. Vet. Med. Assoc. 150:767-71.
13. Brobst, D. F. 1970. Pancreatic function. In: Clinical Biochemistry of Domestic Animals, vol. 1, 2nd ed., J. J. Kaneko and C. E. Cornelius (eds.). Academic Press, New York.
14. Brobst, D., Ferguson, A. B., and Carter, J. M. 1970. Evaluation of serum amylase and lipase activity in experimentally induced pancreatitis in the dog. J. Am. Vet. Med. Assoc. 157:1697-1702.
15. Challis, T. W., Reid, L. C., and Hinton, J. W. 1957. Study of some factors which influence the level of serum amylase in dogs and humans. Gastroenterol. 33:818-22.
16. Coffin, D. L., and Thordal-Christensen, A. 1953. The clinical and some pathological aspects of pancreatic disease in dogs. Vet. Med. 48:193-98.
17. Cooper, G. R., and McDaniel, V. 1966. Workshop Manual of Methods for the Determination of Glucose. Council on Clinical Chemistry, Am. Soc. Clin. Pathol., Washington, D.C.
18. Cornelius, L. M., Cotton, R. B., and Theran, P. 1969. Evaluation of certain biochemical parameters in dogs with naturally occurring diabetes mellitus. In: Advances in Automated Analysis. Technicon Co., Tarrytown, N.Y.
19. Cotton, R. B., Cornelius, L. M., and Theran, P. 1971. Diabetes mellitus in the dog: A clinicopathologic study. J. Am. Vet. Med. Assoc. 159:863-70.
20. Dimbiloglu, E., Howard, J. M., Appert, H. E., and Pairent, F. W. 1967. Changes in serum calcium concentration following the intravenous injection of pancreatic juice in the dog. Surg. Forum 18:408-9.
21. Duncan, J. R., and Prasse, K. W. 1977. Veterinary Laboratory Medicine: Clinical Pathology. Iowa State Univ. Press, Ames.
22. Finco, D. R., and Stevens, J. B. 1969. Clinical significance of serum amylase activity in the dog. J. Am. Vet. Med. Assoc. 155:1686-91.
23. Free, A. H., and Free, H. M. 1975. Urine sugar testing—State of the art. Lab. Med. 6:23-47.
24. Gage, E. D., and Anderson, N. V. 1967. Acute pancreatitis in a dog. Anim. Hosp. 3:151-59.
25. Gilmore, C. E. 1964. Chronic pancreatitis in dogs. Calif. Vet. 18:11-14.
26. Giulian, B. B., Mitsuoka, H., Mansfield, A. O., Trapnell, J. E., Seddon, J. A., and Howard, J. M. 1967. Treatment of pancreatic exocrine insufficiency. II. Effects of fat absorption on pancreatic lipase and fifteen commercial pancreatic supplements as measured by ^{131}I-tagged triolein in the dog. Ann. Surg., pp.571-79.
27. Goetsch, D. D., McDonald, L. E., and Odell, G. 1959. The effects of four synthetic corticosteroids on leukocytes, blood glucose, and plasma sodium and potassium in the cow. Am. J. Vet. Res. 20:697-701.
28. Greve, T., Dayton, A. D., and Anderson, N. V. 1973. Acute pancreatitis with coexistent diabetes mellitus: An experimental study in the dog. Am. J. Vet. Res. 34:947-50.
29. Hardy, R. M., and Stevens, J. B. 1975. Exocrine pancreatic diseases. In: Textbook of Veterinary Internal Medicine, vol. 2, S. J. Ettinger (ed.). Saunders, Philadelphia.
30. Hill, F. W. G., and Kidder, D. E. 1970. The estimation of daily faecal trypsin levels in dogs as an indicator of gross pancreatic exocrine insufficiency. J. Small Anim. Pract. 11:191-95.

31. Holzworth, J., and Coffin, D. L. 1953. Pancreatic insufficiency and diabetes mellitus in a cat. Cornell Vet. 43:502-12.
32. Jasper, D. E. 1954. A simple diagnostic test for pancreatic enzyme deficiency of dogs. North Am. Vet. 35:523-25.
33. Kaneko, J. J., and Rhode, E. A. 1964. Diabetes mellitus in a cow. J. Am. Vet. Med. Assoc. 144:367-73.
34. Kaneko, J. J. 1970. Carbohydrate metabolism. In: Clinical Biochemistry of Domestic Animals, vol. 1, 2nd ed., J. J. Kaneko and C. E. Cornelius (eds.). Academic Press, New York.
35. Kaneko, J. J. 1970. Pancreatic function. In: Clinical Biochemistry of Domestic Animals, vol. 1, 2nd ed., J. J. Kaneko and C. E. Cornelius (eds.). Academic Press, New York.
36. Kaneko, J. J. 1974. Standard values in domestic animals. Univ. Calif., Davis.
37. Kessler, J. I., Miller, M., Barza, D., and Mishkin, S. 1967. Hyperlipemia in acute pancreatitis. Am. J. Med. 42:968-76.
38. King, J. M., Kavanaugh, J. F., and Bentinck-Smith, J. 1962. Diabetes mellitus with pituitary neoplasms in a horse and a dog. Cornell Vet. 52:133-45.
39. Krook, L. 1967. Insuloma in the dog. N. Y. C. Vet. 9:5.
40. Loeb, W. F., and Edge, L. I. 1962. A method for the determination of serum amylase in the dog. Am. J. Vet. Res. 23:1117-19.
41. Lorenz, M. D., and Cornelius, L. M. 1976. Laboratory diagnosis of endocrinological disease. Vet. Clin. North Am. 6:687-722.
42. MacKay, N., Gordon, A., and Neilson, J. M. 1965. Observer error in Dextrostix estimations of blood-sugar. Lancet, pp. 269-70.
43. Mager, M., and Farese, G. 1965. What is "true" blood glucose? Am. J. Clin. Pathol. 44:104-8.
44. Meier, H. 1961. Comparative aspects of spontaneous diabetes mellitus in animals. Am. J. Med. 31:868-73.
45. Nielsen, S. W., and Pocock, E. F. 1953. Chronic relapsing pancreatitis in a dog. Cornell Vet. 43:567-72.
46. Perman, V., and Stevens, J. B. 1969. Clinical evaluation of the acinar pancreas of the dog. J. Am. Vet. Med. Assoc. 155:2053-58.
47. Phillips, R. W., Knox, K. L., Pierson, R. E., and Tasker, J. B. 1971. Bovine diabetes mellitus. Cornell Vet. 61:114-24.
48. Quam, E. F., Westgard, J. O., and Carey, R. N. 1975. Selecting glucose methods that meet your laboratory requirements. Lab. Med. 6:35-39.
49. Rapp, J. P. 1962. Normal values for serum amylase and maltase in dogs and the effect of maltase on the saccharogenic method of determining amylase in serum. Am. J. Vet. Res. 23:343-50.
50. Stackhouse, K. L., Glass, D. D., and Zimmerman, B. 1966. Relationships of lipoprotein lipase and hyperlipemia in pancreatitis. Surg. Forum 17:343-44.
51. Stevens, J. B. 1974. In-office clinical biochemistry. II. Clinical enzymology. Am. Anim. Hosp. Assoc. Proc., pp. 623-32.
52. Tasker, J. B., Whiteman, C. E., and Martin, B. R. 1966. Diabetes mellitus in the horse. J. Am. Vet. Med. Assoc. 149:393-99.
53. Thordal-Christensen, A., and Coffin, D. L. 1956. Pancreatic diseases in the dog. Nord. Vet. Med. 8:89-114.
54. Wilkinson, J. S. 1960. Spontaneous diabetes mellitus. Vet. Rec. 72:548-55.
55. Wilkinson, J. S. 1969. Kidney disease and urine analysis. In: Textbook of Veterinary Clinical Pathology, W. Medway, J. E. Prier, and J. S. Wilkinson (eds.). Williams and Wilkins, Baltimore.
56. Wolff, A., Donovan, E. F., and Nielsen, S. W. 1957. diagnosis and treatment of a dog with acinar atrophy of the pancreas. J. Am. Vet. Med. Assoc. 131:104-6.

Chapter 23

1. Arthur, G. H. 1947. The diagnosis of traumatic reticulitis and pericarditis of bovines. Vet. Rec. 59:69-72.
2. Brown, J. M., Kingrey, B. W., and Rosenquist, B. D. 1959. The hematology of chronic reticuloperitonitis. Am. J. Vet. Res. 20:255-64.
3. Cardinet, George H., III. 1971. Skeletal muscle. In: Clinical Biochemistry of Domestic Animals, vol. 2, 2nd ed., J. J. Kaneko and C. E. Cornelius (eds.). Academic Press, New York.
4. Dunavant, M. L. 1971. Personal communication.
5. Eshenour, R. W., Newberne, J. W., and Burch, G. R. 1958. Accelerated (three-day) treatment with Filcide for canine heartworms. Allied Vet. 29:7-9.

6. Jones, T. C. 1969. Clinical and pathologic features of equine viral arteritis. J. Am. Vet. Med. Assoc. 155:315-17.
7. Kaneko, J. J. 1971. Standard values in domestic animals. Univ. Calif., Davis.
8. Ryff, J. F. 1957. Brisket disease syndrome. J. Am. Vet. Med. Assoc. 131:425-30.
9. Shouse, C. L., and Meier, H. 1956. Acute vegetative endocarditis in the dog and cat. J. Am. Vet. Med. Assoc. 129:278-89.
10. Tilley, L. P., and Wilkins, R. J. 1974. Pericardial disease. In: Current Veterinary Therapy, No. 5, R. W. Kirk (ed.). Saunders, Philadelphia.
11. Wilkins, R. J. 1977. Clinical pathology of feline cardiac disease. Vet. Clin. North Am. 7:285-90.

Chapter 25

1. Bleich, H. L., Berkman, P. M., and Schwartz, W. B. 1964. The response of cerebrospinal fluid composition to sustained hypercapnia. J. Clin. Invest. 43:11.
2. Cornelius, C. E. 1959. Cerebrospinal fluid in large domestic animals. Calif. Vet. 12:22-24.
3. Dixon, E., and Bowie, W. C. 1962. Serum and cerebrospinal fluid: Their diagnostic and prognostic value. Tuskegee Vet. 6:45.
4. Fankhauser, R. 1962. The cerebrospinal fluid. In: Comparative Neuropathology, J. R. M. Innes and L. Z. Saunders (eds.). Academic Press, New York.
5. Fedotov, A. I. 1951. Veterinariya Likvorologia, Leningrad. (Trans. L. Z. Saunders, Cerebrospinal Fluid of Domestic Animals. Distributed by the Russian Scientific Translation Program, NIH, Bethesda, Md.)
6. Hibbs, C. M., and Coles, E. H. 1965. Transaminases in blood, urine and cerebrospinal fluid of normal and unilaterally nephrectomized dogs. Proc. Soc. Exp. Biol. Med. 118:1059-62.
7. Lending, M., Slobody, L. B., and Mestern, J. 1959. Effect of convulsions on cerebrospinal fluid and plasma activity of glutamic oxaloacetic transaminase and lactic dehydrogenase. Neurology 9:672.
8. Roszel, J. F. 1972. Membrane filtration of canine and feline cerebrospinal fluid for cytologic examination. J. Am. Vet. Med. Assoc. 160:720-25.
9. Yeary, R. A., Shannon, I. L., and Prigmore, J. R. 1960. Cerebrospinal fluid electrolytes in the dog. Am. J. Vet. Res. 21:306-7.

Chapter 27

1. Anderson, J. J. B., and Dorner, J. L. 1971. Total serum thyroxine in thyroidectomized Beagles, using ^{125}I-labeled thyroxine, and comparison of T_3 and T_4 tests. J. Am. Vet. Med. Assoc. 159:760-62.
2. Baker, H. J. 1971. Laboratory evaluation of thyroid function. In: Current Veterinary Therapy, No. 4, R. W. Kirk (ed.). Saunders, Philadelphia.
3. Belshaw, B. E. 1968. Hypothyroidism in the dog. Paper presented at Am. Anim. Hosp. Assoc. annual meeting, Las Vegas.
4. Bullock, L. 1970. Protein-bound iodine determinations as a diagnostic aid for canine hypothyroidism. J. Am. Vet. Med. Assoc. 156:892-99.
5. Bush, B. M. 1969. Thyroid disease in the dog—A review. I. J. Small Anim. Pract. 10:95-109.
6. Bush, B. M. 1969. Thyroid disease in the dog—A review. II. J. Small Anim. Pract. 10:185-96.
7. Bush, B. M. 1972. Thyroid function tests in a group of euthyroid dogs. Res. Vet. Sci. 13:177-81.
8. Bustad, L. K., and Fuller, J. M. 1970. Thyroid function in domestic animals. Lab. Anim. Care 30:561-81.
9. Capen, C. C., Belshaw, B. E., and Martin, S. L. 1975. Endocrine disorders. In: Textbook of Veterinary Internal Medicine, S. J. Ettinger (ed.). Saunders, Philadelphia.
10. Ganong, W. F. 1969. The thyroid gland. In: Review of Medical Physiology, 4th ed. Lange, Los Altos, Calif.
11. Hoge, W. R., Lund, J. E., and Blakemore, J. C. 1974. Response to thyrotropin as a diagnostic aid for canine hypothyroidism. J. Am. Anim. Hosp. Assoc. 10:167-70.
12. Irvine, C. H. G. 1967. Protein-bound iodine in the horse. Am. J. Vet. Res. 28:1687-92.
13. Jubb, K. V. F., and Kennedy, P. C. 1963. Pathology of Domestic Animals, vol. 1. Academic Press, New York.
14. Kallfelz, F. A. 1968. The triiodothyronine ^{131}I resin sponge uptake test as an indication of thyroid function in dogs. J. Am. Vet. Med. Assoc. 152:1647-50.

15. Kallfelz, F. A. 1969. Comparison of the $^{125}T_3$ and $^{125}T_4$ tests in the diagnosis of thyroid gland function in the dog. J. Am. Vet. Med. Assoc. 154:22-25.
16. Kallfelz, F. A., and Lowe, J. E. 1970. Some normal values of thyroid function in horses. J. Am. Vet. Med. Assoc. 156:1888-91.
17. Kallfelz, F. A. 1973. Observations on thyroid gland function in dogs: Response to thyrotropin and thyroidectomy and determination of thyroxine secretion rate. Am. J. Vet. Res. 34:535-38.
18. Kallfelz, F. A., and Erali, R. P. 1973. Thyroid function tests in domesticated animals: Free thyroxine index. Am. J. Vet. Res. 34:1449-51.
19. Kaneko, J. J. 1970. Thyroid function. In: Clinical Biochemistry of Domestic Animals, vol. 1, 2nd ed., J. J. Kaneko and C. E. Cornelius, (eds.). Academic Press, New York.
20. Kaneko, J. J., Baker, B., and Mills, R. 1975. Laboratory evaluation of the canine thyroid gland. Am. Soc. Vet. Clin. Pathol. Bull. 4:30.
21. Kuhns, L. J., Tallman, D. F., and Sippel, W. L. 1969. The T_3 values for mares and the effect of age, pregnancy, and fertility on these values. J. Comp. Lab. Med. 3:27-30.
22. Larsen, P. R. 1975. Tests of thyroid function. Med. Clin. North Am. 59:1063-74.
23. Ling, G. V., Lowenstine, L. J., and Kaneko, J. J. 1974. Serum thyroxine (T_4) and triiodothyronine (T_3) uptake in normal adult cats. Am. J. Vet. Res. 35:1247-49.
24. Lombardi, M. H., Comar, C. L., and Kirk, R. W. 1962. Diagnosis of thyroid gland function in the dog. Am. J. Vet. Res. 23:412-21.
25. Lorenz, M. D., and Cornelius, L. M. 1975. Laboratory diagnosis of endocrinological disease. Vet. Clin. North Am. 6:687-722.
26. Mallo, G. L., and Harris, A. L. 1967. ^{131}I triiodothyronine resin uptake, serum protein-iodine and serum cholesterol tests in normal dogs. Vet. Med./Small Anim. Clin. 62:533-40.
27. Mason, R., and Wilkinson, J. S. 1973. The thyroid gland—A review. Aust. Vet. J. 49:44-49.
28. McDonald, L. E. 1975. The thyroid gland. In: Veterinary Endocrinology and Reproduction, 2nd ed. Lea and Febiger, Philadelphia.
29. Quinlan, W. J., Jr., Thomson, R. A. E., and Michaelson, S. 1969. *In vitro* resin sponge uptake test of T_3 and T_4 in animals and man. Am. J. Vet. Res. 30:1471-73.
30. Reid, C. F. 1969. Thyroid function tests in the dog. J. Am. Vet. Med. Assoc. 155:1571-80.
31. Rijnberk, A., and van der Horst, C. J. G. 1969. Investigations on iodine metabolism of normal and goitrous dogs. Zentralbl. Veterinaermed. A 16:495-508.
32. Thomson, R. A. E., and Michaelson, S. M. 1967. A source of false iodine-131 uptake and protein-bound iodine values in dogs. Am. J. Vet. Res. 28:1623-25.

Chapter 29

1. Bach, L. G., and Ricketts, S. W. 1974. Paracentesis as an aid to the diagnosis of abdominal disease in the horse. Equine Vet. J. 6:116-21.
2. Crowe, D. T., Jr., and Crane, S. W. 1976. Diagnostic abdominal paracentesis and lavage in the evaluation of abdominal injuries in dogs and cats: Clinical and experimental investigations. J. Am. Vet. Med. Assoc. 168:700-705.
3. Maksic, D. 1964. Abdominal paracentesis and its use in diagnosis in the horse. Am. Assoc. Equine Pract. Proc., pp. 319-24.
4. McGrath, J. P. 1975. Exfoliative cytology of equine peritoneal fluid—An adjunct to hematologic examination. First Int. Symp. Equine Hematol. Proc., pp. 408-16.
5. Nelson, A. W. 1964. Intestinal infarction. Am. Assoc. Equine Pract. Proc., pp. 35-47.
6. Oehme, F. W. 1969. Cytologic examination of the peritoneal fluid in the diagnosis of cattle disease. J. Am. Vet. Med. Assoc. 155:1923-27.
7. Oehme, F. W., and Noordsy, J. L. 1970. Examination of peritoneal fluid in differential diagnosis of bovine diseases. Vet. Med./Small Anim. Clin. 65:54-59.
8. Perman, V. 1966. Diagnostic cytology in canine medicine. Sixteenth Gaines Vet. Symp., Philadelphia.
9. Schalm, O. W. 1962. New methylene blue stain for the study of cells in pathologic body fluids. Calif. Vet. 16:32-34.

Chapter 30

1. Bloom, F. 1954. Pathology of the Dog and Cat. Am. Vet. Publ., Evanston, Ill.
2. Evans, H. M., and Cole, H. H. 1931. An introduction to the study of the oestrus cycle in the dog. Univ. Calif. Memoirs 9:65-118.
3. Gier, H. T. 1960. Estrous cycle in the bitch: Vaginal fluids. Vet. Scope 5:2-9.
4. Kirk, R. W., Rickard, C. G., and McEntee, K. 1959. The urogenital system. In: Canine Medicine, 2nd ed., H. P. Hoskins (ed.). Am. Vet. Publ., Santa Barbara, Calif.

Chapter 31

1. Conant, N. F., Smith, D. T., Baker, R. D., Callaway, J. L., and Martin, D. S. 1954. Manual of Clinical Mycology, 2nd ed. Saunders, Philadelphia.
2. Georg, L. K. 1954. The diagnosis of ringworm in animals. Vet. Med. 49:157-66.
3. Hoerlein, A. B. 1945. Studies on animal dermatomycoses. I. Clinical studies. Cornell Vet. 35:287-98.
4. Moss, L. C., and Benjamin, M. M. 1959. Dermatomycoses. In: Canine Medicine, 2nd ed., H. P. Hoskins (ed.). Am. Vet. Publ., Santa Barbara, Calif.

INDEX

Abetalipoproteinemia, 124
Abomasum, cattle, 100
Abscess, horse, 119
Acanthocytes, 38, 124
Acetone, 194-96, 221
Acetonemia, cattle, 120. *See also* Ketosis
Acid hematin, 62
Acidosis, 216-19
Acid phosphatase, 10
ACTH, 133
  cattle, 100
  dog, 93
  eosinophils, 87-88
  horse, 98
  pig, 105
Actinomycosis, 316
Adenosine triphosphate, 38
Adenoviral infection, horse, 98
Adrenal corticosteroids
  dog, 93
  eosinophils, 87-88
  leukocytes, 80
Adrenalin, 98, 100
African swine fever, 105
Agalactia, pig, 105
Age
  A/G ratio, 115
  fibrinogen, 119
  globulins, 115
  hemorrhage, 165
  leptocytes, 125
  leukocytes, 77, 81
  PCV, 74-75
  plasma protein, 113
Agglutinins, serum, 101
Agranulocytosis, 38
Albumin, 12, 108, 110
  decreased, 114
  ESR, 64
  liver function, 250, 251-52
  measurement, 109
Albumin:globulin (A/G) ratio, 115, 252-53
Alkaline phosphatase, 9-10, 257, 289
Alkalosis, 216-17, 219-20
Allergies, 87
Ammonia, 10, 254
Ammonia intoxication, sheep, 113
Ammonium and potassium oxalate mixture, 70
Amylase, 10-11, 255-56, 287
Amyloidosis, dog, 93
Anaphylactoid, purpura, 170
Anaplasmosis, cattle, 100, 120
Anemia, 15, 38, 127-49
  aplastic, 133, 158, 170
  autoimmune hemolytic, 136-40, 142, 159, 171
  basophils, 124
  cat, 97, 120
  cattle, 100, 102-3
  causes, 131-32, 134-36
  chronic disorders, 145-46
  classification, 129
  clinical evaluation, 130-31
  diagnosis, 130
  dog, 93-96
  erythrocytes, 125, 127-29, 132-34, 145-46
  ESR, 64
  fibrinogen, 120
  globulins, 115
  hemolysis, 135-36
  hemorrhage, 131, 134-35
  horse, 98-99
  hypoplastic, 39
  infectious, 97-98
  iron finding capacity, 146
  lab evaluation, 131, 134-36
  lymphosarcoma, 152-53, 155
  microcytes, 126
  nonregenerative, 136, 154
  ovalocytes, 126
  PCV, 127, 144
  pig, 105-7
  poikilocytes, 126
  polycythemia, 113
  pyruvate kinase deficiency, 143-44
  regenerative, 134-36, 167
  schistocytes, 126
  sheep, 104
  siderocytes, 127
  spherocytes, 127
  stomatocytes, 127
Anesthesia, dog, 93
Anions, 214
Anisocytosis, 38, 123
Antibodies, anemia, 132, 139
Anticoagulant, 8-10, 38, 70
  blood glucose, 260
  ESR, 64-65
  hemostasis, 165
Antigen-antibody reaction, anemia, 139
Antihemophilic factor, 164
Antinuclear antibody (ANA) tests, 142
Antithyroid compounds, 294
Aplastic, 38
Aplastic anemia, 133, 158, 170
Arginase, 11, 247
Arneth's index, 38
Arthritis, 98, 140, 143
Aspergillosis, 100, 315
Aspirin, 97, 165, 171
Atrophic rhinitis, 105
Aujeszky's disease, pig, 105
Autoimmune disease, 124, 139-40, 159, 171
Azurophil, 38

Babesiasis, dog, 93
Bacillary hemoglobinuria, cattle, 100
Bacterial endocarditis, 68, 265, 268
Band form, 38
Basket cell, 38, 150
Basophils, 38, 88-89, 124
  cattle, 101-2
  dog, 95-96
  pig, 105-6
  sheep, 104
Bicarbonate
  anions, 214
  fluid and electrolyte balance, 222-23, 225
  metabolism, 216-18
Bile, urinalysis, 183, 198-99
Bile-stained cast, 208
Biliary obstruction, 125, 201, 204
Biliary pigments, 233-41
Bilirubin, 12, 14, 304
  BSP, 250
  liver function, 233
  PCV, 73
  serum, 10, 234-38, 287
  urine, 198-99, 238-39
  urobilinogen, 201-2
  values, 237-38
Biopsy, 299, 312-13
Birds, 6, 29
Blastomycosis, 93, 315
Bleeding time, 38, 168
Blood
  ammonia, 10, 254
  cardiovascular disease, 268
  cast, 208
  cell count, 48-59
  cells, 20-21
  coagulation. *See* Coagulation; Hemostasis
  collection, 5-14
  CSF, 276-77
  cultures, 268
  dyscrasia, 38
  enzymes, 230
  fluid and electrolyte balance, 222-24
  pH, 9, 11
  plasma protein, 113-14
  SLE, 140, 142
  stability, 12-14
  urinalysis, 196-98, 204
  volume, 12
Blood smear, 9, 25-37
  fixation, 26-27
  leukocytes, 35-36
  staining, 26-35
  thrombocytes, 36-37
Blood transfusion, 119, 139, 161
Blood urea nitrogen (BUN), 10-12, 175-78
  abnormalities, 286
  autoimmune hemolytic anemia, 138
  interpretation, 177
  methods, 176-77
  pancreatic function, 263
Blood values, 43-47
Bluetongue, sheep, 103-4
Bone
  disorders, 270-75
  enzymes, 231
  fractures, 69, 118-19
  SAP, 244
Bone marrow
  anemia, 134, 145-46
  aspiration, 15-19
  basophils, 88-89
  cells, 19-24
  eosinophils, 86-88
  erythropoiesis, 123
  imprint, 17
  leukocytes, 78
  lymphocytes, 89-92, 154
  lymphosarcoma, 155
  microcytes, 126
  monocytes, 92
  neutrophils, 81-86
  platelet disorders, 170
  pools, 84-85

Bone marrow *(cont.)*
  smear, 17
  thrombocytopenia, 158, 160
  types, 15
Bone marrow depression
  cat, 97
  erythrocytes, 127
  horse, 99
  leptocytes, 125
  PCV, 73
Boric acid, 181
Bracken poisoning, 100, 119
Brain, enzymes, 231
Brisket disease, cattle, 100-101
Bromsulphalein (BSP), 10
  liver function, 247-50
  protein analysis, 109
Brucella, cattle, 101
Buffer systems, 214-16
Buffy coat, 38
Burns, A/G ratio, 115
Butazolidin, horse, 98, 165, 171

Calcium, 12, 155, 164, 257
  abnormalities, 289-90
  blood, determination, 10
  cardiovascular disease, 269
  cations, 214
  CSF, 282
  hyperparathyroidism, 272
  serum, 155, 257
  urinalysis, 203
Calorigenesis, thyroid functions, 293
Candidiasis, 314
Carbohydrates, 194, 228
Carbonic acid, 218-20
Carboxyhemoglobin, 63
Cardiac hemangiosarcoma, dog, 93
Cardiovascular disease, 265-69
Cassia occidentalis, cattle, 101
Casts, urinalysis, 205, 207-9
Cat
  actinomycosis, 316
  A/G ratio, 252
  amylase, 256
  aspergillosis, 315
  autoimmune hemolytic anemia, 136-37
  bilirubin, 234, 237, 239
  blood collection, 5, 6
  blood picture in specific conditions, 97-98
  blood values, 47
  bone marrow aspiration, 15-16
  cholesterol, 250
  coccidioidomycosis, 315
  CPK, 267
  cryptococcosis, 315
  CSF, 280-81
  dermatomycosis, 310-11
  electrolytes, 226
  enzymes, 240-41
  eosinophils, 87
  erythrocytes, 124-26, 129
  ESR, 64-65
  fibrinogen, 118, 120
  glucose, 262
  hemophilia, 172
  hyperparathyroidism, 272-73
  LDH, 268
  leukemia, 154
  leukocytes, 77-80
  lipase, 256
  lymphocytes, 91-92
  lymphosarcoma, 78, 152-53
  maduromycosis, 314
  monocytes, 92
  myeloproliferative disease, 154-57
  neutrophils, 81-82
  nocardiosis, 315
  PCV, 73-74
  phycomycosis, 314
  polycythemia, 147
  protein, 111, 252
  regenerative anemia, 134
  reticulocytes, 122
  SGOT, 243
  SGPT, 241-42
  SLE, 140, 143
  thyroid, 292, 297-98
  urinalysis, 185, 188, 201-3, 212
  urobilinogen, 239
Catarrhal fever, 102
Cations, 213-14
Cattle
  actinomycosis, 316
  A/G ratio, 115, 252
  anemia, regenerative, 135
  arginase, 247
  aspergillosis, 315
  autoimmune hemolytic anemia, 137
  basophils, 124
  bilirubin, 235, 237-39
  blood collection, 6
  blood picture in specific conditions, 100-103
  blood values, 44
  bone marrow aspiration, 15, 17-18
  BSP, 249
  calves, 110, 135
  cardiovascular disease, 265-67
  cholesterol, 250
  CPK, 267
  CSF, 280-81
  dermatomycosis, 310-11
  dermatophilosis, 315
  electrolytes, 226
  enzymes, 240-41
  erythrocytes, 126, 129
  ESR, 64-65, 67, 69
  fibrinogen, 118-20
  GLDH, 247
  globulins, 115
  glucose, 262
  goiter, 294
  hypoglycemia, 263
  hypothyroidism, 295
  immunoglobulins, 110
  LDH, 268
  leukocytes, 77-80
  lymphocytes, 91-92
  maduromycosis, 314
  monocytes, 92
  neutrophils, 83
  PCV, 71, 73-74
  polycythemia, 113, 147-48
  protein, 111, 252
  prothrombin time, 169
  PTA, 173
  reticulocytes, 122
  SGOT, 243
  SGPT, 241
  thyroid, 292-93
  urinalysis, 185, 187, 199, 203
  water, 224
Cells, 20-21
  bone marrow, 18-24
  count, 48-49, 283-84
  disintegrated, 38
  enzymes, 230
  shape, 133
Cerebrospinal fluid (CSF), 276-85
Charcot-Leyden crystal, 150
Chediak-Higashi syndrome, 150
Chemical agents. *See also* Drugs
  anemia, 132
  leukocytes, 79-80
Chicken, 73, 112, 115
Chinchilla, blood collection, 5
Chloramphenicol toxicity, cat, 97
Chlorides, 11-12
  abnormalities, 291
  acidosis, 216
  alkalosis, 217-18
  anions, 214
  blood, 11
  CSF, 282
  fluid and electrolyte balance, 221-24
Chloroform, urinalysis, 181
Chlorpromazine hydrochloride, dog, 93
Cholesterol, 12, 14, 257
  abnormalities, 288
  CSF, 282
  diabetes mellitus, 263
  liver function tests, 250
  normal values, 250
  serum, 257, 263
Christmas disease, 164, 173
Chronic disorders, anemia, 134, 136, 145
Chylomicra, 73
Cirrhosis, albumin, 251
Clotting, 11, 116
Coagulation. *See also* Hemostasis
  anemia, 132
  blood, 164-65
  disorders, 171-72
  plasma, 162-63
  time, 38, 168-69
Coal tar poisoning, pig, 106
Coccidioidomycosis, 315
Colitis, 93, 98
Collagen-vascular disease, 140
Color index, 38
Concentration tests, 175
Contagious bronchopneumonia, horse, 98
Convulsive seizures, leukocytes, 80
Coombs' test, 96, 137-39, 160
Copper
  deficiency, 93, 105, 134
  poisoning, sheep, 104
  sulfate, protein analysis, 109
Corticosteroids
  cattle, 101
  eosinophils, 88
  ESR, 64
  horse, 98
  lymphocytes, 92
  neutrophils, 83-85
Coumarin, coagulation disorders, 172
Creatine phosphokinase (CPK)
  abnormalities, 289
  cardiovascular disease, 266-68
  CSF, 282-83
  values, 267
Creatinine, 9, 11-12, 175, 177-78
  abnormalities, 286
  methods, 178
Crenation, 38, 127
Cryptococcus neoformans, 285
Crystals, urinalysis, 210-11
Cutler ESR, 66-67
Cyanmethemoglobin, 61-62
Cylindroid, urinalysis, 209
Cytology, 299-302, 305
  CSF, 283-85
  lymphosarcoma, 154
Cytoplasm, enzymes, 231

Deer, 237, 314-16
Dehydration, 224. *See also* Fluid; Water
  erythrocytes, 146
  polycythemia, 113
Dehydrogenase, 229
Dermatomycosis, 310-13
Dermatophilosis, 315
Dermatosis, dog, 93

Diabetes insipidus, 186
Diabetes mellitus, 187
  cholesterol, 263
  dog, 93
  glucose, 262
  glucose tolerance test, 263
  glycosuria, 194
  ketosis, 195
  pancreatic function, 259-63
  PCV, 73
  urinalysis, 188, 212
Diagnosis, enzyme tests, 230
Diarrhea, cattle, 100-101
Diet
  ketosis, 104, 195-96
  urinalysis, 187-88, 212
Differential cell count, 38, 305
  anemia, 146
  CSF, 284-85
Digestion, leukocytes, 80
Disseminated intravascular coagulation (DIC), 172
Distemper, 93
  erythrocytes, 124
  ESR, 68
  fibrinogen, 118
  leukocytes, 77
DNA, 58, 133
Dog
  actinomycosis, 316
  A/G ratio, 115, 252
  amylase, 255-56
  anemia, regenerative, 135
  arginase, 247
  aspergillosis, 315
  autoimmune hemolytic anemia, 136-39
  basophils, 88
  bilirubin, 234, 237-39
  blastomycosis, 315
  blood collection, 5-6
  blood picture in specific conditions, 93-96
  blood values, 46
  bone marrow aspiration, 15-16, 18
  cardiovascular disease, 265, 267
  cholesterol, 250
  Christmas factor, 173
  coccidioidomycosis, 315
  CPK, 267
  CSF, 280-82
  cultures, blood, 268
  dermatomycosis, 310-11
  electrolytes, 226
  enzymes, 240-41
  eosinophils, 87
  erythrocytes, 72, 124-27, 129
  ESR, 64-68
  factor VII, 172
  fat, 259
  fibrinogen, 115, 118-20
  globulins, 114-15
  glucose, 262
  goiter, 294
  hemophilia, 172
  hyperparathyroidism, 272-74
  hyperthyroidism, 298
  hypoglycemia, 263-64
  hypothyroidism, 295-98
  LDH, 268
  leukocytes, 77-80
  lipase, 256
  lymphocytes, 91-92
  lymphosarcoma, 154-55
  maduromycosis, 314
  monocytes, 92
  myeloproliferative disease, 157
  neutrophils, 81-83
  nocardiosis, 315
  partial thromboplastin time, 169
  PCV, 71, 73-74
  polycythemia, 95, 147
  protein, 111, 113, 252
  prothrombin, 169, 253
  PTA, 173
  purpura, 170
  pyruvate kinase deficiency, 143
  reticulocytes, 122
  rhinosporidiosis, 314
  SGOT, 11, 243
  SGPT, 11, 241-42
  SLE, 140-41, 143
  sodium, 223, 225
  sporotrichosis, 314
  Stuart factor, 173
  thrombocytopathy, 174
  thrombocytopenia, 159
  thyroid, 292-93
  uric acid, 254
  urinalysis, 182, 185, 188, 192, 195, 199, 201-3, 209
  urobilinogen, 239
  vaginal smear, 308
  von Willebrand's disease, 173
  water, 224
Döhle bodies, 38, 96, 150
Drugs
  BSP, 250
  erythrocytes, 125
  fibrinogen, 120
  hemostasis, 165
  leukopenia, 79
  platelet disorders, 170-71
  SGOT, 243
  SGPT, 242
  thrombocytopenia, 158-59
Duck, protein, 112
Dysentery, cattle, 103

EDTA, 9, 25, 64-65, 70
Electrolytes, 213-14, 226, 269
  balance, 220-24
  determination, 10
  parenteral solutions, 227
  replacement therapy, 224-26
  values, 225
Electrophoresis, 110, 142, 279
Emphysema, cattle, 101
Endocarditis, 94, 119
Endocrine disorders, anemia, 133
Endotoxemia, horse, 98
Endotoxicosis, 94, 105
Endotoxin, platelet disorders, 171
Enteritis, fibrinogen, 119
Enteropathy, plasma protein, 114
Enterotoxemia, sheep, 104
Enzymes, 13, 229-32
  cardiovascular disease, 266-68
  CSF, 282-83
  classification, 230-31
  diagnosis, 230
  fate, 231
  intracellular, 231
  levels, 240-41
  liver function tests, 241-47
  mechanism of alteration, 229
  methods of assay, 229-30
  nature, 229
  pancreatic, 257-58
  reporting activity, 230
  stability, 13
  tests, 10
  tissues, 231
Eosinopenia, 88
Eosinophilia, 38, 87-88
Eosinophilic myositis, dog, 94
Eosinophils, 34, 86-88
  cat, 97
  cattle, 100-103
  count, 53-54
  cytology, 300
  dog, 93-96
  horse, 98-99
  leukemia, 156-57
  pig, 105-6
  sheep, 104
Epinephrine, 104, 264
Epithelial cast, 207-8
Epithelial cells, 205-7, 301,
Erythrocytes, 10, 34-35, 60, 71-72, 74, 121-29
  abnormal, 123-27
  anemia, 136-37, 145-46
  autoimmune hemolytic anemia, 138
  cardiovascular disease, 265-66
  cat, 97
  cattle, 100-103
  count, 48-51
  CSF, 283
  cytology, 300
  destruction, 122
  dog, 93-96
  horse, 98-99
  life span, 121-22
  myeloproliferative disorders, 155-57
  normal values, 129
  pig, 105-6
  polycythemia, 146-49
  pyruvate kinase deficiency, 143-44
  sheep, 103-4
  urinalysis, 197, 205, 207
  urobilinogen, 201
  values, 129
Erythrocyte sedimentation rate (ESR), 41, 64-69, 116, 125
Erythrocytic hypoplasia, 38
Erythrocytopenia, 38
Erythrocytosis, 38
Erythrophagocytosis, 150
Erythropoiesis, 39, 122-23, 127
Erythropoietin, 39, 123, 149
Esophagogastric ulcer, pig, 105
Estrogens, 94, 160, 165
Estrous cycle, vaginal smears, 308-9
Ethylene glycol poisoning, 94, 105
Exudates, 303-6

Factor VII (proconvertin), 172
Factor VIII (hemophilia), 172-73
Factor IX (Christmas factor), 173
Factor XI (PTA), 164, 173
Factor S (Stuart factor), 164, 173
Fat, 258-59, 212
Fatty cast, urinalysis, 208
Feces, 239, 257-58
Ferritin, 39
Fibrin, 39, 87, 164
Fibrinogen, 64, 115-20, 163-64, 170-71, 250, 304
Filariasis, ESR, 68
Fish, blood collection, 6
Fistula, horse, 98-99
Fluid balance, 147, 220-24
Fluoride, 10
Folic acid deficiency, pig, 105
Foot and mouth disease, 120
Formalin, urinalysis, 181
Fragility test, 39
Fungus, 115
  skin lesions, 311-13
  urinalysis, 209

Gaisbock's syndrome, 147
Gamma globulin, 113, 115. *See also* Globulin
Gastroenteritis, pig, 106

Gestation and lactation, pig, 105. *See also* Pregnancy
Globin, 39
Globulin, 12, 108-9. *See also* Albumin: globulin ratio
  CSF, 278-79
  ESR, 64
  increased, 114-15
  liver function, 250, 252
Glomerular filtration rate, 178
Glomerulonephritis, SLE, 140, 142
Glucagon tolerance test, 264
Glucocorticoids, 87, 160
Glucose, 14, 39, 304
  blood, 12, 257, 260-64, 286-87
  CSF, 279
  fluid and electrolyte balance, 221
  pancreatic function, 257
  ranges, 262
  tolerance test, 263
  urinalysis, 191-94, 204
  urine, 262-63
Glutamic dehydrogenase (GLDH), 247
Glycosuria, 193-94
Gmelin test, 199
Goat
  A/G ratio, 115, 252
  bilirubin, 237
  bone marrow, 15
  cholesterol, 250
  CPK, 267
  CSF, 280-82
  dermatophilosis, 315
  enzymes, 240-41
  erythrocytes, 129
  ESR, 64-67
  glucose, 262
  goiter, 295
  hypofibrinogenemia, 173
  LDH, 268
  PCV, 71, 73
  protein, 112, 252
  reticulocytes, 122
  rhinosporidiosis, 314
  urinalysis, 185
  water, 224
Goiter, 294-95
Granular cast, 207-8
Granulocytes, 39, 81
Granulocytic leukemia, 152, 155-57
Granulocytosis, 39
Griseofulvin intoxication, cat, 97
Guinea pig
  blood collection, 5-7
  cholesterol, 250
  PCV, 73
  protein, 112
  reticulocytes, 122
  vitamin C deficiency, 170

Haemobartonellosis, 94, 97
Hageman factor, 164
Hamster, blood collection, 6
Haptoglobin, 39
Heartworms, 94, 265
Heinz bodies, 39, 125
Hematinics, horse, 99
Hematocrit. *See* Packed cell volume
Hematuria, 183, 190-91, 197
Hemocytometer, 39
Hemoglobin, 60-63, 74
  anemia, 127-28, 133-34, 144
  cat, 97
  cattle, 100-103
  dog, 93-96
  erythrocytes, 122-23
  horse, 99
  pig, 105, 107
  sheep, 103-4
  urinalysis, 183
Hemoglobinemia, 39
Hemoglobinuria, 183, 197-98
Hemolysis, 10-11, 39
  anemia, 135-36
  leukocytes, 80
Hemophilia, 172-73
Hemorrhage
  anemia, 131, 134-35
  fibrinogen, 119
  leukocytes, 80
  PCV, 73
  thrombocytopenia, 158
  types, 165
  underlying disease, 165-66
Hemosiderin, 39
Hemostasis, 162. *See also* Coagulation
  clinical evaluation, 165-66
  disorders, 170-74
  lab evaluation, 166-70
Heparin, 9-10, 64, 70, 88, 170
Hepatic insufficiency, 99, 177
Hepatitis, 69, 77, 94, 140
Hepatobiliary conditions, SAP, 244-45
Hepatopathy, 113
High mountain disease, dog, 265
Histamine, 86-88, 99
Histiocytes, cytology, 300
Histoplasmosis, 95, 315
Hog cholera, 105
Hormones, 133, 292-94, 298
Horse
  A/G ratio, 115, 252
  anemia, regenerative, 135
  arginase, 247
  aspergillosis, 315
  autoimmune hemolytic anemia, 137
  bilirubin, 234-35, 237-38
  blood picture in specific conditions, 98-100
  blood values, 43
  bone marrow aspiration, 15, 16
  BSP, 249
  cardiovascular disease, 265, 267
  cholesterol, 250
  CPK, 267
  cryptococcosis, 315
  CSF, 280-82
  dermatomycosis, 310-11
  dermatophilosis, 315
  electrolytes, 226
  enzymes, 231, 240-41
  erythrocytes, 124, 126, 129
  ESR, 64-65, 66-69
  fat, 259
  fibrinogen, 118-19
  globulins, 115
  glucose, 262
  goiter, 295
  hemophilia, 172
  hyperparathyroidism, 273
  LDH, 268
  leukocytes, 77-80
  lymphocytes, 91
  maduromycosis, 314
  neutrophils, 83
  PCV, 71, 73-74
  peritoneal fluid, 306-7
  phycomycosis, 314
  polycythemia, 147
  protein, 111, 114, 252
  prothrombin, 169, 253
  purpura, 170
  reticulocytes, 122
  rhinosporidiosis, 314
  SDH, 246-47
  SGOT, 242-43
  SGPT, 241
  sporotrichosis, 314
  thrombocytopenia, 159
  thyroid, 292-93, 297
  urinalysis, 183-85, 187, 209
  water, 224
Howell-Jolly bodies, 39, 124, 135
Human
  A/G ratio, 115, 252
  amylase, 255
  anemia, autoimmune hemolytic, 137
  arginase, 247
  blastomycosis, 315
  erythrocytes, 127, 129
  ESR, 65, 67
  fibrinogen, 118
  hypothyroidism, 295
  icterus index, 234
  leukemia, 152
  leukocytes, 82
  PCV, 73
  polycythemia, 147-48
  protein, 112
  pyruvate kinase deficiency, 143
  SDH, 246
  SGOT, 11
  SGPT, 11
  SLE, 140
  uric acid, 254
  urinalysis, 185, 188, 203
Hyaline cast, 207-8
Hydration. *See* Fluid
Hydrolases, 229
Hydronephrosis, 94
Hyperadrenocorticism, 88, 94
  ESR, 69
  lymphocytes, 92
  PCV, 73
Hypercholesterolemia, ESR, 64
Hyperchromasia, 39
Hyperchromic, 39
Hyperglycemia, 262
Hyperlipemia, leptocytes, 125
Hyperparathyroidism, 271-75
Hypersegmented, 39
Hypersplenism, 39
Hyperthyroidism, 298
Hypertonic, 39
Hypertrophic osteodystrophy, dog, 95
Hypervolemia, 39
Hyperventilation, 219-20
Hypochromasia, 39, 125
Hypofibrinogenemia, 173-74
Hypoglycemia, 263-64
Hypoplastic anemia, 39
Hypothermia, dog, 95
Hypothyroidism, 69, 73, 295-98
Hypotonic, 39
Hypoventilation, 218-19
Hypoxia, polycythemia, 148

Icterus index, 10-11, 234-35
Idiopathic, 39, 170
Immunity, lymphocytes, 90-91
Immunocyte, 150
Immunofluorescent test, 154
Immunoglobulins, 109-10
Immunosuppressive therapy, thrombocytopenia, 160
Indican, 184, 202
Indices, 39
Indigestion, 101, 119-20
Infectious anemia, 97-98
Infectious peritonitis, 97, 154

Inflammation
  anemia, 145
  fibrinogen, 118-19
  neutrophils, 83-86
Influenza, 99, 106
Inorganic phosphorus, 10, 12, 14, 290
Insulin, 99, 101, 104. *See also* Diabetes
Interstitial nephritis, 68
Intestine, 99, 231
Intoxication, leukocytes, 80
Iodine, thyroid, 292, 294-95
Ionizing radiation, platelet disorders, 170
Iron
  anemia, 145-46
  binding capacity, 39, 146
  calves, 101
  erythrocytes, 123
  pig, 105
Isoenzymes, 232, 268

Jaundice, 239. *See also* Bilirubin
Johne's disease, cattle, 101-2

Ketones
  acidosis, 216
  pancreatic function, 263
  urinalysis, 194-96, 204
Ketosis, 104, 195-96
Kidney, 175-79, 231

Lactation, 101, 105, 113. *See also* Pregnancy
Lactic dehydrogenase (LDH), 10-11, 245-46
  abnormalities, 289
  cardiovascular disease, 267-68
  CSF, 282
  values, 267
Lead poisoning, 95, 101, 105-6
Lee-White method, 168-69
Leptocytosis, 39
Leptospirosis, 64, 95, 125
  ESR, 68
  fibrinogen, 118
  horse, 99
  pig, 106
Leukemia, 15, 39, 151-52, 154
Leukemoid, 40
Leukocytes, 9, 32, 70-72, 76-92
  abnormal, 150-51
  anemia, 138, 146
  cat, 97
  cattle, 100-103
  count, 35-36, 51-52, 152, 154, 156-57
  CSF, 283
  dog, 93-96
  horse, 98-100
  lymphosarcoma, 153-54
  pig, 105-7
  sheep, 103-4
  urinalysis, 205, 207-8
Leukocytic cast, 208
Leukocytosis, 40, 79-80
Leukopenia, 40, 77-79
Lignin test, 203-4
Lipase, 10, 256-57, 287
Lipemia, 11, 73, 88
Listeriosis, 104, 106
Liver
  coagulation, disorders, 171
  cytology, 300-301
  damage, 115, 119
  disease, 73, 114-15
  enzymes, 231, 263
  function tests, 233-54
  platelet disorders, 171
  protein production, 108
  urea, 176
  urobilinogen, 201
Locoweed poisoning, sheep, 104
Lungs, platelet disorders, 171
Lyases, 229
Lymph nodes, 154-55, 301
Lymphocytes, 89-92
  cat, 97
  cattle, 100-103
  cytology, 300
  dog, 93-96
  horse, 98-100
  pig, 105-7
  sheep, 104
Lymphocytic leukemia, 152
Lymphocytosis, 91
Lymphoma, 40, 151-55. *See also* Lymphosarcoma
Lymphopenia, 92
Lymphosarcoma, 19
  cat, 120, 152-54
  dog, 120, 154-55, 265
  platelet disorders, 171
Lysine deficiency, pig, 106

Macrocytes, 40, 123, 144
Macrocytic, 40
Macrocytosis, 64
Macrophages, 92
Maduromycosis, 314
Magnesium, cations, 214
Malnutrition, plasma protein, 113-14. *See also* Diet
Mast cells, 40, 150, 300
  basophils, 88-89
  eosinophils, 87
  leukemia, 151
Mastitis, 102, 104, 119
Mean corpuscular hemoglobin, 128-29
Mean corpuscular volume, 128
Megaloblast, 40
Melanin, 184
Mesothelial cells, 300
Metabolism
  disturbances, 216-18
  erythropoiesis, 126
  leptocytes, 125
  liver function tests, 233-41
Metal poisoning, 79, 124
Metaphosphoric acid, urinalysis, 181
Methemoglobin, 63
Methemoglobinuria, 183
Method. *See* under specific name
Metritis, dog, 95
Microcytes, 40, 64, 126
Microcytic, 40
Microhematocrit, 71
Microorganisms, CSF, 285
Microsomes, enzymes, 231
Millar method, 117
Mitochondria, enzymes, 231
Moldy corn poisoning, pig, 106
Moniliasis, 314
Monkey. *See also* Primates
  blood collection, 5
  dermatophilosis, 315
  hyperparathyroidism, 273
  protein, 112
  uric acid, 254
  vitamin C deficiency, 134, 170
Monocytes, 92
  cattle, 101-3
  dog, 95
  horse, 98
  leukemia, 152
  pig, 105-6
  sheep, 104
Mouse. *See also* Rat; Rodent
  autoimmune hemolytic anemia, 137
  blood collection, 5-6
  PCV, 73
  protein, 112
  reticulocytes, 122
Mucus, urinalysis, 209
Multicentric fibrosarcoma, 154
Muscle, enzymes, 231
Muscular dystrophy, sheep, 104
Musculoskeletal manifestations, SLE, 140
Mycetoma, 314
Mycoses, systemic, 315
Myelocytes, 82
  cattle, 101, 103
  dog, 94
  pig, 105
Myelofibrosis, 155
Myeloid: erythroid ratio, 18-19
Myelophthisic anemia, 40
Myeloproliferative disease, 120, 154-57
Myocarditis, ESR, 68
Myoglobin, 183
Myoglobinuria, 196
Myositis, dog, 95

Neoplasia, 80, 113
Neoplasms, ESR, 68
Neoplastic cells, 301
Neoplastic disease, anemia, 145
Nephritis, 68, 95, 118-19
Nephrosis, dog, 95
Neutropenia, 40, 86
Neutrophilia, 40, 83-86
Neutrophils, 78-80, 81-83, 150
  cat, 97
  cattle, 101-3
  cytology, 300
  dog, 93-96
  horse, 98-99
  pig, 105-7
  sheep, 104
Nitrate, cattle, 102
Nitrogen, 12, 104, 175-76
Nocardiosis, 315
Nonprotein nitrogen (NPN), 175
Normoblast, 40
Normochromasia, 40
Normochromic, 40
Normocyte, 40
Normocytic, 40
Nucleated cell count, 305
Nutrition. *See also* Diet
  anemia, 134
  erythropoiesis, 126
  hyperparathyroidism, 272-73

Obermayer's test, 202
Occult blood, 304
Organic acids, 214, 216
Ornithine carbamyl transferase (OCT), 247
Osteodystrophia fibrosa, 271-75
Osteomalacia, 271
Osteopenia, 270-75
Osteoporosis, 270
Otitis interna, fibrinogen, 118
Ovalocytes, 40, 126
Oxyhemoglobin, 60-61

Packed cell volume (PCV), 10, 65-66, 70-75, 304
  anemia, 127, 144
  cat, 97
  cattle, 100-103
  dog, 93-96
  fluid and electrolyte balance, 222
  horse, 98-99
  normal values, 73
  pancreatic function, 73

Packed cell volume *(cont.)*
  pig, 105, 107
  polycythemia, 113
  sheep, 103-4
Pancreas
  enzymes, 231
  function tests, 255-64
  insufficiency, 257-59
  PCV, 73
Pandy's test, 279
Panleukopenia, 77, 97, 120
Panosteitis, dog, 95
Parasites, 134
  A/G ratio, 115
  blood smears, 31-32
  cattle, 102
  dog, 95
  eosinophils, 87
  horse, 99
  lymphocytes, 91
  pig, 106
  protein, 114
  sheep, 104
  urinalysis, 209
Parenteral solutions, composition, 227
Partial thromboplastin time, 169
Parturition, 102, 106
Pasteurellosis, pig, 106
Pelger-Hüet anomaly, 40, 150
Pericardial effusion, 269, 299
Pericarditis, 103, 119, 265
Peritoneal effusion, 299
Peritoneal fluid, 306-7
Peritonitis
  blood, 14
  cat, 97, 118
  cattle, 119
  dog, 118
  ESR, 69
  fluid and electrolyte balance, 221
  horse, 69
  infectious, 97, 154
  pH, 214-20
  urinalysis, 187-88
Phagocytosis
  eosinophils, 87
  erythrocytes, 122
  monocytes, 92
  neutrophils, 83, 85
Phenol derivatives, 184
Phenolsulfonphthalein (PSP), 175
Phenylbutazone, 165, 171
Phosphate, anions, 214
Phosphorus, 10, 12, 14, 228, 290
Phycomycosis, 314-15
Picornavirus infection, cat, 97
Pig
  A/G ratio, 115, 252
  bilirubin, 234, 237
  blood collection, 5-6
  blood picture in specific conditions, 105-7
  blood values, 46
  bone marrow aspiration, 15
  cholesterol, 250
  CSF, 280-81
  dermatomycosis, 310-11
  electrolytes, 226
  enzymes, 240-41
  erysipelas, 106
  erythrocytes, 126, 129
  ESR, 64-65, 67
  fever, 105
  globulins, 114
  glucose, 262
  goiter, 295
  hemophilia, 172
  hypoglycemia, 263
  LDH, 268
  leukocytes, 77-78
  lymphocytes, 92
  PCV, 71, 73-74
  protein, 112-13, 252
  purpura, 170
  reticulocytes, 122
  SDH, 246
  SGPT, 241
  thyroid, 293
  urinalysis, 185, 188
  von Willebrand's disease, 173
  water, 224
Pingue poisoning, sheep, 104
Placenta, enzymes, 231
Plasma, 70-73
  cells, 150-51, 300
  enzymes, 230
  protein, 98, 108, 113, 293
  protein: fibrinogen ratio, 118
  thromboplastin antecedent (PTA), 164, 173
Plasmocytic leukemia, 152
Platelets, 32, 36-37, 70, 162
  anemia, 138, 146
  cattle, 103
  count, 52, 54-55, 166-67
  destruction, 159-60
  disorders, 170-71
  dog, 94-96
  dysfunction, 167-68
  horse, 99
  numbers, 158, 160
  pig, 105
  sheep, 104
  transfusion, 161
Pleural effusion, 118, 299
Pleurisy, SLE, 140
Pleuritis, 69, 119
Pneumonia
  dog, 95
  ESR, 68
  fibrinogen, 118-19
  pig, 106
Poikilocytes, 40, 64, 126
Poisoning. *See* under substance
Poll evil, horse, 99
Polyarteritis nodosa, SLE, 140
Polychromasia, 40, 123
Polycythemia, 40, 113, 147-49, 265-66
Porphyrins, 102, 133
Potassium, 14
  abnormalities, 290-91
  alkalosis, 217-18
  blood, determination, 10
  cardiovascular disease, 269
  cations, 213-14, 225
  effects, 228
Pregnancy
  cattle, 103
  dog, 96
  ESR, 68
  fibrinogen, 118-19
  leukocytes, 80
  protein, 113
  sheep, 104, 114
Primates. *See also* Monkey
  bilirubin, 237
  blood collection, 6
  cholesterol, 250
  hyperparathyroidism, 272
  SGPT, 241
Primidone, dog, 96
Proaccelerin, 164
Proconvertin, 164, 172
Progranulocyte, 82
Promazine, horse, 99
Prostatic abscess, dog, 96
Protein, 108-15, 251-52, 296, 304. *See also* Enzymes
  cardiovascular disease, 266
  concentration, 266
  CSF, 278-79, 284
  indican, 203
  lymphosarcoma, 155
  malnutrition, 113-14, 177
  metabolism, 250-54
  pig, 106
  plasma, 64, 108-15
  serum, 251-52, 296
  urinalysis, 188-91, 204, 221
  values, 111-12, 251
Proteinate, anions, 214
Proteinuria, 190-91
Proteolytic activity, 258
Prothrombin, 11, 163-65, 169, 171, 253
Protozoan infection, leukocytes, 78
Psittacosis, cattle, 103
Purpura, 15, 99, 165, 170
Pyelonephritis, 96, 118-20
Pyknotic nuclei, 151
Pyometra, 68, 96, 118
Pyridoxine, pig, 106
Pyruvate kinase deficiency, 124, 143-44

Quittor, horse, 99

Rabbit
  bilirubin, 237
  blood collection, 5
  cholesterol, 250
  PCV, 73
  protein, 112
  reticulocytes, 122
Rabies, dog, 96
Radiation, 68, 104, 158
Radioimmunoassay, insulin, 264
Radioiodine uptake, 295-96
Rat. *See also* Mouse; Rodent
  arginase, 247
  bilirubin, 237
  blood collection, 5-6
  cholesterol, 250
  hypothyroidism, 297
  PCV, 73
  protein, 112
  reticulocytes, 122
  thrombocytopathy, 174
Regenerative anemia, 134-36, 167
Renal disease, 177-78, 186-87
  anemia, 96, 133
  dog, 95
  hyperparathyroidism, 273-74
  proteinuria, 190-91
Reserpine, dog, 96
Respiratory disturbances, 97, 216, 218-20
Retained fetal membranes, cattle, 103
Reticulitis, cattle, 103
Reticulocytes, 33-34, 40, 121-23, 146
Reticuloendotheliosis, 151, 155-56
Reticulum cell sarcoma, 151-52
Rheumatoid arthritis, SLE, 140, 143
Rhinosporidiosis, 314
Rhinotracheitis, cattle, 101
Rickets, 78, 86, 270-71
Rift Valley fever, 103-4, 106
Rinderpest, 103, 106
Ring sideroblast, 40
Robert's test, 188-89
Rodent, 310, 314. *See also* Mouse; Rat
Ross test, 195
Rouleaux formation, 41, 126
Rumen impaction, fibrinogen, 119

Salmon disease, 69, 95
Salmonellosis, 106, 119
Salt poisoning, pig, 106
Schalm method, 117
Schilling index, 41, 81
Schistocytes, 126

Secondary polycythemia, 265-66
Sediment
  microscopic, 221
  urinalysis, 205-12
Septicemia, 106, 119
Seroflocculation tests, 109-10
Serotonin, basophils, 88
Serum alkaline phosphatase (SAP), 243-45, 257
Serum glutamic oxaloacetic transaminase (SGOT), 11, 242-43
  abnormalities, 288
  cardiovascular disease, 266, 268
  CSF, 282
Serum glutamic pyruvic transaminase (SGPT), 11, 241-42
  abnormalities, 289
  cardiovascular disease, 268
  CSF, 282
  pancreatic function, 257
Serum iron, anemia, 146
Serum lipase, 10, 256-57, 287
Sheep
  actinomycosis, 316
  A/G ratio, 115, 252
  arginase, 247
  basophils, 124
  bilirubin, 234, 237-38
  blood collection, 6
  blood picture in specific conditions, 103-4
  blood values, 45
  bone marrow aspiration, 15, 17
  BSP, 249
  cholesterol, 250
  CPK, 267
  CSF, 280-81
  dermatophilosis, 315
  electrolytes, 226
  enzymes, 240-41
  erythrocytes, 126, 129
  ESR, 64-65, 67
  glucose, 262
  goiter, 294
  hypoglycemia, 263
  hypothyroidism, 295
  LDH, 268
  leukocytes, 77-78
  PCV, 71, 73-74
  polycythemia, 147
  protein, 252
  reticulocytes, 122
  SDH, 246
  SGOT, 243
  SGPT, 241
  urinalysis, 185, 187, 194
  water, 224
Shift to the left, 41, 81
Shift to the right, 41, 81
Shipping fever, cattle, 103
Shock, leukocytes, 78
Sideroblast, 40-41
Siderocytes, 34, 41, 126-27
Sideroleukocytes, 34
Skin
  ESR, 68
  lesions, 310-16
  SLE, 140
Smears, 11, 301, 308-9
  blood, 25-37
  bone marrow, 17
Smudge cell, 41
Snake venom, anemia, 132
Sodium
  abnormalities, 290
  acidosis, 216
  blood, 10, 11
  cations, 213-14
  CSF, 282
  effects, 228
  fluid and electrolyte balance, 223-25
Sorbitol dehydrogenase (SDH), 246-47
Specific gravity, 184-87, 190
Spermatozoa, urinalysis, 209
Spherocytes, 41, 127
Spherocytosis, 64
Spleen
  erythrocytes, 124
  leptocytes, 125
  platelet disorders, 171
  polycythemia, 147
  thrombocytopenia, 160
Splenectomy, 120, 139, 167
Splenic anemia, 41
Sporotrichosis, 314
Stab cell, 41
Stains
  Camco Quik, 32-33
  Diff Quik, 33
  Field's, 31-32
  Giemsa, 29-31, 305
  Hemal, 33
  Leishman's, 30
  May-Grünwald-Giemsa, 17, 31
  new methylene blue, 32
  Papanicolaou, 300
  Pollak's, 300
  Prussian blue, 34
  reticulocyte, 33-34
  Romanowsky type, 26
  Wright-Giemsa, 30
  Wright-Leishman, 30-31
  Wright's, 17, 26, 28-29, 300, 305
Starch, feces, 258
Steatitis, 97, 118
Stem cell leukemia, 152
Stippling, 41
Stomatocytes, 41, 127
Strangles, horse, 99
Streptococcal infection, cat, 97
Stress, 114, 147
Stuart factor, 164, 173
Subacute leukemia, 41
Subcutaneous mycoses, 314-15
Sulfate, anions, 214
Sulfhemoglobin, 63-64
Sulfonamides, urinalysis, 203-4
Sulkowitch test, 203
Supravital staining, 41
Surgery, 68, 118
Systemic lupus erythematosus (SLE), 139-43, 159
  cells, 40, 141-42, 150
  dog, 96
  platelet disorders, 171

Target cells, 41
Tart cell, 151
Test. *See* under specific name
Tetanus, 96, 99
Thallium poisoning, 96, 97
Thorn test, 93
Thrombasthenia, 171
Thrombin, 116-17, 169-70
Thrombocytes. *See* Platelets
Thrombocythemia, 167
Thrombocytopathy, 167-68, 174
Thrombocytopenia, 158-61, 166, 170
  lymphosarcoma, 155
  purpura, 140, 142
Thrombocytosis, 167
Thymol, urinalysis, 181
Thyroglobulin, thyroid function, 292-93
Thyroid function, 133, 292-98
Thyroiditis, 140
Tissues
  enzymes, 231
  ESR, 68
  fibrinogen, 118
  leukocytes, 80
  thromboplastin, 164
Tolbutamide response test, 264
Toluene, urinalysis, 181
Total protein, 12, 288
Total serum cholesterol, abnormalities, 288
Toxic granulation, 151
Toxic neutrophil, 41, 151
Toxoplasma organisms, 285
Toxoplasmosis, cat, 97
Tracheobronchitis, dog, 96
Transaminase, 10-11, 242-43, 257, 266, 282, 288-89
Transferases, 229
Transmissible gastroenteritis, pig, 106
Transudates, 303-6
Tranquilizers, dog, 96
Trichloroethylene, cattle, 103
Trypanosomes, 285
Trypanosomiasis, ESR, 69
Tumors, cytology, 302
Turbidity tests, 109-10
Turkey, protein, 112

Urea, 12, 176-77
  liver function, 253
  nitrogen. *See* Blood urea nitrogen
Uremia, 171, 177
Urethral obstruction, 98, 118
Uric acid, 10, 12, 254
Urinalysis, 175, 180-212. *See also* specific species
  bilirubin, 198-99, 238-39
  blood, 196-98, 204
  color, 183-84
  fluid and electrolyte balance, 220-21
  glucose, 191-94, 204
  hemoglobin, 183
  ketones, 94-96, 204
  microscopic, 205-12
  oliguria, 182-83
  pH, 221
  polyuria, 182
  protein, 221
  specific gravity, 184-87, 220-21
  urobilinogen, 199-202, 204, 239
Urinary tract infection, dog, 96
Urobilin, 239
Urobilinogen, 199-202, 204, 239
Urobilinoids, 183

Vaginal smears, 308-9
van den Bergh's test, 235-38
Vascular disorders, 170
Venipuncture, 6, 8
Viral arteritis, horse, 99-100, 265
Viral diarrhea, cattle, 100
Virus, 77-78, 86, 171
Vitamin B deficiency, 96, 106, 137
Vitamin C deficiency, 134, 170
Vitamin E deficiency, 107, 134
Vitamin K deficiency, 171
von Willebrand's disease, 173

Wallace-Diamond test, 199-200
Warfarin, hemostasis, 165
Water, 213, 220-24, 228
Waxy cast, 208
Westergren, ESR, 66-67
Winter dysentery, cattle, 103
Wintrobe
  ESR, 65, 67
  hematocrit, 70-71

Yeast, urinalysis, 209
Yellow fat disease, pig, 107